1 MONTH OF FREE READING

at
www.ForgottenBooks.com

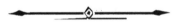

By purchasing this book you are eligible for one month membership to ForgottenBooks.com, giving you unlimited access to our entire collection of over 1,000,000 titles via our web site and mobile apps.

To claim your free month visit:
www.forgottenbooks.com/free543307

* Offer is valid for 45 days from date of purchase. Terms and conditions apply.

ISBN 978-0-428-76699-3
PIBN 10543307

This book is a reproduction of an important historical work. Forgotten Books uses state-of-the-art technology to digitally reconstruct the work, preserving the original format whilst repairing imperfections present in the aged copy. In rare cases, an imperfection in the original, such as a blemish or missing page, may be replicated in our edition. We do, however, repair the vast majority of imperfections successfully; any imperfections that remain are intentionally left to preserve the state of such historical works.

Forgotten Books is a registered trademark of FB &c Ltd.
Copyright © 2018 FB &c Ltd.
FB &c Ltd, Dalton House, 60 Windsor Avenue, London, SW19 2RR.
Company number 08720141. Registered in England and Wales.

For support please visit www.forgottenbooks.com

OF

NAVAL HYGIENE

BY

JOHN D. MACDONALD, M.D. F.R.S.

INSPECTOR-GENERAL R.N.
PROFESSOR OF NAVAL HYGIENE, ARMY MEDICAL SCHOOL, NETLEY

WITH ILLUSTRATIONS

LONDON
SMITH, ELDER, & CO., 15 WATERLOO PLACE
1881

[All rights reserved]

TO

JOHN WATT REID, Esq., M.D.
&c. &c.

DIRECTOR-GENERAL OF THE MEDICAL DEPARTMENT OF THE NAVY

This Work is Dedicated

WITH FEELINGS OF RESPECT AND ESTEEM

AND IN TOKEN OF

OLD AND VALUED FRIENDSHIP

BY

THE AUTHOR

PREFACE.

Of all the departments of science connected with medicine, Hygiene is perhaps that which may be most profitably studied by nonprofessional persons; and it is hoped that the present treatise will be found useful to executive as well as to medical officers on ship-board both in the Royal Navy and in the Mercantile Marine.

Those who regard the espousal of the principles of hygiene as the clearest evidence of the social and intellectual advancement of any community must be gratified to see that in the British Navy, from the Admirals' List downwards, a growing sense of its importance is now so far exhibited as to afford an additional incentive to medical officers to keep pace with the times in their studies. It is satisfactory also for them to know that any sanitary suggestions they may make are now more likely to receive practical attention than could have been expected in former times.

It should be remarked, however, that the memory of Anson, Collingwood, Curtis, Cook, and other illustrious naval officers of the past will always be revered for their humane solicitude, not only for the sick, but for the health and comfort of the crews under their command. Perhaps the first prize in naval hygiene—namely, the gold medal of the Royal Society—was awarded to the great and good Captain Cook, in especial consideration of the excellence of the sanitary measures adopted by him, unprecedented success having attended his hygienic arrangements. Speaking of the system carried out by himself, he says :—'In conjunction with fresh provisions and vegetables, and with a continual supply of fresh water to the men, the most material part of the arrangements was that proper methods were taken to keep their persons, hammocks, bedding, clothes, &c. constantly clean and dry. Equal care was taken to keep the ship clean and dry between decks. Once or twice a week she was aired with fires, and, when this could not be done, she was smoked with gunpowder mixed with vinegar and water. I had also a fire made in an iron pot at the bottom of the well, which was of great use in purifying the air in the other parts of the ship.' Now if we compare the advanced views expressed in this quotation with even anything that the great medical pioneers Lind, Blane, and Trotter could have written, it might well be asked, Who was the father of naval hygiene?

The fundamental questions of ship-structure and ship-ventilation have been dealt with more at length, as the basis, so to speak, upon which the whole superstructure of naval hygiene should be raised; and the other parts will at least form a nucleus around which

CONTENTS.

	PAGE
PREFACE	vii–ix
LIST OF ILLUSTRATIONS	xvi
AUTHORITIES QUOTED	xvii–xviii

INTRODUCTION.

Nature of the Subject, and Plan of Arrangement	1
Division I.—Conservative Hygiene	2
„ II.—Prophylactic, or Preventive Hygiene	5
„ III.—Corrective, or Remedial Hygiene	7
„ IV., or Appendix	8

DIVISION I.

CONSERVATIVE HYGIENE.

CHAPTER I.

STRUCTURE AND ECONOMY OF SHIPS.

Section A.—Introductory Remarks and Historical Retrospect	9
„ B.—Designing and Sheer Drawing	15
„ C.—Construction of the Hull of Wooden Ships	17
„ D.—Construction of Iron Ships	31
„ E.—Internal Economy of Ships	41

CHAPTER II.

THE VENTILATION OF SHIPS.

	PAGE
Section A.—Atmospheric Air, Physical Constitution and Properties	45
" B.—The Physics of the Atmosphere, and Leading Principles of Ventilation	50
" C.—Practical Application of the Foregoing Principles	59
Sub-section A.—Natural Ventilation	Ibid.
" B.—Artificial Ventilation	77
" D.—Special Systems of Ventilation	90

CHAPTER III.

WATER SUPPLY.

Section 1.—General Remarks	134
" 2.—Natural Waters	136
" 3.—Condensed Water	139
" 4.—Storage of Water, and Watering Ship	146
" 5.—Filtration	148
Physical, Chemical, and Microscopical Examination of Water	151
Chemical Tests and Volumetric Solutions required for Hygienic Purposes	157
Section A.—Ordinary Test Solutions	Ibid.
" B.—Special Solutions	Ibid.
" C.—Standard Solutions	158

CHAPTER IV.

CLEANLINESS.

Section A.—Personal Cleanliness	160
" B.—Cleanliness of the Ship—Humidity	162
" C.—Rendering the Deck Planking Impervious to Moisture to Facilitate Drying	164

CONTENTS.

Section I.—The Importance of Dryness and Cleanliness of the Ship to the Health of the Crew 238
„ K.—The Ill Effects of Sleeping on Shore in Malarious Districts 240

DIVISION III.

REMEDIAL OR CORRECTIVE HYGIENE.

CHAPTER I.

Section A.—The Treatment of Bilges and Bilge Effluvia . . . 243
„ B.—Conservancy, Water-closets, Heads and Bow-galleries, Deodorants and Antiseptics 245
„ C.—Infected Ships 256

CHAPTER II.

Section A.—Segregation of the Sick on the First Appearance of Infectious Disease 259
„ B.—Disinfection of the Bedding, Clothing, and Effects of the Sick 261
„ C.—The Fumigation of Ships with Disinfectant Gases . . 262

DIVISION IV., OR APPENDIX.

CHAPTER I.

Section A.—The Physique of the Sailor 270
„ B.—The Natural Character and Habits of the Sailor . . 272
„ C.—The Daily Duties of the Sailor 276

LIST OF ILLUSTRATIONS.

PLATE		PAGE
I.	Sheer Drawing	16
II.	The Tabled Scarph	17
III.	Construction of the Bilge	18
IV.	Framing of Wooden Ships	20
V.	Stern of a Frigate with Screw Port and Sole Plate	24
VI.	Midship Section of a Frigate	26
VII.	Bow of a Frigate and Knee of the Head	29
VIII.	Construction of Iron Ships	32
IX.	Body Section of H.M.S. 'Bellerophon'	37
X.	Body Section of H.M.S. 'Devastation'	39
XI.	Trade and Prevalent Winds and the Law of Storms	51
XII.	Different Forms of Wind-Sails	61
XIII.	Application of the Simple Cowl to the Ventilation of Frigates ('Lord Warden')	63
XIV.	Up- and Downtakes	67
XV.	Several Ventilating Systems	79
XVI.	The Twin-Fan Ventilator of the Author	81
XVII.	Up- and Downtake in Combination	84
XVIII.	Improvement in the Ventilation of H.M.S. 'Racoon'	92
XIX.	Dr. Edmonds's Ventilating System	94
XX.	System of Ventilation in H.M.S. 'Undaunted'	100
XXI.	Ventilating System with Tubular Shelf-pieces	102
XXII.	Ventilating System, with Tubular Shelf-pieces, and the addition of Ventilating Trusses	104
XXIII.	Thier's Automatic Ship Ventilator, Bilge-pump, and Fog-horn	110
XXIV.	Ventilation of H.M.S. 'Devastation'	121
XXV.	The Ventilation of the Fore Magazine, H.M.S. 'Duncan'	127
XXVI.	Dr. Normandy's Condensing, Aërating, and Filtering Apparatus	144
XXVII.	Body Section of H.M.S. 'Victor Emanuel'	219
XXVIII.	Bow Gallery of H.M.S. 'Egmont'	247
XXIX.	Ambulance Lift for Ship or Shore	288

AUTHORITIES.

THE more important works more or less bearing on the subject of Naval Hygiene are the following:—

ENGLISH WRITERS.

Dr. Lind *On the Health of Seamen. On Scurvy. On Hot Climates*, and other writings, published towards the close of the last century.

The Dissertations of Sir Gilbert Blane, Bart., 3rd Edition, 1803.

The works of Trotter, Fletcher, Turnbull, and Finlayson may also be consulted with advantage; but from that remarkable epoch onwards to the present time, but few original writers on the subject of Naval Hygiene have made their appearance in this country.

Hygienic, Medical, and Surgical Hints for Young Officers of the Royal Navy and of the Merchant Navy. By W. M. Saunders, M.D., Surgeon, R.N. London, 1856.

Observations on Naval Hygiene and Scurvy. By Alexander Armstrong, M.D., R.N. London, 1858.

The Annual Reports of the Health of the Navy, Merchant Shipping Acts, and Admiralty Instructions for Transports, &c.

AMERICAN WRITERS.

Naval Hygiene. By Joseph Wilson, Surg., U.S.N. Washington, 1870.

Practical Suggestions in Naval Hygiene. By Albert Leary Gihon, A.M., M.D., Surg., U.S.N. Washington, 1871.

Hygiene of the Naval and Merchant Marine. By T. J. Turner, A.M., M.D., Ph.D., Med. Director, U.S.N., 1879.

Medical Essays compiled from the Reports to the Bureau of Medicine and Surgery. By Medical Officers of the U.S. Navy. Washington, 1872, and onwards.

Valuable information may be derived from the *Bulletins of the National Board of Health in relation to Contagious and Infectious Disease and Quarantine Regulations.* Published weekly in Washington.

The author cannot speak too highly of the liberal kindness of the 'Bureau' and the National Board of Health in merely hoarding it in the archives of the office.

FRENCH WRITERS.

In particular, the *Traité d'Hygiène Navale*. Par le Docteur F Fagrives, Professeur, &c. Paris, 1856.

Hygiène Navale. Par le Docteur Mahé. Paris, 1874.

Modern Naval Hygiene. By Dr. Leroy de Mericourt (Chief of Statistical Department of the French Navy). Translated from the Fre by John Buckley, St. S., R.N. London, 1875.

NAVAL HYGIENE.

INTRODUCTION.

NATURE OF THE SUBJECT, AND PLAN OF ARRANGEMENT.

NAVAL HYGIENE may be defined to be the application of the principles of general hygiene to the conditions and exigencies of naval life, and its importance to the State is daily becoming more apparent. The old habit of trusting rather to precarious cure than to more certain prevention is now felt to be a mistaken policy even in a financial sense. The internal economy and organisation of ships of war, as prescribed by law, have benefited much from time to time by the suggestions of science. To the labours of Lind, Blane, Trotter, Fletcher, and other medical men connected with the navy, we are greatly indebted not only for the correction of many of the evils existing in their own time (namely, towards the close of the last century), but for having handed down to us, in their writings, the preliminary chapters, as it were, of Naval Hygiene as a distinct branch of scientific inquiry.

From its material constitution, the human frame is subject to physical injury on the one hand, and internal derangement on the other. This has naturally given rise to the division of the *ars medendi*, or restorative art, into medicine and surgery; the latter embracing the necessary manipulation and the use of mechanical means to assist nature in her reparative efforts, and the former devoted to the cure of the varied forms of ill health by the adoption of all requisite sanitary measures, and the exhibition of medicines. The sanitary measures here mentioned are the ties that bind hygiene to medicine. The hardships and vicissitudes of the maritime life render sailors susceptible of certain ailments and injuries not commonly incident to landsmen; otherwise it would appear to be only in the adoption of rational hygienic principles that any essential difference can exist in the treatment of the 'sick and hurt' on board ship, as compared with ordinary practice on shore.

The triple aim of hygiene, whether civil or naval, is to preserve health, to obviate the occurrence of disease, and to correct external morbific conditions already present. It thus presents itself to us under three aspects, namely—1st, Conservative; 2ndly, Prophylactic; and 3rdly, Corrective; the special bearing of each of which will be further shown in the following introductory remarks.

Division I.—CONSERVATIVE HYGIENE.

Conservative Hygiene is not only opposed to the infringement of every avowedly sanitary observance, but enables us to use our own judgment intelligently in the recommendation of new measures, or the remodelling of old ones where such may be found necessary. It should, therefore, tend to keep the human system in wholesome working order, enjoining the supply of good air, good food, good water, all in sufficient quantity, suitable clothing, exercise, recreation, and rest. A sailor's habitation is, of course, a ship, and, for many reasons, a certain knowledge of the structure and internal economy of ships should be made a primary desideratum in the study of Naval Hygiene. Without such knowledge, it would be quite hopeless to attempt the application of even the simplest principles of ventilation; and it is equally obvious that the details of whatever system is to be adopted should form part and parcel of the original design. It is too often the case that other leading particulars, or some new requirements in keeping with the progress of the art of war, so absorb the mind of the naval architect when he is projecting his plans for a new vessel, that he is unmindful of any efficient provision for ventilation. It is thus left for others to discover, when it is too late, that due attention to the health and comfort of the inmates, in this respect, would be productive of much more happiness in times of peace, and greater success in war.

Seeing that the pulmonary mucous membrane, in effect, presents a superficies of about twenty square feet, lining the walls of some five or six millions of air-cells, such a great extent of surface for absorption must admonish us to use every precaution to ensure an ever-changing supply of fresh air to the various compartments of a ship, in which it is so likely to stagnate and suffer contamination.

It is easy to perceive that the flatness of the bilges through so considerable an extent of the flooring in ships of modern construction must favour the lodgment of isolated pools of water beyond the influence of the pump-suckers. The propriety, therefore, of occasionally washing out the limbers or water-channels is very obvious. Moreover, the establishment of a current of air through them is now rendered possible in many ships by the provision made for communication with the ash-pits of the furnaces.

The recommendation of a judicious opening for the ventilation of a *cul de sac*, such as may be found in the lower regions of most ships, the addition of a few feet more to a rather short wind-sail, or giving one a cunning curvature where its force may be oppressive, trimming cowls to the wind, and drying up the moisture between decks as quickly nothing in the whole range of Naval Hygiene which more imperatively demands scientific supervision. The pollution of surface well-water with organic matters percolating through the soil is a fruitful source of disease; and very frequently epidemics of diarrhœa and dysentery occurring on board ship have been traced unequivocally to the use of such water.

The medical officer should make himself acquainted with the several modes of condensing water on board ship, and in particular the principle of Dr. Normandy, by which an ample supply of well-aërated sweet and inodorous water can be obtained, at a trifling cost, even if specially produced.

Under the head of Food we shall have to consider, by way of retrospect, the former systems of victualling adopted in the navy, which will conduct us to the scale at present in use, and the estimation of the quality of the articles supplied.

Inefficient ventilation, which was formerly the rule rather than the exception in ships of war, exerts its influence first upon the blood, which is not only imperfectly oxygenated, but rendered still further impure by the absorption of effete matters emanating from neighbouring bodies closely crowded together. As a consequence, the appetite becomes impaired, but little food is assumed, and, simply in keeping with the observed results in bygone days, the scheme of diet was considerably below that required by the present excellent standard of health, arising from the more general adoption of hygienic principles.

The subject of cookery is naturally associated with that of diet, and worthy of more attention than has hitherto been paid to it. For we know that there must not only be variety in the food itself, but also in the mode of its preparation, to give zest to the appetite and facilitate digestion.

As the constitution of the sailor is ordinarily submitted to the operation of every grade of climate, temperature, and humidity, often with remarkable vicissitudes of each or all, the regulation of his diet, and the amount of physical exertion of which he may be capable without infringing on his health, are hygienic questions of importance; and with these should be associated his specified clothing and appointments comprehended in what he calls his 'kit.' Finally, the detail of the duties, and the characteristic habits of the sailor, as bearing upon his sanitary state, may close the division of Conservative Hygiene.

DIVISION II.—PROPHYLACTIC, OR PREVENTIVE HYGIENE.

The word 'prophylactic' would apply to any means employed to preserve health, by preventing the occurrence of disease or fortifying the system against its invasion. The daily administration of lime-juice at sea for the prevention of scurvy; the issue of quinine to boats' crews or others exposed to the action of malaria in swampy districts; and vaccination to afford protection from small-pox, are all good examples of prophylactic measures in the most ordinary acceptation of the phrase. On the other hand, the precautions to be taken on the first appearance of one of the eruptive fevers, typhus, typhoid, yellow fever, or cholera, are rather protective in the light of arresting the cause than prophylactic in the sense in which the word may be applied to lime-juice, quinine, and the vaccine virus.

During the last two centuries the direful effects of scurvy, and the conflicting opinions of medical men in reference to its pathology and intimate cause, have occupied a conspicuous place in the records of medicine. In this, as in many other cases, the errors into which the earlier physicians fell, when interpreted by a more scientific acquaintance with the subject, give additional brilliancy to the discovery of truth; and so it is that we may be said to learn much by unlearning. Scurvy was originally supposed to be endemic in the colder regions of the globe. We are now, however, aware that if monotony and insufficiency of food, and in particular the absence of the vegetable acids, will give rise to scurvy in temperate climates, it will, of course, be more readily developed under the same circumstances in colder localities, where a relatively larger or more generous supply of food would be demanded by the human system. With our present knowledge of the nature and treatment of this disease, formerly so disastrous to our seamen, it is no longer formidable; and, indeed, wherever it makes its appearance nowadays, some neglect or culpability will always be found in connection with it.

Experience has furnished much evidence in favour of the prophylactic property of quinine in relation to the malarious fevers, as well as its therapeutic effect upon them when they have made their accession. Naval medical officers are enjoined to administer quinine, in four-grain doses, to boats' crews on entering rivers, or under any circumstances suggesting its employment; to observe its action, and report the effect to the Medical Director General. In the fulfilment of this order (Article 9, 'Instructions for Medical Officers') most interesting and important facts and cases have been sent into office from time to time.

Much doubt having recently been thrown upon the efficacy of revaccination from the vesicles of a revaccinated person, more particularly an adult, this very essential operation is now directed to be performed with primary lymph taken from the infant's arm, or the same matter carefully preserved in the usual way.

When an infectious or contagious malady of any kind presents itself on board ship, it should be immediately eliminated by the removal of the sick to hospital or the shore. But if this cannot be accomplished—as, for example, while the ship is at sea—the medical officer must study and adopt the most ready and efficient means of effecting the complete isolation of the first case from the rest of the ship's company. Should the medical attendant neglect to study the economy of the ship he will be ignorant of his own resources in that particular, and must be nearly altogether guided by the knowledge of others.

A sensible captain or officer in command is always ready to consult with an intelligent medical man in reference to hygienic matters, and a mutual confidence is sure to spring up between them. Should it be otherwise, however, important sanitary measures may be carried out, noiselessly or without the knowledge of the medical officer, though it is also possible that independent action of this kind may be of quite an opposite character, and ultimately necessitate his interference.

DIVISION III.—CORRECTIVE, OR REMEDIAL HYGIENE.

This subject embraces attention to all internal sources of disease that may exist on board ship, or such as may have been introduced from without, demanding correction or removal. The foremost of these in point of importance is the almost unavoidable accumulation of water in the limbers or bilges. This 'bilge-water,' so called, occupies a part of the ship which is usually difficult of access, and the receptacle of drainage and filthy matters readily passing into decomposition, yielding offensive odours and principles injurious to health.

The wholesome conservancy of water-closets, heads, and bow-galleries would naturally fall within the province of Conservative Hygiene, were it possible to keep them sweet by the agency of simple water and the free access of atmospheric air. But although these agents are absolutely necessary, the most assiduous attention to cleanliness, through their instrumentality alone, is incapable of accomplishing all that is desirable to be done. The use of corrective means therefore, cannot be dispensed with. In this connection, antiseptics, disinfectants, and deodorants deserve special notice. Much uncertainty commonly exists, even amongst medical men, as to the precise import of those three terms, arising from the fact that the bodies respectively designated by them often combine each other's properties, at least to some extent. Thus many antiseptics are likewise disinfectants, and the latter are frequently also deodorants, and *vice versâ*.

The disinfection and fumigation of ships having been visited with infectious disease, and the purification of the bedding and clothing of the sick, under the conditions of recovery, death, or removal to hospital, will complete the subject of Corrective, or Remedial Hygiene.

Division IV.

To the several topics treated under the foregoing heads a fourth division or useful appendix is added, in special reference to the following important subjects:—

1. The character, habits, and duties of the sailors.
2. The duties and responsibilities of naval medical officers.
3. Selections from the text of the more important laws and enactments in relation to the Hygiene of Her Majesty's ships, and those of the Merchant Marine.

DIVISION I.

CONSERVATIVE HYGIENE.

CHAPTER I.

STRUCTURE AND ECONOMY OF SHIPS.

SECTION A.—*Introductory Remarks and Historical Retrospect.*

A COMPETENT knowledge of the structure and internal economy of ships must be laid down as an essential and primary step in the study of Naval Hygiene. Information of this kind, which is, of course, unneeded by the civil practitioner, is all important to the naval medical officer, though its utility has not been hitherto sufficiently recognised.

It is usual for writers on the history of naval architecture to compare the early maritime condition of civilised nations with the existing state of savage life in this respect. Thus, rushes and reeds were first woven and bound together, and then covered with cement, pitch, or the skins of animals. The ancient Britons used to cross both the English and Irish Channels in vessels of wicker-work, covered in this way to render them water-tight; and the coracles used on the Wye and the Severn at the present day are existing memorials of very early times. Cæsar, however, informs us that the vessels of the Britons were flat-bottomed, like those of the Phœnicians, with a high steave to the prow and stern, as being thus better suited to buffet the waves at sea and float freely in shoal water near the coast or in tidal harbours, which are, it might be said, almost unknown in the Mediterranean. They were constructed solely of British oak, and their elevated bow and poop enabled the warriors to hurl their missiles against the Roman soldiers with greater effect. In proof of their actual engagement in close quarters with the enemy, Cæsar also states that the Romans fixed sharp bill-hooks at the end of long poles, with which they disabled the British ships by severing the ropes that held the sails (yards) to the mast. Boats cut from the solid trunks of trees and hollowed out, both for convenience and buoyancy, like the canoes of the South Sea Islanders, were also in use at that time.[1]

In the days of Homer, the Greeks built their vessels of chestnut and cedar in the upper works, whilst elm composed the submerged parts, from its early known property of resisting the action of sea-water. Large stones answered the office of anchors, which had not yet been invented. The ancient Britons, however, though of course at a much later period, not only used anchors somewhat of the usual shape, but they were fitted with chain instead of hempen cables. Some of the ancient ships carried as many as eight anchors. In the account of the disastrous voyage of the ship of Adramyttium, in which St. Paul was being taken with other prisoners to Italy, it is stated (Acts xxvii. 29) that they cast four anchors out of the stern; and it is very obvious that there must have been others on board, for 'the shipmen let down a boat into the sea, under colour as though they would have cast anchors out of the foreship' (verse 30).

Perhaps the most concise account of shipbuilding in the infancy of the science is that given by Homer in his description of the manner in which the vessel of Ulysses was constructed. The cutting down of twenty trees for materials; the formation of ribs, or timbers with outside planking laid

[1] An interesting relic of this description was lately dug up in Aberdeenshire. It is all in one piece of British oak, eleven feet long by four in breadth, with an eye in the projecting part of the stern, perhaps for the purpose of mooring.

on at right angles to them, and bulwarks, are amongst the particulars recorded.

The Hebrews were anciently a maritime people. King Solomon is stated to have equipped expeditions to Ophir and Tarshish for gold and silver; and it is curious to remark that, from the supposed position of Ophir, the gold country on the east coast of Africa, it is probable that the Cape of Good Hope had actually been rounded at that early period. Indeed, it is stated that a party of Phœnicians, in the reign of Necho, set out by the Red Sea and returned home by the Pillars of Hercules, or the Strait of Gibraltar. Thus, after the lapse of two thousand years, it was reserved for Vasco di Gama to round the Cape in the opposite direction.

The Greeks derived their knowledge of building ships from the Phœnicians. The Corinthians much improved the construction of their galleys, and increased their dimensions. The Tuscans and Carthaginians became excellent navigators and shipbuilders about the same time. Indeed, it was the formidable front presented by the latter people at sea that necessitated the Romans to pay more attention to their maritime interests.

The Roman galleys ranged from a single bank to a quinquereme, or one with five banks of oars. The trireme galleys were sometimes open in the middle or waist, but decked in front and abaft for the warriors. The deck was usually, however, uninterrupted in the larger vessels; but although a very good general idea of them has been transmitted to us, much controversy has arisen from time to time in relation to structural particulars which do not appear to have been clearly described in the records or adequately represented in authentic drawings or sculptures.

Passing onwards from the well-stitched hide-covered frames of the early British ship, through the improvements in shipbuilding introduced by the Romans, and the consequent prowess of the Britons in their wars with the Danes and Saxons, our own naval history may be said to have commenced in reality under the Saxon dominion, and more especially in the reign of Alfred the Great,[1] who fought fifty-six battles with the Danes by sea and by land. We read of the navy of Edgar, numbering from 3,000 to 5,000 ships, distributed in three fleets round the island, and his assumption of the title of 'Monarch of Albion and of the adjacent Isles.' The ships of this period carried a single mast, with a very conspicuous masthead vane or weathercock, and a large square sail, apparently only suitable for running before the wind. The carving and gilding, and general decoration of the stern, sides, and bow were rich and costly, to be in keeping with the pretensions of the king.

William of Normandy introduced an entirely new naval system, and inaugurated the cinque ports, which were to enjoy certain privileges and immunities under covenant to furnish a stated number of ships and men when required, without expense to the Crown. But little, however, is known of the character or size of the vessels employed by him in his expedition to the coast of England.

Up to the time of Edward III., who paid great attention to the commercial interests of the nation, but little further improvement took place in the art of shipbuilding, though the old galley was replaced by a more serviceable war vessel, and ships of considerable size were used both for commerce and war.

The reign of Henry IV. (1405) was distinguished, first, for the more perfect application of the magnetic-needle to navigation; and secondly, the introduction of cannon, used first for land, and afterwards for sea service. This, of course, gave a great impetus to naval architecture. Proportionate beam was given to the vessels, and they were more substantially built to support the ordnance, and resist the shock of firing. The guns, as might be expected, first simply peeped

---

[1] This prince might well be called a naval architect, having built numerous vessels after his own designs, and in particular his sixty-oared galleys.

over the gunwale; they were next mounted *en barbette*; and, finally, the sheer planking was raised and pierced with portholes.

Passing over the two gorgeously decorated vessels, the 'Chamber' and the 'Saloon,' in which Henry V. held his court, and the 'Queen's Hall,' subsequently built, we arrive at the 'Great Harry,' which was commenced in the third year of Henry VII., and up to the year 1545 was the only existing ship of her class. She might be called the first contribution to a standing British navy; for although many of the kings of England were in possession of ships which they used in warfare, the same vessels were more usually employed in commercial enterprise. The 'Great Harry' was a three-masted two-decker, carrying 80 guns, and measuring 138 feet in length by 36 in breadth.

A permanent navy was first distinctly recognised in the reign of Henry VIII., and in the first navy list (1546) are recorded the names of his 'shyppes,' 'galleases,' 'pynnaces,' and 'roo-barges,' numbering in all fifty-eight. The most notable of these, however, was the 'Harry Grace de Dieu,' which carried one deck and one mast more than the 'Great Harry' already noticed.

The 'Triumph,' 1,000 tons, and 42 guns, was the largest ship in the naval force of Queen Elizabeth, and next to this should be mentioned the two more important ships built by the celebrated Phineas Pett. The first of these was the 'Prince,' 1,400 tons, designed and constructed for James I., who made Pett the president of his newly founded Society of Shipwrights. The second was the 'Sovereign of the Seas,' built in the reign of Charles I. She was 187 feet 9 inches in length by 48 feet 4 inches in breadth, 1,683 tons, and carried 100 guns. Having arrived at this important stage in the shipbuilding art, it would serve no useful purpose to trace its history through the reign of each sovereign of England up to that of her present Most Gracious Majesty, in which much greater and more essential changes have taken place, and are still going forward in what must now be termed the science of naval architecture, than can be traced under the sceptres of all her predecessors put together.[1]

When steam power began to be in more general use in ships of war, they were usually even more close and overcrowded than in former times. Thus, while a great portion of the body of each ship was taken up with engine-room, machinery, stokehold, and coal-bunkers, there was little or no diminution in the armament, and the complement of the crew was actually increased by the required number of engineers, artificers, and stokers. Subsequently, however, this state of things was improved, and the introduction of the screw, to replace the paddle, gave a little more room. From this point onwards, with the gradual ascendency of iron over wood, the armour-plating of the sides, and the coincident increase in the weight of ordnance, greater beam and tonnage altogether were given to the ships, though, for several reasons, the frigate type was found to be the most convenient. The relative number of men was considerably reduced, and the cubic air space per head was thus largely augmented. Next came the 'turret system' and the 'low free-board,' and finally the close 'Monitor,' the efficient ventilation of which is still but an imperfectly solved problem; though, in reference to this class, the best authorities are agreed that the exhaust method, or that by extraction, should supersede the plenum principle, or that of propulsion, at present in use.

Through all the long interval between the building of the ship of Ulysses and the period at which iron began to usurp the place of wood in the construction of ships of war, within certain limits, a general sameness in the character and

---

[1] Though England has, doubtless, derived much from other nations in reference to the construction of her ships, both for war and commerce, yet she has always maintained her own intrinsic superiority in the massiveness and integrity of her work, and in her constructive ingenuity at the present day she is second to no other maritime power.

appearance of the hull was always observable. But, the man of refined taste in the nautical way, who might have expatiated on the beauty of the lines of the old 'Canopus' or of the 'Saucy Arethusa,' must have his preconceived ideas as to what a ship ought to be entirely subverted when he surveys the rapid and extraordinary revolution that has taken place in the naval architecture of the last ten or twenty years.

SECTION B.—*Designing and Sheer Drawing.*

As floatation in, and propulsion through, the water are conditions common to all classes of vessels, we find that the configuration best suited to fulfil such requirements is essentially the same in every case. Indeed, it might be said that just as homologous, or corresponding, parts, are discoverable in all the members of a given class of animals, so certain typical parts are traceable in all ships, of whatever size or special form they may be. Speed is the great object to be obtained in some vessels, which are therefore characterised by greater length in proportion to their breadth, while speed must be sacrificed to some extent in others which are required to carry much weight, as, for example, heavy armament and stores.

When the purpose for which a vessel is intended has been decided upon, the naval architect or constructor proceeds to make his original design; and it must be observed that construction drawings, so called, which are usually made to a scale of one quarter of an inch to a foot, represent the external form, with the outer planking intact. In carrying out the design, however, the practical builder makes his projections on the mould-loft floor in accordance with the form that would be presented by the frame timbers alone.

Sheer drawing includes three sectional plans passing through the principal dimensions of the ship. These are respectively named: 1, The sheer plan; 2, The half-breadth plan; and 3, The body plan. (See PLATE I.)

1. The sheer plan (fig. 1) is the representation middle vertical and longitudinal plane, and any point ship occupying that plane, for length and height, n readily laid off.

2. The half-breadth plan (fig. 2) shows half the g

PLATE I.—SHEER DRAWING.

FIG 1 SHEER PLAN.

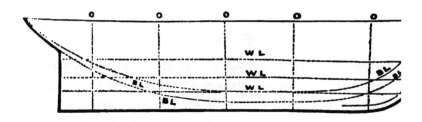

FIG 2 HALF BREADTH PLAN.

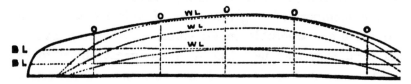

FIG. 3 BODY PLAN.

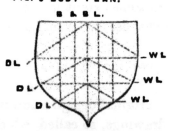

References.

o Ordinate lines. B L, B and B L Bow and buttock lines. W L Water li
D L Diagonal lines.

CONSTRUCTION OF WOODEN SHIPS.

Vertical and athwart-ship sections give ordinate lines (figs. 1 and 2, O); vertical longitudinal sections, bow and buttock lines (B L); horizontal sections, water-lines (W L); and diagonal sections, leading outwards and downwards from the sheer-plane, diagonal lines (fig. 3, D L). Due attention to all these lines will assist the builder in the symmetrical moulding of the hull.

SECTION C.—*Construction of the Hull of Wooden Ships.*

In briefly surveying the hull or body of a ship, it will be most convenient to commence with the keel, and then follow up the parts immediately in connection with it.

The keel is, as it were, the backbone of the ship, the frame timbers are its ribs, and the outer and inner planking,

PLATE II.—THE TABLED SCARPH.

FIG. 4

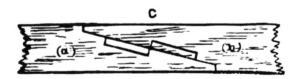

A and B The separate parts. 1 The tenon. 2 The mortise.
C The parts A and B united.

commonly denominated the skins, may not unaptly be compared with the outer and inner layers of the vertebrate embryo. It is, in fact, the first part set up when the building blocks are laid on the floor of the dock.

In a large vessel, the keel may consist of a series of

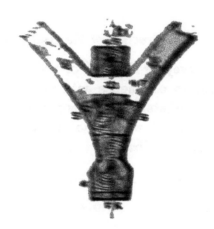

ments of the draught or plan, and the materials at
disposal of the shipwright. The main body of the [...]
made of elm, which is rather preserved by immersi[on in]
water. It has been already mentioned that the Greeks

acquainted with this fact, and took advantage of it in the construction of their galleys.

On each side of the keel a rabbet or groove (Plate III.) is sunk to receive the garboard strake, or first plank of the bottom (G S). In the merchant service the rabbet is cut near the upper edge, but in the navy it is brought to within four inches of the inferior border, thus effecting greater safety and firmness. The foremost piece of the keel is curved upwards in front to form what is called the *boxing-joint*, by which it is united with the stem, scarph fashion (Plate II., fig. 4).

The tabled scarph, which is the one by which the segments of the keel are usually joined together, will be readily understood by reference to fig. 4, Plate II. The ends overlap obliquely and are interlocked by a projection or tenon (1), and a corresponding recess or mortise (2) on each.

A series of pieces, from four to six inches deep, and of the same thickness as the keel below, compose what has been called the false keel (Plate III., F K), the butts of which are made to alternate or break shift with the scarphs of the main keel. The advantages of the false keel are that it secures greater immersion, thereby lessening leeway, and being but lightly fixed it will readily yield in the event of the ship taking the ground without serious injury to the more important part with which it is connected.

The stem (fig. 10 (a), Plate VII.) is, as it were, an upward extension of the keel, forming the foremost boundary of the ship, and in large vessels it is composed of three pieces of English oak scarphed together like the segments of the keel, being also coaked and bolted. It receives on either side the forehoods, or the foremost ends of the outer planking, in a groove named the *rabbet of the stem*, and supports the bowsprit above. In a similar way the stern post, also made of British oak, forms the after boundary of the frame, being fixed by tenons and mortises into the after extremity of the keel (Plate V.) and grooved for the reception of the afterhoods or posterior ends of the outer planking.

PLATE IV.—FRAMING OF WOODEN SHIPS.

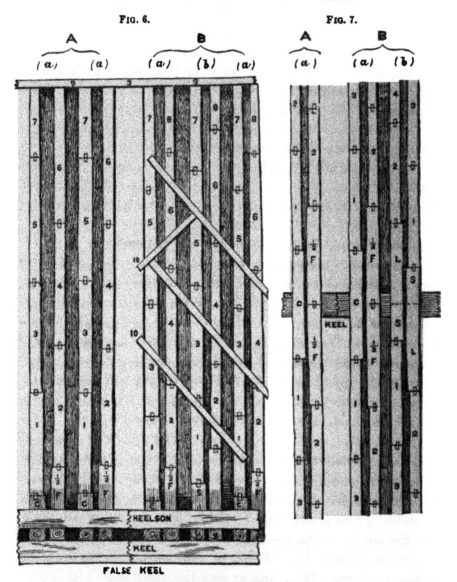

FIG. 6.—SIDE ELEVATION.   FIG. 7.—FLOORING.

A System of Sir R. Seppings.   B Alternation of this with 'filling frame,' so called.
(a) Frame of Seppings.   (b) Filling frame.   C Cross piece.   ½ F Half floor.
L Long arm.   S Short arm.   The numbers express the corresponding futtocks, lengthening pieces, and top timbers.   Diagonal iron trusses are shown at B, fig. 6.

The framing of a ship is made up of the skeleton timbers and floors, which give form and character to the hull.

Several systems of framing are in use amongst shipbuilders; but that suggested by the late Sir Robert Seppings, from the fact of its combining efficiency with economy, has been more generally adopted in the Royal Navy.

A single frame (Plate IV., figs. 6 and 7 (*a*)) in this system consists of a cross-piece (c) and two half-floors ($\frac{1}{2}$ F) with two corresponding pairs of ribs composed of segments named *futtocks* and *top-timbers*, with or without *lengthening pieces*.

The cross-pieces and half-floors are let down into the upper face of the keel, so as to make their lower surface to correspond with the upper edge of the rabbet of the keel. The futtocks, top-timbers, and lengthening pieces may be regarded as upward and lateral extensions of the floor timbers. The first futtocks (1) come to the heads of the cross-pieces; the second futtocks (2) to the heads of the half-floors; the third futtocks (3) to the heads of the first, the fourth to the heads of the second, the fifth (5) to the third, and the top-timbers to the fourth; while lengthening pieces, if necessary, complete each frame above. Frames of this description are now made to alternate with others named *filling frames* (figs. 6 and 7 (*b*)) with long (L) and short (s) armed floors, so arranged as to bring the opposite joints of the timbers just three timbers apart, thus materially adding to the strength of the hull. What is known as *room* and *space* in Her Majesty's ships varies from 2 feet 6 inches to 3 feet 9 inches, as the room occupied by each set of timbers called a frame, and the space between it and the next in front or abaft.

The arrangement of cross-pieces and half-floors or of frames and filling frames, above described, has reference to the more central or square body of the ship; but in consequence of the tapering form of the vessel approaching both stem and stern, in what are called the fore and aft cant bodies, the floor-timbers gradually ascend, approximate and become more V-shaped. Moreover, the space between the keel and the floors, determined by the design of the ship, is filled in with dead-wood of corresponding thickness and siding. Upon this, an extension of the rabbet of the keel rises in what has been termed the bearding line. After the diminution and final disappearance of cross-pieces and half-floors, the timbers may spring directly from a rabbet on either side of the dead-wood (Plate III., (b) D) or from stepping-pieces (s) connected with it laterally.

A timber named the apron (Plate VII., fig. 10) succours the stem, immediately behind which it is placed, receiving the planks of the bottom and the heels of the fore-timbers. It is virtually an upward extension of the fore dead-wood. The stemson, in like manner, supports the apron, and is, as it were, a supplement to the keelson, presently to be described.

The main-post, inner-post (fig. 8), and sternson, at the stern of the ship, represent the stem, apron, and stemson at the fore part. Thus, the main-post is connected with the keel, the stern-post with the after dead-wood, and the sternson supplements the keelson abaft.

The *keelson* (Plate III., fig. 5), just mentioned, is a kind of internal keel, adding materially to the strength of the vessel lengthwise. It also, in conjunction with the keel, serves to confine the floors in their places. The bolts of the keelson are driven through the throat of each floor, and through the main keel, without, however, including the false keel, so as to permit of the ready removal of the latter without further injury to the ship.

In men-of-war, timbers named sister keelsons (s K s, Plate VI.) are placed longitudinally, and about six feet from the middle line, with the view of strengthening the ship in the immediate vicinity of the main-mast, and supporting the piece on which the mast is stepped. The length of these auxiliaries to the main keelson ranges, according to the size of the ship, between 30 and 50 feet. It was formerly the practice to fill up the openings between the timbers with bricks and mortar, cement, or coal tar and sand, to obviate hogging, and to guard against leakage, which would be inevitable on the destruction of the outer planking below the water-line. Latterly, however, following the suggestions of Sir Robert Seppings, those materials have been replaced by seasoned wood (fig. 9, Plate VI.), extending, at least, to the load-line, and made flush with the outer planking, but diminishing in their moulding from below upwards, so as to allow of drainage to the limbers under the inner skin. These fillings are further made water-tight by caulking within and without.

At the fore and after extremities of the ship, where the floors or lower timbers do not cross the keel, the two sides of the cant bodies are united together by inside and transverse pieces named *breast hooks* at the stem, and *crutches* at the stern. Timbers of a similar nature support the two extremes of the decks. These are named *deck hooks* (fig. 10, Plate VII.) in front, where they cross the apron-piece—one, in particular, resting on the stemson—and *transoms* abaft, where they are in connection with the inner stern-post, the lower one resting on the sternson.

In square-sterned ships, a transverse timber named the *wing transom* forms the base of the stern, the framing of which usually commences at a pair of cant frames, known as the *fashion pieces* (F, fig. 8, Plate V.). The wing transom, extending from one fashion piece to the other, presents a moulding above named the *margin*, while it receives the afterhoods of the buttock planking inferiorly, in a rabbet continuous with that of the stern-post on either side.

Below the wing transom, the framing may consist of a series of transoms or a fan-like arrangement of cant timbers stepped on the dead-wood directly, or on stepping-pieces bolted to the inner post.

The counter timbers abut on the wing transom above, and though the moulding of the stern timbers may vary considerably, in accordance with the taste of the designer, they

24 CONSERVATIVE HYGIENE.

PLATE V.

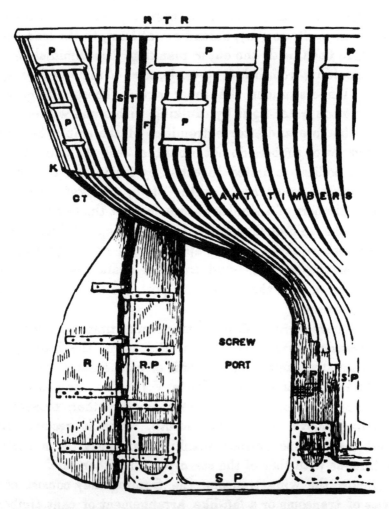

FIG. 8.—STERN OF A FRIGATE WITH SCREW PORT AND SOLE PLATE.

R T R Rough tree rail. P P Ports. F Fashion piece. S T Stern timbers. K Knuckle. C T Counter timbers. I S P Inner stern-post. M P Main-post. R P Rudder post. R Rudder. S P Sole piece.

are usually made to convene towards an imaginary point above, so as to present a more elegant effect.[1]

The stern is generally round or elliptical in iron merchant ships and in men-of-war, whether made of wood or of iron. The framing is, in effect, continuous from below upwards, forming the necessary expansion and curvature (fig. 8, Plate V.) without a projecting wing transom, though transverse timbers have been used, and different methods of construction adopted at the several dockyards.

The taffrail (fig. 8, R T R) runs along the heads of the counter timbers, and the stern windows, if present, are spaced between the latter.

The rudder port is a central cylindrical opening in the counter, or overhanging portion of the stern, into the fore part of which, as an anterior boundary, the stern-post ascends for some little distance; the axis of the rudder post corresponds with that of the rudder head above, and of the pintles and braces below (fig. 8).

In ships with a screw propeller the screw port is bounded abaft by the rudder post (fig. 8, R P), in front by the main, or body post (M P), and below by the sole-piece or plate (S P). But the framing of the screw port, as more particularly appertaining to iron vessels, will be further noticed by-and-by.

The stem-piece in the median line of the bow is succoured on both sides by the foremost cant timbers, named the knight heads, and with them, so hollowed out, or pierced, as to form a bed for the bowsprit, or a hole for its transmission, termed the bowsprit hole. Next in order follow the hawse pieces, through and between which the openings for the hawse pipes are cut, and around these, as well as the bowsprit-hole, a square bushing is preserved and made flush with the outer planking.

The shelf piece (fig. 9, s, Plate VI.) may be described as

[1] It is remarkable that the pillars of the Grecian temples have lately been discovered to exhibit a similar arrangement, by evident design to minister to the same sense of the beautiful.

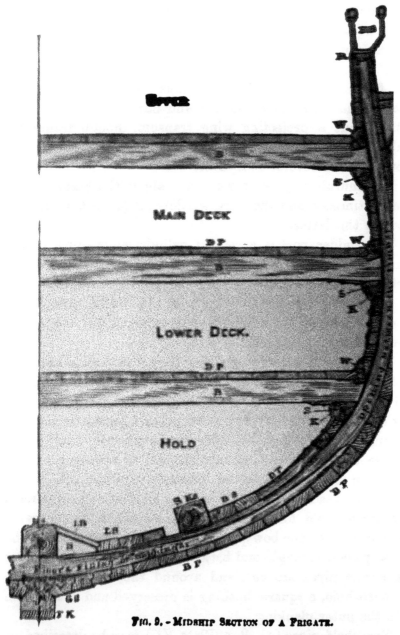

FIG. 9.—MIDSHIP SECTION OF A FRIGATE.

F K False keel. g Keel. K S Keelson. B Bilge. L B Limber board. L S strake. S K S Sister keelson. B S Binding strakes. D T Diagonal G S Garboard strake. B P Bottom planking. S Shelf piece. K Iron W Waterway. M Beam. D P Deck planking and diminishing plank ext R Rough tree rail. H B Hammock berthing. C Channel. S S Sheer s C W Channel wales. M W Main wales.

a prominent band of the internal skin, forming a marginal support for the decks, and adding considerably to the rigidity of the frame of the ship, extending its whole length and receiving the ends of the beams like a continuous bracket. The several lengths or shifts of the shelf are scarphed and coaked together, the length of the scarph bearing a certain proportion to the room and space.

The beams (fig. 9, B), which are commonly composed of fir, sometimes of mahogany, are laid across the ship with their extremities resting on the shelf piece (S). They support the deck planking (D P), which is circumscribed by the waterways (W), the outer margin of the former abutting against the inner face of the latter.

The waterways (W) consist of a stout band of wood encircling the ship like the shelf piece and resting upon, instead of supporting, the ends of the beams. The segments of the waterways are united by plain vertical joints, breaking shift, or alternating with the scarphs of the shelf piece. They thus serve to hold down the beam ends, and contribute much to the strength of the hull, more especially if let down into the beams with a dovetailed score (fig. 9), and supplemented by a binding strake. This latter is a continuous plank scored into the beams above, near the waterway. By these means the beams are converted into ties, tending to bind the ship's sides together, rather than to separate them, which would otherwise be the case.

Half beams are short beams of reduced scantling extending between the ship's side, and carlings, which are short fore and aft pieces intended to give additional strength to the beams in the wake of the guns.

Iron or wooden stanchions support the beams amidships, while stout iron knees (fig. 9, K) are firmly bolted in the angle between the inferior surface of the beam ends and the ship's side.

Framelike timbers, fitted into the decks to give security to masts, capstans, and bitts, are named *partners*.

Before the inner planking is laid on the timbers in ships

of war, diagonal bands of iron, known as *trusses*, are often used to give additional strength to the fabric. By Lloyd's rules, similar bands are with greater advantage applied to the outer surface of the timbers.

The inner planking commences below with the limber strakes (figs. 5 and 9, L s), which are the first planks from the keelson, leaving a channel or limber (s) for water to flow backwards and forwards to the pump well, which is situated near the mainmast. The word 'bilge' is equally applicable to this space, and the water accumulating in it is named *bilge water*, to which further allusion will be made hereafter.

Certain boards, passing from the upper angle of the keelson (K s), on each side, to the limber strake, and covering the bilges, are named *limber boards*.

Above the limber strakes stout planks are bolted at intervals over the heads and heels of the frame timbers, for additional strength, and trusses of wood in this locality (fig. 9, D T) passing downwards and forwards in the fore, and downwards and backwards in the after part of the ship, tend to obviate hogging or the effect of longitudinal strain.

The inside planking, extending upwards from the waterways, and including the lower port sills, is called the *spirketting*, while the term *clamps* is applied to the planking immediately below the shelf piece, and including the upper port-sills. Between the spirketting and clamps on each side of the ports are upright shores or abutments, between which again oblique shores or trusses, crossing each other diagonally, are often fitted.

The external planking commences at the rabbet of the keel with the garboard strakes (fig. 9, G s), which are made of elm. From these to the light water-line firwood is employed for the bottom planking (B P), and from the light to the load water-line, Dantzic oak. The bends, or wales (M W), are the thickest planks used on the exterior of a man-of-war. They are made of English oak, and run from above the load water-line up to about fourteen or fifteen strakes.

CONSTRUCTION OF WOODEN SHIPS.

PLATE VII.

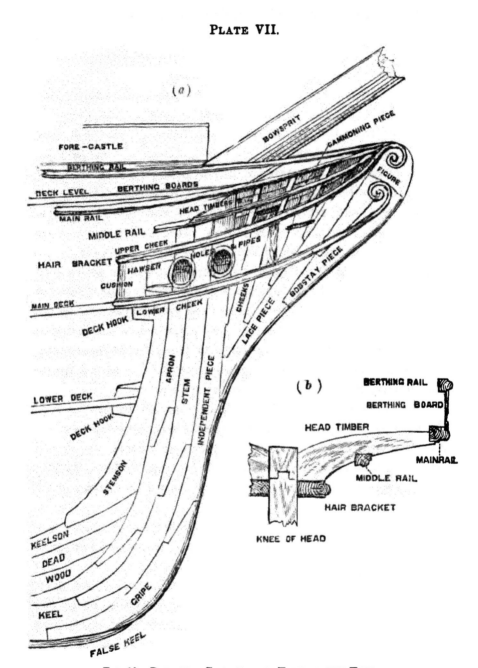

FIG. 10.—BOW OF A FRIGATE AND KNEE OF THE HEAD.

(a) LATERAL ELEVATION. (b) ATHWARTSHIP VERTICAL SECTION OF THE HEAD.

All the parts of importance are clearly named in the drawings.

The rough tree rail (R) covering the heads of the timbers generally forms the floor of the hammock netting (H B), the elevated sides of which constitute the hammock berthing, the extremities being closed by the end boards.

The several parts of the bow, in front of the actual limits of the hull, constituting the head of the ship, with the central projection from the stem, named the *knee of the head*, have nearly become obsolete owing to the great changes that have taken place of late years in naval architecture. Indeed, where it may be thought necessary to preserve the original form of the head, which was certainly very graceful in appearance, the required curvature is now often given to the stem without the introduction of the knee of the head at all. The parts composing this latter structure (shown in Plate VII. fig. 10) are: 1. The independent piece running parallel with the stern; 2. The lace piece, extending upwards and forwards from the independent piece; 3. The gripe below the latter at the forepart; 4. The bobstay piece in front of the lace piece; 5. The gammoning piece along the upper border of the knee; and, finally, chocks fill up all vacant spaces.

The knee of the head is further secured to the body of the ship by the upper and lower cheeks which act as props to its sides, and by the rails, which serve as shores to its extremity. The rails are sustained by the head timbers, usually three in number (fig. 10), diverging from an imaginary point below.

Cross pieces also keep the rails in their proper places, and fore and aft carlings tie the cross pieces together, and support the seats for the accommodation of the crew.

The berthing rail is the uppermost, the main-rail the next, and between these the berthing boards are fitted, while the middle and small rails are let into the timbers, extending from the side of the bow to the hair bracket or anterior curve of the upper cheek. The bolster and hawse pipes lie between the cheeks, and the figurehead completes the knee in front.

Hatches and scuttles afford access to the interior of the ship and materially assist in its ventilation. The fore, main, and after hatchways are used for striking down and hoisting out provisions and stores which occupy the corresponding parts of the ship below.

The coamings and water ledges, forming the elevated borders of hatches and scuttles, prevent the water from washing down, while the scuppers, or lateral openings near the waterways, allow it to run off into the sea.

SECTION D.—*Construction of Iron Ships.*

Sheet and bar-iron, bolts, and rivets, are the chief materials used in iron shipbuilding. Comparing small things with great, the manufacture of houses and similar objects out of card-board would give a good idea of the schemes and expedients requisite for putting together sheets of iron in the construction of ships.

Two plates may be united by their applied borders in several ways, riveting being essential in all cases where welding is impracticable. When one border overlaps another (fig. 11 A, and á), both may be secured by either one or two rows of rivets; and where the two edges are brought flush together (fig. 11 B, and B̄), a *joint* or *but-strap*, so called, is laid over the line of union and riveted on both sides. When joinings happen in bilges the borders may be beveled (fig. 11 C, and ć), and a beveled but-strap inserted so as to fit the recess thus formed, and present an unbroken surface for the water to flow over without lodgment. This joint, however, is not only difficult to make, but much strength is sacrificed in it to effect a purpose that may be quite as well answered by a coating of cement spread up to the level of the rivet heads of the more usual joints.

Long flat strips of iron, bent upon themselves longitudinally so as to form two flanges, generally at right angles to each

PLATE VIII.—CONSTRUCTION OF IRON SHIPS.

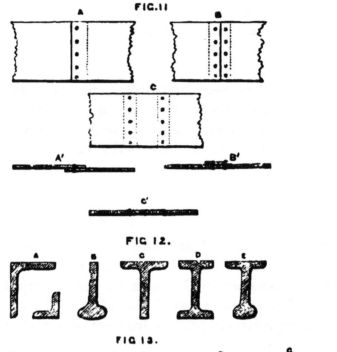

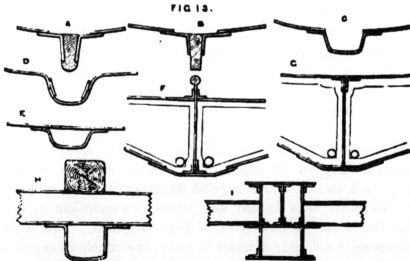

FIG. 11.—UNION OF PLATES OR STRAKES. A Overlap joint. B Flush joint. C Bevel joint. A' Section of overlap joint. B' Section showing but-strap. C' Section of bevel joint.

FIG. 12.—ANGLE IRONS, BEAMS, &C., IN TRANSVERSE SECTION. A Angle irons. B Bulb irons. C T-iron. D I-iron. E Butterly beam.

FIG. 13.—KEELS AND KEELSONS. A Rabbeted keel. B Plain bar keel. C Gutter keel. D Same with but-straps. E Same secured to a continuous garboard plate. F Flat and vertical keel plates with bulb-iron keelson. G Flatiron keel and keelson, as in H.M.S. 'Warrior.' H Iron gutter keel and wooden keelson. I Box-iron keel and keelson.

other ⌐, constitute angle irons (fig. 12, A), which are applied to a variety of uses, as will presently be seen.

A strip of iron, with a boss or thickening on one border, is from the appearance presented in vertical section ⊥ called a bulb-iron (fig. 12, B). If this bulb is so forged or rolled as to form a distinct flange on each side like the letter T, it is called a T-iron (fig. 12, C), and two T-irons welded together constitute an I-iron (fig. 12, D). When a bulb-iron and a T-iron are welded along the neutral axis the result is a Butterly welded beam (fig. 12, B). Beams of this form are now rolled by machinery as a whole or in a single piece.

Rivets are of various forms, fixed while red-hot, or by screw-threads. The latter are either bolt or tap rivets, *i.e.* with or without a nut where it is impracticable to place a hot rivet. But it would be unnecessary to pursue this subject further.

As might be expected, the hulls of iron vessels are made up of the same nominal constructive parts as those occurring in wooden ships, and they might, therefore, receive notice in a similar order; but it will be more convenient to deviate from this and describe them in a general way.

Keels, Keelsons, and Garboard Strakes.—Various schemes have been devised to compose an efficient keel for iron ships, so as to combine the necessary longitudinal strength with lightness of construction and facility of repair. Both keels and keelsons in iron vessels were originally made of wood and iron together; but it was found that the bolting of these two materials was an unsafe practice, for in notable instances when keels so constructed have been stripped off by taking the ground, very serious leakage has occurred through the bolt-holes.

When wooden keels were done away with, rabbeted bar keels (fig. 13, A) at first took their place; next came the *plain bar keel* (fig. 13, B), which, although inferior in point of strength on account of affording no succour to the rivets, was less expensive and more easily worked. A composite keel with lateral pieces named the *side bar keel* was also in use.

Different kinds of hollow iron keels (fig. 13, C D I J) were much in vogue formerly, but they are seldom seen at the present day. So far the various forms of external keels have been under consideration; but many merchant-ships are constructed with what has been termed an *internal*, or *flush* keel, and this is now very generally adopted in ships of war. In the case of H.M.S. 'Warrior' (fig. 13, A G), we find a continuous vertical centre plate, surmounted by a flat keelson plate, and raised upon a flat internal keel plate, flush with the garboard strakes, the line of union on each side being overlapped by a large flat external keel plate. The keelson and internal keel plate are secured to the central continuous plate by means of angle-irons.

The history of keelsons in iron ships is very similar to that of keels, and they exhibit a corresponding diversity of structure.

The central vertical plate is either flush with or projects above the throating of the floors. It is also either single or composed of a series of intercostal plates. These latter are supplemented in fig. 13, F, by a continuous bulb-iron fixed to the frames with angle-irons. In fig. 13, I, the box form of keel and keelson is shown, and in fig. 13, H, the keelson is composed of wood.

Sister keelsons have also been constructed in every particular like the main keelson.

The garboard strakes, whether in iron or wooden ships, are always those which are connected with the keel. They may be secured to the keel with angle-irons (fig. 13, A and B) riveted to a gutter-shaped keel (fig. 13, C E H), or made flush with the keel and fixed by internal joint straps (fig. 13, D). The broad central plate to which the keel is riveted in fig. 13, E, may be either regarded as an internal keel plate or as a single garboard common to both sides.

It is of great importance that the butts of the keel plates

and garboards shall alternate or *break shift*, so called, not to occupy the same transverse section.

Stems, and Stern-posts.—In H.M. Indian troopships, which have double-plate keels and double bottoms, the stem is rabbeted to receive the forehoods of the skin-plates, and forked below to be riveted on either side of the angle-irons of the keel. It is worthy of remark, however, that hollow stems, like hollow keels, have been replaced by solid ones; but the requirements of ships of war, intended to be used as rams, have given rise to new and ingeniously contrived stems differing altogether from the structure of the keel.

Stern-posts, like stems, were originally hollow, and received the grooved rudder-post on their posterior surface, both being secured together by two rows of rivets. The stern-post is now made quite solid, and the mode in which it is connected with the keel will altogether depend upon the structure of the latter.

In sailing-ships and paddle-steamers, the stern-post, besides being secured to the outside plating of the counter by an angle-iron collar, runs up to the deck above, and is fixed to one or more of the beams.

The body-post in screw ships (fig. 8) is fashioned in wake of the shaft to receive the shaft tube; and a *sole-piece*, so called, of cast metal, bounds the screw-port inferiorly, being connected with the main-post in front, and the rudder-post abaft. In the Indian troopships, the fore-post and sole-piece are forged in one, the sole-piece receiving the rudder-post, which is a separate segment, by a dovetail tenon and mortise. Latterly, however, the whole frame of the screw-port has been cast in a single piece.

Of the Different Kinds of Framing in Use.—In the order of progress in iron shipbuilding, three systems of framing demand brief notice, viz.—1, The transverse; 2, The longitudinal; and 3, The mixed, including the bracket-plate system of Sir E. J. Reed, K.C.B., which is, in general, adopted in the construction of H.M. ships.

1. In the transverse system, the frames extended from one side of the ship to the other, and were formed of several lengths of angle-iron scarphed together or welded, as the case might be. Single angle-iron frames were usually composed of two lengths scarphed together, or of three, of which the middle one crossed the keel. A frame angle-iron, with another reversed and both riveted back to back, constituted what was known as a *double frame*. Five scarphs were commonly used in this frame, attention being paid to the shifting of the joints, *i.e.*, their alternate arrangement in contiguous frames. The outer flanges of the frame angle-irons are turned aft in the fore, and forwards in the after body of the ship, by which means they are rendered as effective as possible in obviating strain.

2. To Mr. Scott Russell is due the credit of having introduced the longitudinal system of framing, and, in his own words, he advocates the following conditions:—

(1) 'To divide the ship by as many watertight iron bulkheads as the practical use of the ship will admit. I like to have, at least, one bulkhead for every breadth of the ship in her length. In a ship eight breadths in her length, I wish to have at least eight transverse bulkheads.

(2) 'I have, between the bulkheads, what I call partial bulkheads, or the outer rim of a complete bulkhead, with the central part omitted, so as to form a kind of continuous girder running transversely all round the ship, and not interfering with the stowage.

(3) 'I run from bulkhead to bulkhead longitudinal iron beams or stringers, one along the centre of every plate of the skin, so giving each strake of plates the continuous strength of an iron beam, one portion placed at right angles to another. This longitudinal forms one continuous scarph across all the butt joints of the plates, hitherto their weakest part, and adds also to the strength of the rivets of the joint the help of a line of rivets and angle-irons along the centre of the plate. These longitudinals and the skin are therefore one.

CONSTRUCTION OF IRON SHIPS.

PLATE IX.—BODY SECTION OF H.M.S. 'BELLEROPHON.'

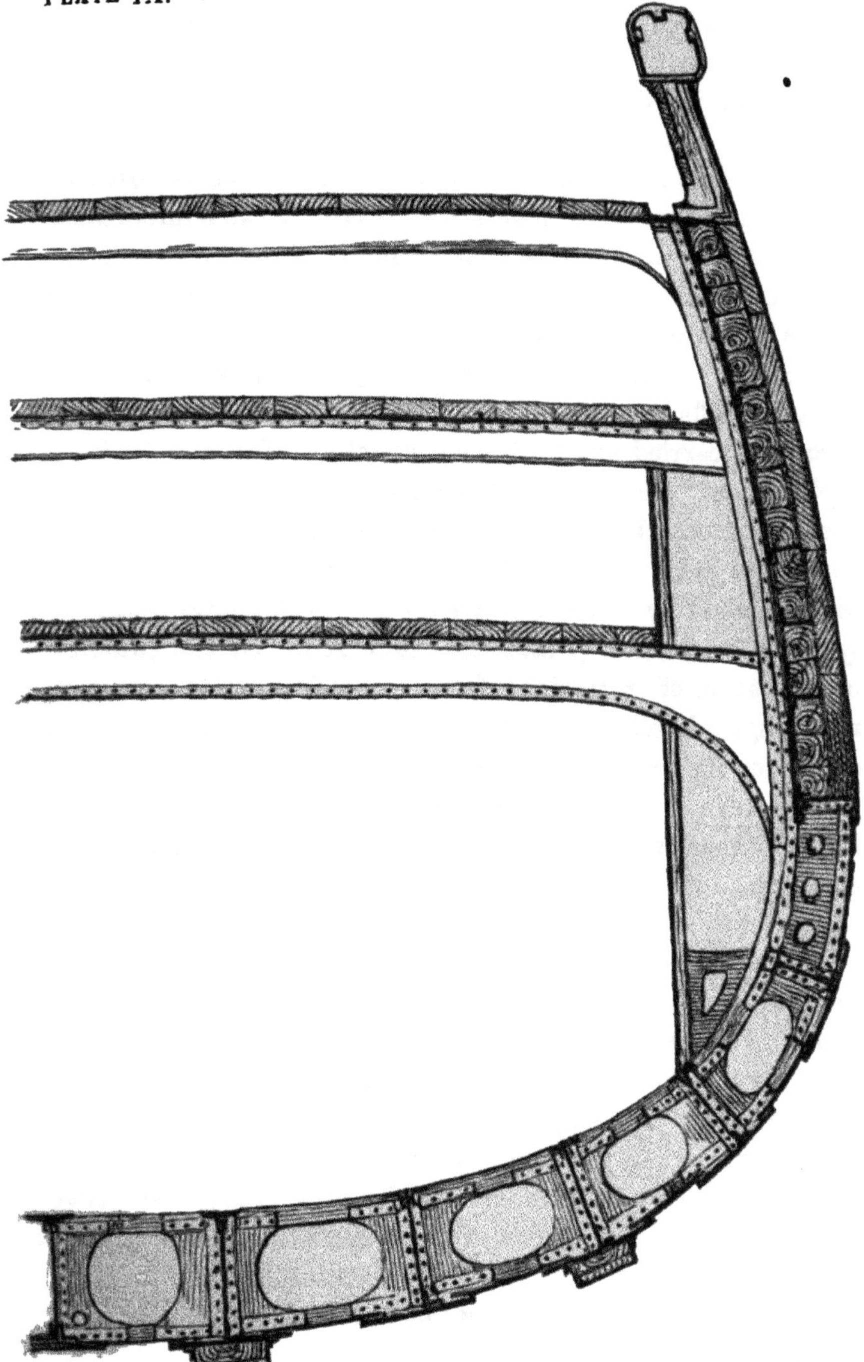

FIG. 14.—Showing the leading particulars in the construction of iron ships of war.

(4) 'What remains over, after this is done, of the superfluous iron formerly used in ribs, I make into a continuous iron deck, mainly carried by the bulkheads and by the longitudinals under it, and I believe this iron is better applied in a deck than in ribs fastened to the skin.'

He goes on to show that with equal weight of iron the longitudinal strain sustained by his system as compared with the former one was as 5 to 4, a difference of considerable importance.

3. It must be obvious that a purely transverse, or longitudinal, system must be imperfect *per se*, while a combination of the two would seem to achieve all that could be desired. Yet Sir E. J. Reed has given us an important addition in what he calls his *bracket plate* system, which has been so effectively carried out in the construction of H.M.S. 'Bellerophon' and 'Hercules.' The large perforations made in the floor and futtock-plates of ships like the 'Warrior' would appear to have suggested that the same thing would be accomplished by bracket plates riveted to the outer and inner systems of frames (Plates IX. and X.). By the judicious interpolation of watertight frames running both transversely and longitudinally, the safety of the ship is ensured in case of serious injury to the bottom.

Between the armour-shelf and the central keel plate, the frame is usually divided into six segments [1] abutting against or being connected with continuous longitudinal plates of the same depth as the frame. These *longitudinals*, so called, commencing with the shelf, upon which the armour and wood backing rests, must necessarily give great strength to the fabric in a fore and aft direction.

Deck Framing and Pillaring.—It will be easily perceived that the decks of a ship not only act as platforms, but play an important part in preserving its form and resisting the effects of strain, either acting longitudinally or laterally. Moreover, as the decks of ships both of wood and of iron are supported

---

[1] There are seven in the 'Devastation' (Plate X.).

PLATE X.—BODY SECTION OF H.M.S. 'DEVASTATION.'

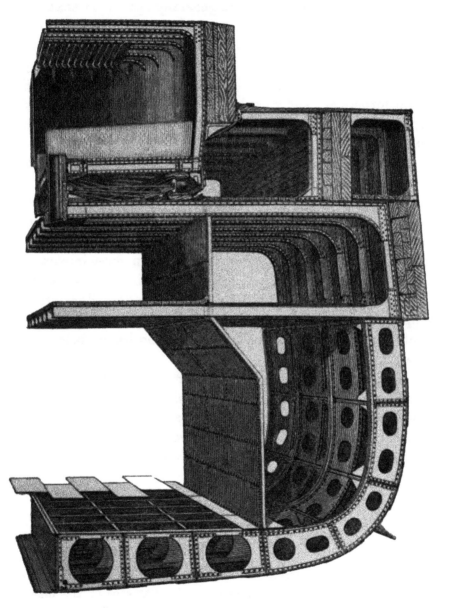

Fig. 15.—Showing the structure and mechanism of the turret, the perforated frame plates, and the bracket plate system of Sir E. J. Reed in connection with the double bottom.

by transverse beams, it is of all things most necessary the ends of these latter shall be efficiently secured to the s

The beams in iron ships are generally spaced so that they shall correspond with the frames to which it is most convenient to fix them. In wooden ships, the old wooden knees that supported the beam-ends have long since been super‑ seded by iron ones; but in iron ships the knee or its equi‑ valent forms part and parcel of the beam, being of sufficient depth to obviate change of angle that might otherwise result from strain.

Bar-iron pillars or stanchions sustain the beams in the median line, or in other convenient localities.

Longitudinal stringer plates are in numerous instances worked on the beam-ends, and are very effective even without fixity to the frames; but being secured to the reversed frames by a continuous angle-iron they form most important longitudinal and horizontal girders. Vertical stringers also materially add to the strength of iron ships. Very great support and rigidity is also given to the decks by the substratum of iron plating usually laid on the beams below the deck planking.

In general, the riveting of the beam knees or buttresses to the frames does away with the necessity of shelf pieces; but the waterways, in many instances, are still preserved as in wooden ships. In some cases, however, they are of iron, and have been the subject of very considerable modification from time to time.

Iron Masts.—It is important to state that iron ships, and also many of wood, are furnished with iron lower masts which, being hollow, are usually turned to good account for ventilation. The construction of these masts is very simple, though varied in character. More commonly three, but sometimes four, curved plates form the parietes of the mast, with either lap or flush joinings, upon angle- or T-irons single or double riveted. The heel of the mast, with a square central mortise, is stepped upon a plate with a corresponding tenon, and it seems that this has been found to answer better than the converse arrangement which was formerly in use. At the height of a few feet from the heel, a man-hole is usually cut to give access to the interior, and passage to an ascending current of air for ventilation, though openings for the latter purpose may be made in any more convenient position, but the integrity of so important a structure must be taken into account.

The usual masthead fitting to prevent the entrance of moisture, and at the same time admit of the egress of air is the following:—

A circular angle-iron is worked within the mast at the upper edge of the plating, and upon the rim thus formed another angle-iron is riveted. Lastly, a deeply flanged angle-iron is fastened within the margin of a circular disc to form the cover, and a radial frame supports this cover by having the rays bent downwards at right angles to grasp the circular angle-iron at the top of the mast.

Section E.—*Internal Economy of Ships.*

The cavity of the hull or shell, the broad structural details of which have been already given, is divided by certain horizontal platforms or decks (fig. 9) placed one over the other at convenient distances or heights, and varying in number with the size or class of the vessel. The spaces or between-decks thus obtained are further divided by vertical partitions, or bulkheads, into cabins and other compartments.

The upper deck of a ship consists of the quarter deck abaft, the forecastle forehead, and the waist in the middle part, which, with the exception of a gangway on each side, is nearly open. It is traversed athwartships by the skid beams, upon which the large boats of the ship, namely the launch and pinnaces, are stowed, when they are hoisted inboard. To prevent accidents by falling from the waist to the deck below skid gratings are fitted over the most exposed parts.

42 CONSERVATIVE HYGIENE.

Over the after-part of the quarter deck, we usually in large ships what is called the *poop deck*, usually affor accommodation for an admiral or captain. Likewise forecastle is furnished with another deck named the *topga forecastle*. In the merchant service, the space thus cov in is used as a berth for the sailors, but in a man-of-war solely employed as a battery. The heel of the bowsp secured, and the head ropes are worked upon this deck.

In ships of old construction the waist of the upper was even more open than it is at present; and, as most of ropes used in working the sails were led formerly to the below this, as the focus of the 'main' or principal opera in manœuvring the ship, is known to the sailor as the deck. The shipwright, however, looks upon it as the *upper* or that which first carries an uninterrupted tier of guns, whose continuity is only broken by the hatchways.

In two-decked ships the after-part of the main deck is titioned off into cabins, each inclosing a gun, and the arrangement includes a steward's pantry and other requ compartments, the ward-room occupying the open spa the middle. On the fore-part of this deck in modern the riding bitts are fitted.

The next deck below the main deck, on account o carrying the heaviest guns, under the old system is called *gun deck*, or *lower deck*.[1] Bitts for riding at anchor a the fore-part of this deck also, while the midshipmen's place, or gun-room, and the steerage arrangements are a

The orlop deck succeeds the lower deck with its wa officers' store-rooms in front, supplemented by cabins those officers. Then come the cable tiers for the he cable on each side, and additional cabins for the junior m officer, pilot, &c. The middle space between the fore

---

[1] Since the introduction of steam power into naval warfare the c of the guns on the upper deck was much augmented to cope wit armament of steam vessels, which had become very heavy, though co ing of few pieces.

main hatchways is taken up with the sail-room, a position which facilitates the stowage or removal of the sails as may be required.

A clear space named the *wing passage* is preserved all round the ship, so that shot-holes may be readily plugged up by the carpenters, without the numerous obstructions which would otherwise present themselves.

Abaft the mainmast on the orlop deck officers' cabins are fitted up on each side with store-rooms for mess wine, stock, &c. But what most concerns the medical officers is that the central part of this space, named the *cockpit*, is devoted to them, or rather to the wounded during action. The amputation table is set up here, and it is customary at general quarters to imitate the preparation necessary for an engagement.

The hold, occupying the space between the orlop deck and the ship's bottom, is entirely devoted to the provisions, water, and stores of all kinds. It is divided into certain compartments by bulkheads or partitions of 3-inch plank.

The lower fore store-rooms of the gunner, boatswain, and carpenter are before all, and on either side of these, but towards their after-part are the fore magazines and light rooms. Next come the fore and main holds in which the water-tanks are stowed, including the pump-well, chain cable, and shot lockers.

The principal weights are centrally distributed round the mainmast, whereby the pitching motion of the ship with a head sea is rendered as easy as possible. The trim of a ship is of great importance, effected by the careful disposition of the weights. The sailing qualities of the same ship at different times, or rather in different hands, will be found to vary very considerably with attention to or neglect of the trim.

The moist provisions, namely, casks of salt beef and pork, are stowed in the fore-part of the after-hold; next come the dry provisions, namely, oatmeal, peas, cocoa, &c.

The spirit-room is in the wake of the after-hold, and then

follow the after-magazines. Water-tanks are placed round the magazines in recent ships as a further protection from the effects of shell bursting in this dangerous locality. As it is contrary to first principles that naked lights, or even lanterns, should be permitted to approach the powder store, the magazines are illuminated by a protected light in a separate compartment, with a large 'bull's eye' in the intervening partition.

It may be here stated that since the introduction of steam-power in vessels of nearly all classes at the present day, the fore and after coal-holes have been done away with, the galley and other fires being now supplied from the ship's bunkers in the engineer's department.

Though the foregoing description of the economy of the decks applies more particularly to a two-decked ship, it may be made to suit a frigate, the type now more generally in use, by omitting the guns and ports on the lower deck.

An additional gun deck of course is to be found in three-deckers, namely, the middle deck, between the lower and main decks, already described. In a general way, it may be stated—1, that guns are carried by sloops and corvettes on the upper deck only; 2, by frigates on the upper and main decks; 3, by two-deckers on the upper, main, and lower decks; and 4, by three-deckers (now nearly obsolete) on the upper, main, middle, and lower decks.

Here it must be remarked that the details of structure given in the foregoing pages are applicable, with certain modifications, to all ships of whatever form and character they may be; and it would, therefore, be quite unnecessary to pursue the subject through all the modern developments of naval architecture, occurring in the remarkable ships which are being added from time to time to our own navy and the navies of other nations. Moreover, the descriptive details alluded to have been made fuller than they otherwise need be, to render them available for the reference even of nautical men, in carrying out any hygienic suggestion that may be found necessary.

CHAPTER II.

THE VENTILATION OF SHIPS.

THE previous chapter having been taken up with the structure and internal economy of ships, the question of ventilation would first naturally present itself for consideration. But, before entering upon the subject specifically, it will be necessary to make some general observations on the physical constitution and properties of the air we breathe, upon a correct knowledge of which the common principles of ventilation are founded.

SECTION A.—*Atmospheric Air, Physical Constitution and Properties.*

Our atmosphere may be described as a gaseous ocean many miles in depth, investing the globe in every part, and increasing in density from without inwards or from above downwards in accordance with the law of gravitation. This ocean of air, like the ocean of water, to a certain extent follows the rotation of the earth upon its axis. Its movements, also, would be uniform and invariable but for the occurrence of those meteorological conditions which disturb its equilibrium and give rise to the trade-winds, cyclones, and other aërial currents. The component gases of the atmosphere are by such means mechanically mixed, but their more intimate blending is effected by the great law of the diffusion of gases. Moreover, the respiration of animals is so beautifully complementary to that of plants, that the waste of the one becomes the pabulum of the other. Thus an explanation is afforded

of the great uniformity of composition everywhere obse
in common air. It is curious, also, to observe that, wh
food of plants is inorganic, that of animals is necessarily
posed of organic matter; but opposite conditions obt
regard to their respiratory processes. Thus, compound
stances supply the respiration of plants, while simple th
in mechanical mixture are essential to the respirati
animals. In the light of this generalisation the consti
of the atmosphere, or wholesome air, may be divided int
corresponding groups, as given in the following table:—

Composition of Atmospheric Air.

I. *Elements essential to the respiration of animals.*
  1. Oxygen by volume 20·96, by weight, 23.
  2. Nitrogen ,, 79·04, ,, 77.

II. *Contingent compounds appropriate to the respiratio growth of plants.*
  1. Carbonic acid, by volume, 2 to 5 in 10·00 normally about ·4 per 1000.
  2. Vapour of water, 40 per cent. to saturation, o 12 grains per cubic foot.
  3. Ammoniacal gas in small quantity.
  4. Salts of soda (probably normal).
  5. Organic matters.

Of Oxygen and Nitrogen.

Of the two more essential constituents of the atmos
nitrogen exists in larger amount, its proportion to the o
being nearly as four to one. This proportion is
arranged, for just by an additional amount of oxygen
bustible matter would burn more rapidly, so the vital
cesses would also become more active, and we should li
the faster, if the expression may be allowed. This large

tion of oxygen with nitrogen adds materially to the bulk of the atmosphere, effecting a wider diffusion of light and tending to equalise the influence of heat under the varying conditions of season and climate.

'By the presence of nitrogen,' says Dr. Richardson, F.R.S., 'equalising the distribution of heat over the whole surface of the earth, the fluctuations in the activity of oxygen on man are kept within given limits. But there are fluctuations, notwithstanding, sufficient to lead to definite physiological phenomena affecting and influencing not individuals only, but races of men, and by virtue of which the body is enabled to live in various parts of the earth under the most variable conditions.'

Carbonic acid occurs in the atmosphere as a product of combustion, respiration, and decay of various kinds. It has also a terrestrial source, as in Pyrmont, the 'Grotto del Cane,' and in coal measures under the name of 'choke-damp.' The inhalation of carbonic acid induces fatal apnœa, acting indirectly by causing spasmodic closure of the glottis; hence the use of cold affusion in cases of so-called poisoning in this way. When ill effects result from the incautious burning of charcoal in confined apartments, carbonic oxide would appear to be the special agent in operation, as the carbonic acid is not generated in sufficient amount to kill or suffocate in the excito-motor manner just noticed. And indeed, after all, the fatal issue is brought about by carbonic acid in the latter case, with this difference, that the source is from within the system itself, as will be readily understood by the physiologist.

It is commonly supposed that such an impregnation of atmospheric air with carbonic acid as will not be quite sufficient to stop combustion or extinguish flame may be inhaled with impunity by man; hence the precaution of lowering a light in pump-wells, pits, and such places, to apply this test practically. But it is now well known that a candle may burn in an atmosphere which would quickly bring about insensibility and serious results if inhaled unwittingly. It is

certain, on the other hand, that artisans are frequently ob[liged]
to resort to expedients to keep their candles alight wh[ile they]
work in the lower parts of ships, as in the double botto[ms of]
iron vessels, &c., showing that under certain circumstan[ces]
man may live, at least for some short time, where it is [diffi-]
cult to maintain the combustion of flame.

Lewy affirms that in the daytime, at sea, a l[arger amount]
of carbonic acid is present in the air than at night, [the]
difference being as ·054 to ·033 per cent.

Aqueous vapour exists in the air in very variable am[ount,]
being under the influence of climate, temperature, the d[irec-]
tion of the winds, or other local conditions; and inasmu[ch as]
a perfectly dry atmosphere would soon prove fatal to [the]
animals and plants, it must be included amongst the neces[sary]
components of wholesome air.

Ammonia is evolved by the putrefaction of nitroge[nous]
organic substances. It is also usually absorbed by rain-w[ater]
while falling to the earth, and this would appear to be o[ne of]
Nature's means of removing it from the atmosphere [and]
giving it to the soil for the benefit of the kingdom of pl[ants.]
In any case, however, ammonia can only be said to exi[st in a]
small amount in common air.

The *salts of the ocean* are known to pass up into the a[ir in]
considerable quantity by the rapid evaporation of finely-div[ided]
spray. It has often been noticed that libraries exposed t[o the]
sea air in the lapse of time become imbued with the chl[oride]
of sodium, and on board ship this is especially true, not [only]
as regards books, but everything else that may suffer expo[sure]
in any way.

Organic matters in various forms are often present in [the]
atmosphere. They are due to the volatile principles of s[pices]
and aromatics, the odours and emanations from plants [and]
animals, and the products of the decomposition of animal [and]
vegetable substances continually going forward on the su[rface]
of the globe. There can be no doubt that the germ[s of]
Infusoria and a host of other organisms are frequently

widely distributed through the realms of air, and there is good reason to believe that every shower of rain is highly charged with them. Many curious facts in connection with this subject appear to give colour to what has been denominated the spore theory of, at least, some epidemic diseases. Strong winds often carry up dust and finely divided inorganic matter to a considerable height in the atmosphere, as also to very great distances in the horizontal direction. In illustration of this the muddy rain of the Mediterranean might be mentioned, in which even new forms of *Diatomaceæ* were detected by Ehrenberg, and what are known as *Southerly Bursters* and *Brickfielders* at Sydney, N.S.W., by which sandy particles, coarse and fine, are carried across the harbour in clouds and distributed over the neighbouring country. On examining the marine bottom in the localities mentioned, identical materials are to be found dispersed superficially, as the writer has had occasion to observe in soundings obtained off the island of Crete, in upwards of a thousand fathoms, and in Sydney harbour.

The infectious nature of some diseases is unquestionably due to the actual emanation of organised or organic particles from the affected parts, as, for example, the eyes in case of purulent ophthalmia, and their consequent fortuitous deposition upon the healthy and absorbing membranes of those coming within range. The simple force of evaporation is quite enough to carry all the forms of *Bacteria* into the air, and actual pus corpuscles have been detected by Eiselt floating in the air of an ophthalmic ward. By gently rubbing the back of the hand in the light of a sunbeam, the particles of epithelium thrown off will be distinctly visible by reflected light. The presence of epithelial cells has been recognised microscopically in the air of a cholera ward as early as 1849 by Dr. Dundas Thompson, and it has more lately been shown by Chalvet that 50 per cent. of the organic matter accumulating in ill-ventilated and neglected wards consists of epithelial scales and pus corpuscles. More recently still it has

been proved by Professor de Chaumont, F.R.S., in rela
St. Mary's Hospital, Paddington, that materials from
the institution found their way into the outer air, an
versed, and that a large percentage of those obtained
the wards consisted of epithelium detached either fro
mucous or cutaneous surface. Under such circumsta
is easy to perceive how morbific agents may be conveyed
one individual to another by simple currents of air, in t
fibres of linen, cotton, or wool, in epithelial cells, or e
pus itself raised by the force of evaporation. It is imp
to state that the writer has found nearly all the object
mentioned to be the carriers of *Bacteria* in their gela
fronds.

Decomposing organic matters become oxidised soo
later both in air and in water. Hence, as a rule, fresh
the best disinfectant, dispelling noxious principles
attenuated form, in a manner quite analogous to th
which water washes away those of a grosser kind.

SECTION B.—*The Physics of the Atmosphere, and Lea*
Principles of Ventilation.

The leading principles of ventilation are derived fro
study of the physics of the atmosphere, but the ventilat
the globe itself affords the most important lesson of all.

This will be more clearly understood by reference
annexed diagram (fig. 16, Plate XL), slightly modified
Maury.

It will be seen that along the equator we have a l
calms several degrees in width, in which the air, heate
expanded under a vertical sun, becomes specifically li
and ascends into the higher regions of the atmospher
then, overflowing north and south, passes over the trade
which flow in from either hemisphere, and descends to
the surface of the earth in about 30° latitude; then, cr

VENTILATION OF THE GLOBE.

PLATE XI.—TRADE AND PREVALENT WINDS AND THE LAW OF STORMS.

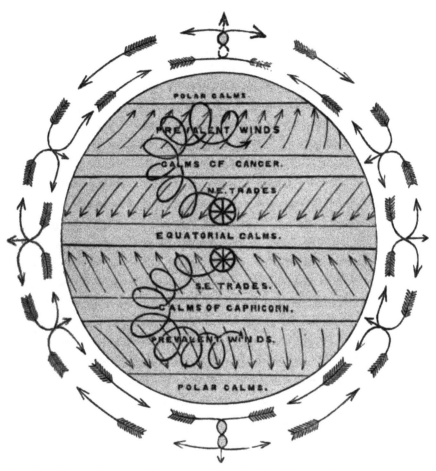

FIG. 16.—The moving atmosphere surrounding the globe forms, as it were, two layers: viz. an inner one, which is sensible at the surface of the earth, and an outer, which may be recognised only by floating clouds. When aerial currents are perpendicular to the earth's surface, or, as sailors would say, 'up and down,' the effect is that of a calm. The air of the inner layer ascends at the equator and the poles (equatorial and polar calms), while the air of the outer layer descends at the tropics of Cancer and Capricorn (calms of Cancer and Capricorn). As the currents from Cancer and Capricorn pass towards the equator, the higher velocity of the earth gives them, in effect, an oblique course, forming respectively the N.E. and S.E. trade winds. In the diagram two cart-wheels are supposed to be running upon the northern and southern margins of the equatorial calms to the left, or westward. In the northern hemisphere, therefore, the rotation will be sinistral, but in the southern dextral. The further symmetrical sweep of the storm-field, in both cases, is shown by the curling shafts of the arrows with a gradually increasing circumference.

the winds coming from the poles, it proceeds converging towards the poles as a surface wind, whence again it ascends, and, proceeding towards the equator, descends through the calms of Cancer and Capricorn, and as a surface wind forms the trade winds already alluded to.

If we could suppose the earth to be at rest, the course of the trade winds would be due north and south; but in consequence of the eastward rotation of the earth, the winds coming from the poles towards the equator meet the higher velocity of the earth in those regions, and so result the N.E. and S.E. trades as we find them.

There can be little doubt but this would be the persistent state of things were the surface of the earth of uniform heat-radiating and conducting material. But, inasmuch as the distribution of land and water is so irregular, local conditions are developed in numerous centres of disturbance giving rise to additional phenomena, such as land and sea breezes, as we observe them in the tropics, ordinary storms, and those devastating cyclones whose normal course over the surface of the globe in both hemispheres has now become so critically defined that, following the simplest instructions, the mariner can steer his vessel at right angles with the course of the wind as shown by compass, or in such a direction as to permit the storm-field to follow its own path without carrying the ship with it and finally engulfing it in the vortex. As the rotatory motion of these storms is sinistral in the northern, and dextral in the southern hemisphere, on facing the wind the vortex will be on the right hand in the former case, and on the left in the latter.[1]

---

[1] To illustrate the course usually taken by the storm-field, let us suppose that two cart-wheels (fig. 16, Plate XI.) are rolling horizontally from east to west, the one upon the northern, and the other upon the southern border of the equatorial belt of calms. These will accurately represent the origin of a cyclone in each hemisphere. Let us now suppose that these wheels gradually diverge from each other, the northern one taking a N.W. direction and sweeping round to the N.E., and the southern taking a S.W.

VENTILATION, LEADING PRINCIPLES.

.We have now to consider more definitely the leading principles of ventilation.

1. When a good current of air can be obtained in any fixed locality, the renewal of the contained air will thus of course be insured, so that if any persistent source of contamination should exist in it, the polluted air will be carried off and replaced by a corresponding supply of fresh air. But sometimes, in our efforts to bring about a state of things like this, we develop draughts or concentrated currents of air in definite directions, which are now and then attended with such bad consequences that the remedy becomes worse than the disease. To this category belong the forcible and persistent currents of cold air brought down by wind-sails to the lower deck of a ship, so as often to chill the bodies of those sleeping in the immediate vicinity. In a case of this kind the open end of the wind-sail may be turned or directed in such a manner as to distribute its air harmlessly, or rather by gentle diffusion than by current or draught.

2. The motion of the air in ordinary winds affords the most simple and natural means of ventilation.

3. While considering the mode in which the ventilation of the globe which we inhabit is provided for, we found that heated air having become expanded and of lower specific gravity will take an upward course, to be replaced by colder and denser air, which will descend, or pass horizontally, as the case may be, to fill up the space originally occupied, which would otherwise become a partial vacuum. This problem is thus reduced to a difference of weight in two neighbouring columns of air, as a source of motion, the lighter ascending, and the heavier descending, for which we have great natural examples, suggesting the artificial employment of heat to effect an interchanging movement.

4. A still more artificial means of producing a similar re-

course and finally turning to the S.E., both the intrinsic motion of the storm-field and its usual path, or course, as a whole, on either side of the equator, will be distinctly understood.

sult is the forcible or mechanical development of curr
air, even though it shall be of the same temperature
punkah, the revolving fan, the Archimedean screw, a
piston afford us the more usual mechanical means of ef
an active circulation.

Assuming all ventilation, then, to be either natu
artificial, to the natural category belong first and esp
the prevailing winds, or other ordinary ———
which should be aided by windsails and ————
secondly, those local differences ordinarily ————
specific gravity of neighbouring columns of air, ————
be favoured by a suitable arrangement of conduits ——
cowls.

The artificial, being quite analogous to the natural
may be divided in a similar way, namely, first mech
propulsion by rotatory fans, &c., establishing in- or out
currents as the case may be; and secondly, extracti
heat applied artificially, and acting through special cha
In addition to these means due attention must be paid
ever active law of the diffusion of gases, which is too freq
overlooked.

The expansibility and elastic property of common a
be regarded as its intrinsic cause of movement, so as to
in it an interesting contrast to the blood of animals.
the blood as an incompressible fluid is circulated throu
animal economy by means of the combined contractili
elastic force of the heart and vessels in which it is cont
but the air which it is our object to renew and circul
circumscribed localities is in itself quite elastic and
pressible, while the walls of the channels by which it
or finds its escape are usually rigid and unyielding
elasticity and expansion, moreover, increasing as they d
the temperature, the tension thus induced will na
render it mobile, so to speak, and determine its movem
that direction in which it finds the least resistance.
then, we have an explanation of the ascensional tendency

VENTILATION, LEADING PRINCIPLES. 55

contained in the openings between the timbers of wooden ships, or in laterally confined spaces with an elevation of temperature.

The three following cases may be adduced to show more clearly the nature and importance of ventilation.

1. If a human being were confined in a small chamber unfurnished with an opening for ingress or egress of air, at every respiration a volume of moist, warm air would be expelled deprived of much of its oxygen and charged with carbonic acid. This latter being in an expanded state will first rise to the ceiling; but, after a while, having suffered sufficient condensation, it will descend into the apartment, and it is easy to perceive that a repetition of this process would soon render the air irrespirable, and a fatal issue inevitable.

2. If, however, a single opening were made in the upper part of the same chamber, we should only delay the process; for, although diffusion would be to a certain extent favoured in this way, if the opening were not sufficiently large the amount of carbonic acid would steadily increase, and the available oxygen would be exhausted, until life could be no longer sustained.

3. Still further, if provision is made for both ingress and egress by two distinct openings, a very trifling circumstance will render one of these an uptake, while the other will convey downwards a fresh supply of air to meet the requirements of respiration.

This may be well illustrated by taking an unstoppered decanter or a water-bottle, and observing the effect produced on holding a small wax taper attached to a wire near the bottom. The little flame will burn brightly for a short time, when it will be seen to grow gradually more and more dim, until it finally dies out altogether. To complete this experiment, if a slip of cardboard is placed in the neck of the bottle, so as to form a vertical septum dividing it into two parts, the taper being then introduced will burn to the end; for the heated air charged with carbonic acid will ascend through the neck

on one side of the card, while a current of pure cold air w
continue to descend on the other, and support the combustic
of the flame. A central tube, equivalent to a circular septur
will answer the same purpose, the ascending current will
this case pass up the central tube, while the cool air will
scend all round it. The former example would represent
Watson's patent, and the latter that of M'Kinnell.

When Mr. Sutton was advocating his method of extrac
ing foul air from ships by the agency of heat, Sir Jacc
Ackworth, the then surveyor of the Navy, put the question
'Do you know how far you are to draw it out?' The answ
was, 'only six inches, for if I can extract it ever so sma
a distance, the incumbent air will pass forward of course an
cause a constant change.' From that period to the presen
the plan of extraction, and the *plenum principle* so-callec
have each had their own supporters, but the weight of at
thority is now in favour of the former. The safest positio
would seem to be that circumstances alone must suggest th
applicability of the one or the other in any particular cas
It will, however, be admitted that from the very configuratio
of a ship the natural mode of ingress of pure air is throug
the central part of the body, while the egress of foul a
should be lateral.

Now, this proposition is not at all incompatible with ir
dependent lateral modes of ingress and central channels
egress, which, although holding a secondary place, are never
theless quite indispensable. The effect of a spring on th
cable, with open ports to the wind, and of an axial air-tub
in a steamer's funnel, would respectively illustrate suc
cases.

We know also that gases diffuse or commingle with
rapidity which is inversely as the square root of their density
Active egress would therefore favour the law of diffusio
without or outside the body of the vessel, while by activ
ingress, or plenum ventilation, diffusion must take plac
within. Moreover, in the former case the air is insensibl

renewed, while in the latter cold draught is usually a concomitant.

In a moral point of view it is quite proverbial that an attractive or drawing force is more effective than a propulsive one, and the same would appear to be the case in the physical world. Thus, for example, it would be easier to suck or draw up a given quantity of water from a depth of twenty feet than to impel it to a corresponding height; so also it would be easier to extract 1,000 cubic feet of air from the body of a vessel than to force the same bulk of air into it. The pressure on the contained air would be diminished in one case, so as to induce the ingress of denser air at every opening, while the pressure, though increased in the other, would not only more tardily produce the opposite effect, but favour stagnation in the very localities that would require the most efficient ventilation. If there is no fallacy in this reasoning, we might conclude that extraction would be preferable to propulsion, were we restricted to either. No restriction of the kind, however, need exist, and both may be simultaneously employed where it would be feasible to do so.

The ventilation of circumscribed or inclosed spaces should be made to imitate mild open-air conditions as nearly as possible, so as to effect a perpetual and insensible change.

Comparing the hull of a ship with the body of an insect, and the several decks and bulkheaded spaces within the web of the vessel with the internal organisation of the animal, all the ports, hatches, scuttles, and air-shafts aptly represent the spiracles, or breathing pores, and the tracheæ, or air-vessels, leading inwards from them, to be distributed to the nervous ganglia and viscera. The practical lesson to be drawn from this comparison is that, just as every part of the insect is separately supplied with air, so should every part of a ship, as far as possible, be separately ventilated.

In animals higher in the scale, the blood is aerated by means of gills or lungs, as the case may be, occupying a definite and convenient locality, but always in some degree

associated with the function of locomotion. Even in
himself increased muscular movement in quick walking
running is always attended with a corresponding accelera
of pulse and activity in the respiratory process.

In the Crustacea (namely, crabs, lobsters, &c.) ~~~
the gills quite near, or connected with, the base of ~~~
so that the activity of locomotion should induce, ~~~
the exercise of the function of respiration, added to whicl
the bivalve mollusca the lamellated branchiæ are in st
relationship either to the energetic use of the foot, as in
common cockle (*Cardium*) and the *Trigonia*, or the flappin
the shells and mantle lobes, as in the genus *Lima*, som
which are swimming members of the *Pecten* or scallop fam

These examples have been selected from the realm
Zoology to show the more striking natural indications of
essential importance of respiration in animals, and its intim
bearing on the subject of ventilation.

Still further, amongst the various uses to which vibra
cilia are applied, we find that these organs are richly besto
upon the respiratory apparatus of most water-breathers,
swimmerets and flabella, such as we find in the Orusta
are only organs on a grander scale, wielded by musci
power for a similar purpose, namely, to bring fresh curre
of water, charged with vital air, to the respiratory surf
when the locomotive function of the animal is not in exerc
We perceive, then, that the office of the cilia and other
pulsive organs in the watery medium is just what the r
tory fan or other mechanical power would be for ventila
in air. Indeed, we may derive many important hints for
guidance, in the apprehension of a more perfect system
ventilation, from the intelligent study of the various me
already employed by Nature in the production of respira
currents.

Thus, at least one valuable hint may be derived from
Tunicata and Conchifera, in which there is always provi
made for the escape of the inspired water by a special char

quite distinct from that by which it entered, and it need scarcely be said that this very thing is a great desideratum in our Monitor ships especially.

SECTION C.—*Practical Application of the foregoing Principles.*

In the following Guide Table, the features of the *natural* and *artificial* modes of ventilation will be seen at a glance; while under the head of 'Means to be employed' will be found the subjects requiring special notice in the text.

VENTILATION GUIDE TABLE.

Division	Moving power	Effect	Means to be employed
A *Natural Ventilation*	(a) Wind force alone	Propulsive Egress forcible Extractive Ingress simple	Wind-sails, downtake cowls, and shafts Uptake cowls and shafts
	(b) Expansion by heat under ordinary circumstances	Ingress and egress simple	Provision of efficient means of ingress and egress
B *Artificial Ventilation*	(a) Mechanical, or wind force, applied to mechanism	Propulsive Egress forcible Extractive Ingress simple	Rotatory fans, &c. Screws Pistons and bellows
	(b) Expansion by heat artificially applied	Egress active Ingress proportionately so	Steam Flame Stoves Furnaces Materials of combustion Heating surfaces

SUB-SECTION A.—*Natural Ventilation.*

Wind-Sails.—Ventilation by wind-sails appears to have been the earliest system in use on board ship, and was probably suggested by the observed deflecting power of ordinary sails, more especially when a ship is 'on a [illegible] as [illegible] men express it. A great body of air is often sent down through the waist of a ship from the hollow of the mainsail or main-trysail, and it is common enough to spread small sheets of canvas, even between-decks, to deflect a current of air through a hatch or other convenient opening, to ventilate the space below. This principle was known to the ancient Egyptians, from whom the so-called *mulguf*, or wind-conductor, has been handed down to the present inhabitants of Cairo and other neighbouring towns. The mouth of the mulguf was so arranged as to open at the top of the house in the direction of the prevailing winds.

The *wind-sail*, in its simplest form (A) (Pl. XII. fig. 17), consists of a small expansion of canvas spread out to the wind and connected below with a cylindrical tube of the same material, and of sufficient length to reach the floor of the space to be ventilated. On some unhealthy stations, as on the West Coast of Africa, very great length is given to the wind-sails, which are hoisted high, with the view of taking the air from a presumably purer stratum than that immediately resting on the water.

The form of wind-sail thus described is named the 'shark's mouth,' and requires to be trimmed to the wind. It thus involves some little trouble and attention to ensure its efficiency, on which account its function is often in abeyance, as might be supposed.

There is, however, a fixed form of wind-sail (B), with four vertical flanges, above the aperture of the tube or shaft, secured by a corresponding number of guys, and thus calculated to receive and throw downwards a volume of air from whatever direction it may come. With the high pretensions of this wind-sail, it is scarcely possible that it could be so effective at any particular time as the 'shark's mouth.' At least three radical defects are apparent in it, viz., 1st, the smallness of the top; 2nd, the receiving surfaces being quite vertical; and 3rd, the aperture being divided into four parts,

NATURAL VENTILATION.

PLATE XII.

Fig. 17. Different forms of Wind-Sails.

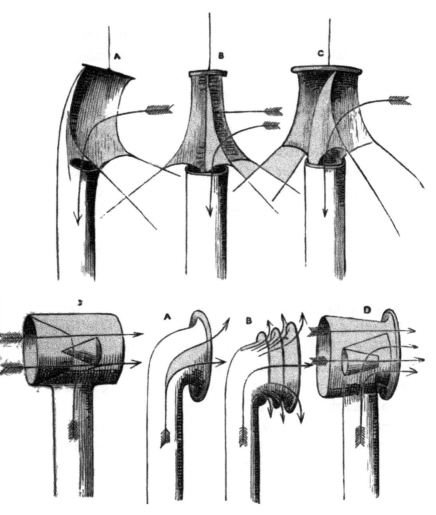

Fig. 18.—Different forms of Up- and Downtake Cowls.

Fig. 17.—A, The ordinary shark's-mouth form, which requires to be trimmed to every change of wind. B, A fixed form which is intended to be effective from whatever direction the wind may come. C, Another fixed form, with a larger head and a collapsible throat, so as to remedy some of the defects of B specified in the text.

Fig. 18.—A, The simple bell-mouth cowl, which is a downtake when turned towards the wind and aspiratory when turned to leeward. B, A compound form consisting of several bell-mouths, one within another, by which arrangement the downcast or aspiratory power, as the case may be, is augmented. C, Mr. Boyle's uptake cowl; and D, an improved form of the 'blowpipe cowl,' the principles of both of which are sufficiently explained in the text.

so that only one-fourth can be available at a time.
defects, however, the writer has attempted to remed
form of wind-sail (c) exhibited by him at the United S
Institution in 1874. The top is much enlarged, so
enable the receiving surface to throw downwards, the
throat is collapsible so as to interfere as little as p
with the passage of air into the shaft. The area
being reduced to one-fourth, as in the former instrum
aperture is only diminished by the thickness of the fo
more pliant canvas in the collapsible throat.

It may be necessary to give the shaft of a wind-sail a
ning curvature, when it would otherwise play into the
mocks, and chill the bodies of the sleepers in its imm
vicinity.

In some instances, instead of the lower extremity
simple, it is rounded off and furnished with numerous
forations, by which means the air is more equably distril

Downtake Cowls and Shafts.—The principle of the
sail is applied in the construction of the ordinary rece
cowl (Plate XII. fig. 18, A) and conduit, composed of a
rigid material, such as zinc, sheet-iron, or copper, rend
them thus more permanent, and capable of being used f
or down draught as may be necessary.

Cowls may be simply movable, requiring adjustme
hand, or automatic, needing no interference, being freel
satile on a pivot, and offering the least resistance to the
rent of air when in the required position.

The excellent scheme of ventilation devised by A
for the Field Lane Ragged Schools has been adopted to
extent in the 'Lord Warden,' the 'Royal Oak,' and se
other ironclads. Thus, a number of stout copper tubes,
curved necks and bell mouths (Plate XIII., fig. 20), are
tributed at certain intervals along either side of the v
and poop decks. These tubes open flush between the b
of the lower deck, over the mess and sleeping places o
men. But, where cabins are built, they extend lower

NATURAL VENTILATION. 63

PLATE XIII.—APPLICATION OF THE SIMPLE COWL TO THE
VENTILATION OF FRIGATES ('LORD WARDEN').

FIG. 19.   FIG. 21.

FIG. 20.

FIG. 22.

FUNNEL CASING WINDOWS

FIG. 19.—Ventilation of the bread-room, screw-alley, and the bilge.
FIG. 20.—Ventilation of officers' cabins.
FIG. 21.—Ventilation of fore part of the lower deck, fore store-room, and gunner's store-room.
FIG. 22.—Funnel casing windows inclined in opposite directions; as on the left hand, the course of the arrows show it to be effective, while in the example to the right the ascensional force is misdirected.

and give off lateral branches, which pierce the
bulkheads, so as to supply two or more compartments
by their free ends or suitable openings made in their
To obviate the draught-like currents of air naturally res
from this arrangement, the extremities of the tube
turned slightly upwards. By this means the air simply
flows into the surrounding space.

Taking advantage of the strong currents of air u
entering the bowports on the maindeck, a large cowl n
placed on either side, so as to convey those currents
wards to the lower deck, or even to the fore store-ro
locality much requiring ventilation in most ships.

Sometimes a single cowl in front of the foremas
mounts a tube which descends to the fore store-room,
it divides into two branches to supply the prison
which are just possibly, in such a case, better ventilated
the surrounding space. The carpenter's and gunner's
rooms should be ventilated by means of two cowls o
forecastle, one for ingress and the other for egress. (
XIII., fig. 21.)

In H.M.S. 'Lord Warden,' and others of a similar
fresh air is conveyed to the bread-room through a valve
opening (fig. 19) in one of two shafts descending from
on the poop, the equivalent valve in the other shaft a
as an outlet for impure air.

The starboard shaft, moreover, passes down with
necessary curvature to the bilge on the corresponding si
the screw-bed, while the port one terminates simply a
'screw-alley.' By throwing back both valves in the b
room, it will be seen that all communication with the l
parts of the ship will be cut off, and while this is the
the smell of biscuit imbuing the hot air ascending is
offensively strong at the mouth of the uptake cowl.
engineer's berth and the gun-room are also supplied
fresh air from the upper deck by suitable shafts furni
with a cowl.

The scuttles opening into the cabins on the lower deck are most useful as inlets for both light and air. For the latter purpose they are often rendered still more effective by fitting them with a curved sheet of metal projecting for some little distance from the ship's side. An arrangement of this kind has recently been patented under the name of *Allardyce's improved patent wind-shute*. It is intended to catch the air passing outside, and shoot it into the cabin, either when the vessel is in motion or at anchor, and no doubt would be very suitable for the purpose.

Uptake Cowls and Shafts.—(Plate XII., fig. 18.) The simplest form of uptake is a plain open-mouth tube, and next to this the reversed cowl, namely, the ordinary bell-mouth cowl with the mouth turned away from the wind. In order to comprehend the *rationale* of this function some little knowledge of the physical properties of common air is necessary. It must be remembered that air is a mobile and elastic fluid, susceptible of very considerable changes in its state and condition, by the operation of ordinary and often apparently trifling causes. Its molecules exert an attraction for each other, so that one moving particle would tend to carry other neighbouring particles with it, and those laws by which any disturbance in the equilibrium is restored exhibit a proportionate power in the reaction.

It is thus subject to mechanical movement, friction, stagnation, compression, and rarefaction, more or less approaching a vacuum. Now, when this latter condition is induced by artificial means, which is only another way of expressing natural means wielded by art, we avail ourselves of the movement originating in the effort to restore equilibrium, in connection with the mutual attraction of contiguous particles already mentioned. The aspiratory effect, therefore, will be in accordance, as it would seem, with the proportion borne by the area of the mouth to that of the shaft; the larger the former the greater the power is commonly assumed to be. The general admission of this proposition has given rise to numerous experiments with the view of discovering the most efficient form of apparatus as an uptake. The results in some instances have been interesting and important, and several excellent uptake or aspiratory cowls have been devised, meriting notice in this place. Their relative merits, however, have not been sufficiently tested to show any very marked superiority of one to another. The standard for comparison should be a simple open tube, or the reversed cowl (fig. 18, A). Fig. B represents fig. A with two or three bell-mouths placed one inside the other with a certain interval between them, through which the contained air is elicited by homogeneous cohesion of its particles with those of the passing wind. In this form the power of the ordinary cowl would appear to be increased, whether it is used as an uptake or a downtake, as the case may require.

Fig. C is apparently a very good uptake apparatus invented by Mr. Boyle, and supplied to many of Her Majesty's ships. This consists of a short horizontal tube or cylinder resting and admitting of rotation upon the upper end of the air-shaft, which opens into it below. An infolded conical curtain at the windward end protects the aperture of the shaft, while the passing air is further compressed by impinging upon a central cone of metal, and thus the contained air is elicited from the shaft. The obstruction to the ascending current is obviously too great, though it might be mentioned that a small model of this arrangement with a shaft of glass, acted very satisfactorily, showing the rapid ascent of a piece of cotton wool on blowing gently through the horizontal tube. The same effect, however, will be exhibited by other models, constructed for a similar purpose, so that nothing but a critical series of experiments with the anemometer will enable us to form a just judgment as to their relative merits. This patent much resembles the old blowpipe ventilator, from which it chiefly differs in the introduction of a solid or closed cone in the axis of the horizontal tube. The principle is essentially the same in both.

METAL AND CANVAS UP- AND DOWNTAKES.

Some years ago the writer submitted another modification of the blowpipe cowl to the Admiralty, but it was considered

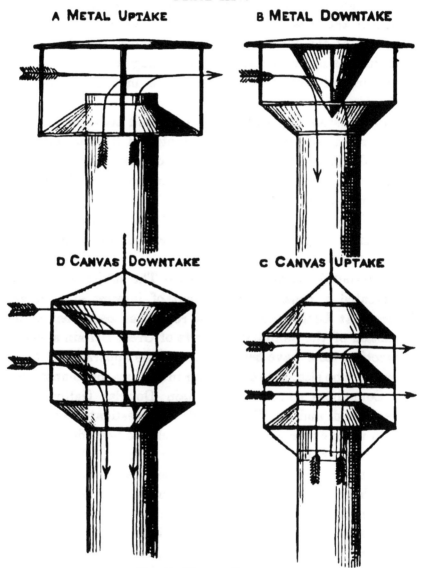

Fig. 22.—Up- and Downtakes.
A and B of metal, and C and D of canvas.

rather too complicated for general adoption. Practical trial, however, has proved its utility. This arrangement (fig. D), may be simply described as an ordinary cowl representing the mouth of the air-shaft, carrying the blowpipe tube in its axis, and being included in an outer conical sheath, sufficiently large to allow of the passage of air between it and the mouth of the cowl within. A current of air entering the large end of the outer cone is thus divided into two parts, with increasing velocity, the one being central, and the other circumferential, as respects the mouth of the air-shaft.

Notwithstanding all that has been said above, some very important experiments lately conducted at Kew would seem to cast doubt on the efficacy of all so-called uptake mechanism in the cowl form and to give preference to the simple open-mouth tube.

The following extract from the 'Standard,' of June 7, 1878, gives a good general statement of the experiments alluded to and the results obtained :—

'TESTING VENTILATORS AT KEW.—The subject of ventilation created a considerable amount of interest at a recent congress at Leamington, and the result has been that under the action of the Sanitary Institute of Great Britain a series of practical tests have been applied to the apparatus of those patentees who elected to enter their inventions for competition. The Committee consists of Captain Douglas Galton, Mr. Rogers Field, and Mr. Eassie, and the investigations are carried on in an experimental house which has been fitted up for the purpose at the Royal Observatory at Kew. The systems competing are only three, but these have been put in comparison with two very simple means—namely, an open pipe, and a pipe terminated by a very slight but effective modification of the common lobster-back cowl. The makers are Mr. Boyle, who has a large fixed cylindrical apparatus, consisting of an internal tube, divided longitudinally by vertical partitions at right angles to each other into four ways, the external to which is a hood of angulated plates, forming a sort of maze ; Mr. Scott, who has a horizontal cone-cowl, open at both ends, the larger end receiving the wind, which passes in through an interior cone, and then through a second one, the principle being not unlike that of a Giffard injector; the cowl is very nicely balanced and slung, turning very easily and steadily with the wind, however light; Mr. Lloyd, who has a circular ventilator, with surrounding rings and spaces for entrance of air, and a flat covering or cap, considerably overhanging all round—almost exactly like the common Dutch chimney pots. The experimental house has five six-inch metal pipes passing through the roof, and extending from about four feet above the floor inside the building to about two feet above the roof ridge outside. At the top of each pipe, at the same level, the apparatus is fitted on; and at the lower end, which is contracted to an orifice three inches in diameter, for adjustment with the current-measuring instrument. An ordinary Robinson's anemometer is also fixed outside to give the velocity of the wind, and the temperatures are taken within or without. The results have so far shown that there is little, if any, gain for the cowl or the hood over the natural draught created in an open pipe; and, further, that the common cowl constructed with the discharge orifice raised to an angle of 45 degrees is an improvement on the mere open pipe. In the experiments which were witnessed yesterday there was only a very little wind travelling, not more than one and a half mile per hour, and the readings of the rates of the currents passing up the tubes were—with Boyle's apparatus, 866 feet in five minutes; with Scott's, 881; with the Lloyd, considerably less; with the open tube, 872; and with the lobster-back cowl, 914 feet in the like period.'

In Plate XIV. are shown some good and simple forms of up- and downtake apparatus, constructed either of metal or of canvas, and requiring no special adjustment.

Air-openings and shafts, intended for ingress or egress, as the case may be, are too frequently of insufficient size to be effective. Moreover, when any obstruction or difficulty presents itself, curving, bending at angles, and subdivision of tubes is resorted to, with apparently little idea as to the results of such a practice.

The proper size of inlets and outlets will, of course, depend upon the capacity of the apartment or space to be ventilated, and the number of times renewal of its air may be required in each hour, such renewal to be without sensible draught, as a first principle.

Currents of air may be estimated, either as moving at so many miles per hour, or as amounting to so many cubic feet in the same time. A current of one mile per hour is scarcely perceptible, but being in constant movement, it will supply 1,800 cubic feet in that space, through an aperture of eight inches in diameter. The delivery of 1,800 cubic feet per hour through apertures diminishing in size must be proportionately quicker, until at length it will become a disagreeable draught.

Ample means of egress for vitiated air is one of the most important points to be effected in ship ventilation. In contemplating the ventilation of a frigate, for example, our first question should be, what provision can be made for the regular escape of impure air, which is but too often pent up between-decks under the ordinary principles of construction. Indeed it might be said that the means of egress are generally unsatisfactory on board ship, and are either permitted to remain so, or a compensation is attempted by introducing what might be called ventilating mechanism or appliances. Thus we seem, as it were, to distrust nature while we practically repudiate her own laws.

1. The necessity for special channels of ingress to cabins of ships arises from the fact that these compartments, each inclosing or confining a body of air, are themselves, so to speak, inclosed. Thus, in order to secure the supply of primary air, or that which has not been already partly used, to such localities, downcast shafts must be furnished. In order to show the value of fair provision for the escape of

CALCULATION OF LOSS BY ANGLES.

vitiated air, and how much greater this should be than is commonly supposed, a very ordinary case may be chosen for comment. Let an officer live in a cabin with 200 cubic feet of available air-space, and if there has been no movement in the air the percentage of carbonic acid from respiration will be 3 per cent., requiring 2,800 cubic feet of fresh air for the first hour, and 3,000 cubic feet for each hour following, to keep the air of the cabin up to the standard of ·06 per cent., or ·6 per thousand volumes. Now, there is commonly no upper outlet to such an apartment, so that the removal of the impure air can only be effected by the law of diffusion. But, should there be also a pouring in of bilge air, over the shelf-piece into the sleeping-place of the occupant, the question becomes much more complicated, and nothing but an accurate analysis could enable us to determine how much more than the 3,000 cubic feet of fresh air per hour would be necessary to keep the air of the place up to the before-mentioned standard. On the other hand, if the removal of the products of respiration and the emanations from the body takes place freely, just as they are formed, through an ample uptake system, the whole case is altered. The law of diffusion has scarcely time to operate inboard, and the supply is equivalent to the demand, without necessarily creating draught. In this latter connection, let us suppose finally that the ventilation is on the plenum principle; then, to furnish the required 3,000 cubic feet of air per hour, with a delivery-pipe of twelve square inches sectional area, which is much larger than the inlet openings of H.M.S. 'Devastation,' the velocity of the current would equal ten feet per second or seven miles an hour!

2. Should it be necessary to give angles to tubes, it must be remembered that the more open the angles are the better. The estimation of loss produced by angles may be approximately made by means of the following formula devised by Professor F. S. B. F. de Chaumont, M.D., F.R.S.

In an air tube

Let v be the velocity of air in feet per hour.

„ A „ actual area of the tube in square feet and decimals.

„ θ „ angle of deflection of the tube.

„ U „ amount of air (utilisable) delivered through A.

When $\theta = 0°$ U = unity, and if we represent this by an equation $U = vA \times \left(1 - \frac{\sin \theta}{2}\right)$, thus we shall have U $= 0.5$ when $\theta = 90°$.

If there be more than one bend in the tube, and the angles be represented successively by θ_1, θ_2, $_m$, then we have

$$U = vA \times \left\{ \left(1 - \frac{\sin \theta}{2}\right)\left(1 - \frac{\sin \theta_1}{2}\right)\left(1 - \frac{\sin \theta_2}{2}\right)\left(1 - \frac{\sin \theta_m}{2}\right) \right\}$$

$$U = vA \times \left(1 - \frac{\sin \theta}{2}\right) m.$$

TABLE.

Angle θ	Sin θ	$1 - \frac{\sin \theta}{2}$	Remarks
0°	0·00000	1·000	
5°	0·08716	0·956	
10°	0·17365	0·913	*Example.*—A tube delivering,
15°	0·25882	0·870	when straight, 1000 cubic feet,
20°	0·34202	0·829	will, if bent at an angle of 50°,
25°	0·42262	0·789	deliver only 617 cubic feet. If
30°	0·50000	0·750	bent twice at 50° it will give
35°	0·57358	0·713	only 617 × 0·617 = 380 cub. feet.
40°	0·64279	0·678	If bent first at 50° and again
45°	0·70711	0·646	at 70° it will give 1000 × 0·617
50°	0·76604	0·617	× 0·530 = 328 cub. feet.
55°	0·81902	0·590	
60°	0·86608	0·567	*Corollary.*—If a tube be bent
65°	0·90601	0·547	at 70° it must be widened in the
70°	0·93969	0·530	proportion of $1 \div 0.530 = 1.88$;
75°	0·96593	0·517	so that A at 0° = A × 1·88 at 70°.
80°	0·98481	0·508	
85°	0·99619	0·502	
90°	1·00000	0·500	

3. Equally important is the method of estimating the loss occasioned by dividing the sectional area of an air-tube into

CALCULATION OF LOSS BY DIVISION.

a number of smaller apertures, as devised by the same authority.

Let v, A, and u be as before.

Let (a) be the sectional area of a division of A, so that $na = A$. Then we have

$$u = vA \times \sqrt{\frac{1}{n}}.$$

If the divisions be unequal in area and be represented respecively by (a), (b), (c), ... (m), so that $a+b+c \ldots +m = A$,

Then $u = \frac{v}{\sqrt{A}} \times (\sqrt{a^3} + \sqrt{b^3} + \sqrt{c^3} + \ldots + \sqrt{m^3})$.

TABLE WHERE THE DIVISIONS ARE EQUAL (i.e. $na = A$).

No. of divisions (i.e. n=)	Square root $\sqrt{}$	Effect $\sqrt{\frac{1}{n}}$	Remarks
1	1	1·000	*Example.*—If a tube of A sectional area deliver 1000 cubic feet of air, it will, if divided into seven (7) small tubes each of (a) sectional area (so that $7a = A$), deliver only 380 cubic feet. Conversely, to obtain 1000 cubic feet through several tubes of (a) sectional area each, we should require $7 \times 100 \div 38 = 18·4$ tubes of (a) sectional area each. If a tube of A sectional area be divided into seven smaller tubes, each of (a) sectional area, and be also bent at an angle of 50°, we shall obtain only $1000 \times ·380 \times ·617 = 235$ cubic feet.
2	1·42	0·704	
3	1·73	0·578	
4	2	0·500	
5	2·24	0·446	
6	2·45	0·408	
7	2·65	0·380	
8	2·83	0·353	
9	3	0·333	
10	3·17	0·316	
16	4	0·250	
25	5	0·200	
36	6	0·166	
49	7	0·143	
64	8	0·125	
81	9	0·111	
100	10	0·100	

To the preceding tables may be added the two following, showing, at a glance, the sectional area, and the number of cubic inches in a linear foot in square and cylindrical tubes respectively. They will be found to facilitate calculation when the anemometer is used. Thus, if we multiply the sectional area by 12, we get the number of cubic inches in a linear foot, and this again, being multiplied by the number of linear feet obtained per hour, will give the whole number of cubic inches, which are converted into cubic feet by dividing by 1728, the number of cubic inches in a cubic foot. Or, to use a short factor, let A = sectional area and L = linear feet, then $A \times L \times 0\cdot00694$ = cubic feet. This factor converts the square inches of the sectional area into feet and decimals.

TABLE FOR SQUARE TUBES.   TABLE FOR CYLINDRICAL TUBES.

Inches square	Sectional area	Cubic inches in a linear foot	Inches in diameter	Sectional area	Cubic inches in a linear foot
1	1	12	1	0·7854	9·4248
2	4	48	2	3·1416	37·6992
3	9	108	3	7·0686	84·8232
4	16	192	4	12·5664	150·7968
5	25	300	5	19·6350	235·6200
6	36	432	6	28·2744	329·2928
7	49	588	7	38·4846	461·8152
8	64	768	8	50·2656	603·1872
9	81	972	9	63·5174	762·2088
10	100	1200	10	78·5400	942·4800
11	121	1452	11	95·0334	1140·4008
12	144	1728	12	113·0978	1357·1726
13	169	2028	13	132·7326	1592·7912
14	196	2352	14	153·9384	1847·2608
15	225	2700	15	176·7150	2120·5800
16	256	3072	16	201·0704	2412·3448
17	289	3468	17	226·8806	2724·5672
18	324	3888	18	254·4696	3053·6352

As a principle, it is found to be much better, whether for propulsion or extraction, to increase the size of the tubes as they undergo subdivision. This will be seen at once on comparing an outline of a gradual diminution with one of a gradual increase in the size of the branch tubes as they are given off. Internal reflection must occur largely in one case, while it will be comparatively little in the other.

We sometimes find an uptake placed within a downcast

shaft, the former having a small reversed cowl which surmounts the larger one, connected with the outer shaft. This arrangement, or the converse of it (Plate XVII., fig. 29, *a*), is very ingenious, but the relative size of the tubes requires some little calculation, as the friction between the two tubes is so much greater than that of the inner tube alone. Let the inner tube (2) be 8 inches in diameter, and the outer tube (1) 11, the frictional area of 25 inches in circumference is all that can affect the inner tube, with a sectional area of 50 square inches; while to 25 we must add 34 inches, or the circumference of the outer tube, to make up the frictional area of 45 square inches. Now, in order to compensate for this difference, the outer tube must be at least three times the diameter of the inner one, or 24 inches, having a most disproportionate effect. A better scheme than this is the division of a tube into two parts by a central longitudinal septum (fig. 29, *b*), so that both shall have the same sectional and frictional area. Two cylindrical tubes, however, even of smaller circumference, would each have a larger cavity than the D-shaped half of a tube of any given diameter divided by a septum. Thus, for example, one-half of an 8-inch tube so divided would give 8 inches for the septum, and 12·5 inches for the rest of the circumference, 20·5 together, and the sectional area would be 25 square inches. Now, a cylindrical tube of 6 inches in diameter would be 18·8 in circumference with a sectional area of 28 square inches.

The advantage of a cylindrical tube over a square one will be seen in the following instance. A cylindrical tube 15 inches in diameter is 47 inches in circumference with a sectional area of 176 square inches; on the other hand, a tube 1 foot square is 48 inches in circumference, and only 144 square inches in sectional area.

An equilateral square tube is better than any other form of square or triangular tube. A square tube divided into two by a septum parallel with one of its sides is superior to the same tube divided by a diagonal septum.

The Siphon System.—In this place might be noticed the inverted siphon of Mr. Tredgold, and a similar thing patented by Dr. Chowne. Mr. Tredgold says: 'If an inverted siphon be placed with one leg in the chimney, so near to the fire that the air in that leg will be warmer than the air in the other leg, motion will take place, for the air will ascend in the warmer leg and go up the chimney, and a descending current in the cool leg will take the air from the room. To render the application of this principle successful, the mouth of the tube should be at the ceiling of the apartment; the lowest part of the curve should be, as much as convenient, below the point where the heat is applied; and the aperture through which the air flows into the chimney should be formed so that the soot may not fall down the tube; also, the mouth should have a register to close it, or regulate the ventilation.' Contrast with this Dr. Chowne's account of his own invention: 'I have found', he says, 'that if a bent tube or hollow passage be fixed with the legs upwards, the legs being of unequal lengths, whether it be in the open air, or with the shorter leg communicating with a room or other place, that the air circulates up the longer leg, and it enters and moves down the shorter leg; and that this action is not prevented by making the shorter leg hot, whilst the longer leg remains cold, and no artificial heat is necessary to the longer leg of the air-siphon to cause this action to take place; thus is the direction of the action of air in a siphon the reverse of that which takes place in a siphon or like bent passage or tube, when used for water and other liquids, wherein the water or other liquid enters and rises up the shorter leg and descends or moves down into the longer leg. And my invention consists of applying this principle when ventilating rooms or apartments, such as those of a house or ship or other building or place.'

Whatever there may be of truth in the analogy thus contended for by Dr. Chowne between the ordinary siphon for liquids and his air-siphon, the action would appear to be too feeble for ordinary purposes, unless assisted by the application of heat, after the manner provided for in Mr. Tredgold's plan, or by external pressure, as in Mr. Tobin's patent, and other systems with such trifling differences, *inter se*, as are permitted by patent law.

SUB-SECTION B.—*Artificial Ventilation.*

(a) MECHANICAL FORCE, OR WIND-FORCE APPLIED TO MECHANISM.

Rotatory Fans and Screws.—What is commonly known as the Rotatory Fan was invented by Desaguliers, in 1734. The purpose of the original fan was stated to be 'for changing the air of the room of sick people in a little time, either by drawing out the foul air or forcing in fresh air, or doing both successively, without opening doors or windows.'

The wheel employed by Desaguliers in 1736 for the ventilation of the House of Commons was seven feet in diameter and one foot in width, having twelve radii or blades approaching to within nine inches of the axis, leaving a circular opening eighteen inches in diameter. This fan was inclosed in a concentric case, furnished with a blowing-pipe above and a suction-pipe communicating with the central opening in the wheel, which was turned by a handle attached to the axis which passed through the case. This was the early form and character of the machine, but it has since been the subject of very important improvement in every particular of its construction, and has thus survived all rival systems of ventilation by propulsion. 1. The diameter of the wheel has been reduced, while the size of the blowing-pipe is proportionately increased. 2. The originally centric axis is now made slightly eccentric, with a corresponding decrease in the length of the fan blades, which are, moreover, reduced to four or five in number, and so rendered much more effective.

When Desaguliers was engaged in the ventilation of the House of Commons, the attention of the Government was directed to the want of ventilation in our ships, in consequence of the bad health of the troops that were embarked at Spithead to proceed on an expedition against the Spaniards. Numbers were re-landed and sent to hospital, and the ships were said to be in such a state that they infected one another. After exhibiting his fan and air-pipes to the Lords of the Admiralty, Desaguliers was ordered to make a blowing-wheel to be tried on board H.M.S. 'Kinsale,' at Woolwich, but smaller than that of the House of Commons, that it might not take up too much room in the ship. But though the principle was good, Sir Jacob Ackworth, who was then the surveyor of the Navy, did not seem to approve of it, and the trials were not conducted with that fairness which the inventor expected. Indeed, the rotatory fan was condemned by Sir Jacob without having once been present to witness its operation. 'Thus ended my scheme,' said Desaguliers, 'which I hoped would have been of great benefit to the public.' In those days the great objection to mechanical ventilation would naturally be the hand-labour required to make it effective. Desaguliers called his machine *a centrifugal blowing-wheel*, and the man who turned it a *ventilator*. The place of the ventilator, however, may now be supplied by steam-power to give rotation to a much better description of blowing-wheel. Up to the present time the rotatory fan has chiefly been employed for plenum ventilation on board ship, as in the case of our monitors 'Devastation,' 'Glatton,' &c.; but in devising the arrangement of tubes for the supply of air by propulsion, at least five essential particulars must be taken into account, viz.:—

1. The manner in which the external air is conveyed to the fan-box.

2. The size of the original shaft in relation to the required supply.

3. The number of divisions and subdivisions of the shaft.

4. The angle at which these divisions and subdivisions are given off.

ARTIFICIAL VENTILATION.

PLATE XV.—SEVERAL VENTILATING SYSTEMS.

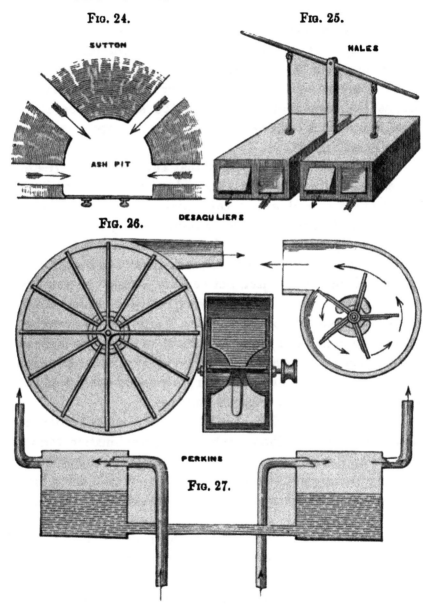

FIG. 24.—Sutton's scheme of extraction by heat, turning the galley fire and ash-pits to account.

FIG. 25.—Dr. Hales's double-lever bellows apparatus, or 'ship's lungs,' so named.

FIG. 26.—Desaguliers' original rotatory fan to the left, and the more modern and improved form of the apparatus on the right.

FIG. 27.—Scheme of Mr. Perkins, identical in principle with Thier's patent automatic ventilator (Plate XXIII.).

5. The calibre of these latter as compared with that of the primary trunk.

All the above particulars have already received notice in a passing way. Their full consideration would occupy more space than would be convenient to devote to it in this work.

Both screws and fans were used for propulsion or extraction, as the case might require, in the ships of the Niger Expedition, which were ventilated under the superintendence of Dr. Reid, F.R.S.

'The larger the fanner,' says that authority, 'the greater the economy with which a given supply of air can be obtained; small fanners turned with great rapidity, as when they have 1,000 to 2,000 revolutions per minute, usually make a penetrating and oppressive noise. In using the fanner for ventilating purposes, it cannot be too particularly recollected that quantity of air is the object, not velocity, except in situations where the small size of the channels permitted renders it impossible to obtain the requisite quantity without great velocity. I have always found it most economical to use large fanners, moving with a comparatively slow velocity, and these have varied, in public buildings requiring a considerable supply of air, from ten to twenty feet in diameter.'

The Patent Twin-fan Ventilator and Double Ventilating Shaft of the Author.—These appliances, in combination, form a complete apparatus for ventilating purposes, but they require separate description in order that the principle upon which they are constructed may be properly understood. (See Plate XVI., fig. 28.)

1. *Of the Twin-fan Ventilator.*—This consists of three essential parts, viz., a *motile fan* (1) revolving with the wind, by which motion is communicated to an *aspiratory fan* (2) placed beneath it on the same axis, and a *self-adjusting cap* (3) so contrived as to direct the wind upon the motile fan to the best advantage.

(i.) The 'motile fan' is composed of several concave blades or cups, upon a transverse circular plate, or fixed at

ROTATORY FANS.

PLATE XVI.—THE TWIN-FAN VENTILATOR OF THE AUTHOR.

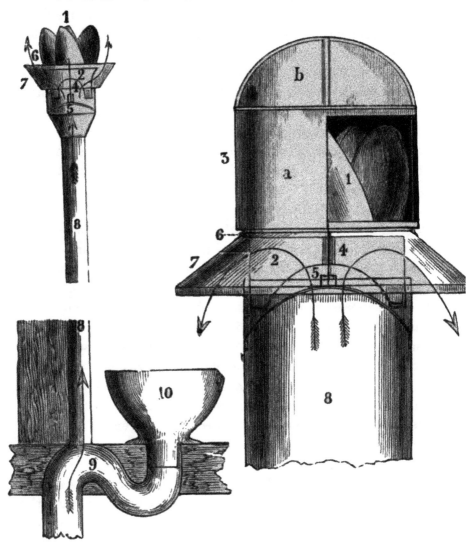

FIG. 28.—This mainly consists of three parts, viz.: 1, The motile fan; 2, The aspiratory fan; and 3, The versatile cap, with alternate quarters closed and open so as always to bring an open quarter on the concave side of the fan-blades, and thus favour the action of the wind in giving rotation. 4, The spindle or common axis of the fans. 5, The lower bearing of ditto. 6, Circular plate between the fans. 7, Conical band round the aperture of 8, The shaft (the current being thrown upwards in the left-hand drawing and downwards in the right). 9 Shows the ordinary siphon of a w.c.; and 10, The receiver. The ventilating shaft (8) is connected with the upper convexity at the drain-pipe end. An escape is thus made for reflex air.

equal distances around the axis. In the amount of resistance offered to the wind, the concave side of each blade exceeds the convex by about one-fourth, so that motion in one direction is determined by this difference, as in the anemometers in ordinary use.

(ii.) One side of the lower or 'aspiratory fan' is turned downwards over the mouth of the air-shaft, while the other side is cut off from the external air by the before-mentioned circular plate between it and the upper or motile fan. The exhaustive action of the aspiratory fan is therefore confined to the air within the shaft, which is thus elicited and thrown off in all directions by centrifugal force.

(iii.) The 'self-adjusting cap' is constructed with the view of still further counteracting the resistance of the convex side of the motile blades by interrupting the wind which would otherwise tell upon them to a disadvantage. To effect this the alternate quarters (a) of the cap are closed and held in the necessarily oblique position by a transverse symmetrical vane (b) at the top; by which also the cap is hung upon a central pivot. The concave side of each motile blade is thus alone exposed to the wind, while the convex side comes up under one of the closed quarters of the cap (a) with much diminished resistance. Moreover, the closed off-quarter of the cap is so arranged as to reflect the current of air in the direction of the movement, and thus supplement the primary force.

The accessories worthy of notice are two cross-rods, bent twice at right angles, which form a framework carrying the pivot for the cap in the centre above, and beneath this the socket for the upper pivot of the fan spindle. The lower pivot of the latter works in a socket (5) on a transverse piece within the shaft. Of course a propulsive effect will be produced by inverting the aspiratory fan and making other suitable arrangements.

2. *Of the Double Ventilating Shaft.*—The more we study the subject the more we perceive it to be necessary to make

provision for the ingress of fresh air, as well as for the escape of that which has been rendered impure. Allusion has already been made to the Bivalve Mollusca, which breathe in water, their respiratory currents entering and passing out by distinct channels or siphon tubes, while the movement is effected by mechanical means, namely, the action of vibratile cilia. Several attempts have been made to obtain this result in a single apparatus. Thus, in some cases, as in the ventilation of mines, a longitudinal septum in a tube divides the incoming from the outgoing current. In other instances, an inner tube serves as an uptake, while an outer one conveys fresh air to the space to be ventilated.

The plan (see Plate XVII., b) which has now to be explained, however, differs from all others in having a central aperture of ingress (2) as well as of egress (1), the intermediate portion of the main shaft (8) being divided by a longitudinal septum (10) into two equal parts. By this arrangement a larger area is made both for the escape of foul and the entrance of fresh air, so as to facilitate the process of interchange, the aperture of ingress above and that of egress below being nearly equal to the whole circumference of the main shaft (8).

The lower inlet (2) may be expanded and perforated or furnished in some simple way, so as to bring it under control and moderate its effect. This scheme would answer well, even without the aspiratory fan, and would be especially suitable for small vessels and passenger steamers. c, fig. 29, represents another form of apparatus to effect the same purpose, the construction of which will be understood by observing the direction of the arrows and following the constructive drawings from $c1$ to $c4$. If, however, the upcast and downcast tubes were quite distinct and perfectly cylindrical, with free inlet and outlet, and as little as possible to obstruct the currents of air, the effect would be more satisfactory still. This is the whole secret of the advantage which cowls of

PLATE XVII.—UP- AND DOWNTAKE IN COMBINATION.

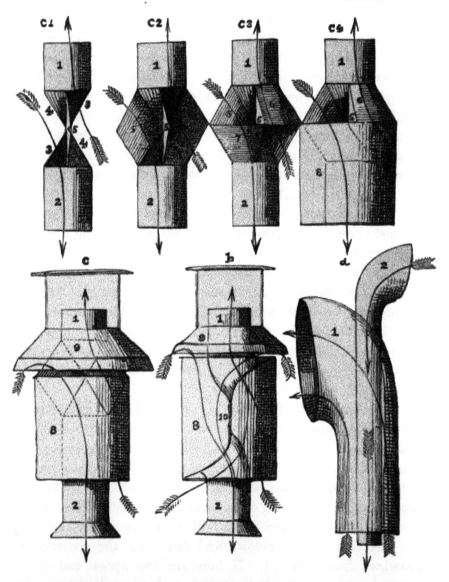

FIG. 29.—*a*, The double cowl and shaft apparatus. The cowls 1 and 2 are turned in opposite directions, and the shaft of 2 is received within that of 1. (The same references will apply to all the remaining drawings.) *b* and *c*, Two forms of double-acting apparatus in which both central and circumferential inlets and outlets are provided. 1, The upper central outlet. 2, The lower central inlet. In *b* the main shaft (8) is divided into two by a vertical septum (10), while in *b* and *c* the upper inlet is covered by a circular hood (9). *c1 c2 c3 c4* show

simple construction are usually found to possess over more complex ones.

The ventilator of Souchon, used for aspiration, consists of an eccentric fan wheel with collapsible blades, in a case which is only open at the circumference for the aspiratory pipe below and the discharge pipe above. An apparatus invented by M. Sochet, founded on the same principles, has been used with advantage, both for propulsion and extraction by reversing the valves, in the frigate 'La Gloire' (Fonssagrives).

The Archimedean screw has long been in use as a moving power in the smoke-jack, and just as it can give rotation, so when motion is given to it by machinery it will develop a current in the air. In 1834, M. Motte substituted it for the rotatory fan, and received a prize for his application of the principle. Subsequently, Mr. Day obtained a patent for a single-threaded screw, to be applied in the same way. Mr. Combe, of Leeds, appears to have been the first to introduce the double-threaded screw in this country, though, strange to say, a gentleman of nearly the same name, M. Combes, in Belgium, employed a similar screw in some of his experiments.

Dr. Reid had a double-threaded screw made for the ventilation of the ships of the Niger Expedition, and found that it propelled the air backwards or forwards according as it was worked to the right or left, but he had no accurate means at the time of testing its power with other instruments. Screws,

---

(*Continuation of Description of Plate XVII.*)

stages in the construction of *c* which would be otherwise rather difficult to comprehend or even describe. In *c*1, 1 and 2 represent two tubes with conical ends united by the apices. 3, Open alternate quarters of the cones. 4, Closed ditto. 5, Rhomboidal plates, arranged radially so as to fit the re-entering angle between the cones internally, and meet the upper border of the outer shaft (8) externally. 6, Two upper covering plates connecting the margins of two opposite pairs of rhomboidal plates with the upper margin of the outer shaft (8). 7, Two lower covering plates alternating with the former and similarly connected. *c*4 shows the completion of the arrangement so far, leaving only the rain plate shown in *b* and *c*, and the circular hood (9) to be added.

however, as compared with fans, are very feeble on account of the obstruction which they must present to the passage of any air but that immediately in contact with the propelling surface. Great velocity must therefore be given to the screw in order to obtain quantity, while great quantity may be supplied by a large fan with comparatively little velocity.

The so-called *Windmill Ventilator*, unless its blades partake more of the character of those of the fan, will offer the same resistance to the passage of the current created by itself that has just been noticed in relation to screws. It has, however, been used with advantage by Mr. Combe and others in certain cases.

Bellows and Pump Ventilators.—Under the pretentious name of the *ship's lungs*, Dr. Stephen Hales, F.R.S., rector of Farringdon, in Hampshire, introduced a large double-acting machine on the bellows principle (Plate XV., fig. 25), which he evidently thought would supersede the rotatory fan of Desaguliers. His paper on the subject was read before the Royal Society in May 1741, and afterwards published in a more extended form in 1743. The 'ship's lungs' consisted of two long boxes with a movable diaphragm within and valvular openings at the ends; the diaphragms being moved by vertical rods communicating above with a transverse two-handled lever working on a central pivot.

As this machine required the physical labour of two men, the Doctor seemed to have been awake to the difficulty, and in advocating his system he reasoned thus:—'If two men can hold to work the ventilators for a quarter of an hour, four men, by changing hands, spell and spell, as they term it, may well work for an hour; and suppose there be 500 or 480 men in the ship, and every one takes his share of the work, then once in five days it will come to every man's turn to work the ventilators for half an hour.' He then asks: 'Is not the benefit proposed thereby, viz., the saving yearly of the lives of thousands a sufficient reward for so small a pittance of labour?'

Dr. Lind speaks very highly of Dr. Hales's machine, but it very soon fell into disuse, not being self-acting in the first instance, and the passage of air, as Dr. Arnott has since very satisfactorily shown, met with too much resistance in consequence of the narrowness of the openings. Mr. Tomlinson, who gives a very concise account of the construction of this ventilator, states that 'Dr. Hales calculated that his machine would expel a tun of air at each stroke, or six tuns per minute ; and that the air issued from the aperture with a velocity of twenty-five miles an hour. This estimate,' he further remarks, 'is far too high, and the machine itself is far inferior to that of his amiable rival, Dr. Desaguliers ; indeed, the use of the rotatory fan at the present day, and the total practical oblivion of the "ship's lungs," is a sufficient commentatory on the respective merits of the two inventions.'

Arnott's Ventilating Pump.—With the view of improving or quite superseding Dr. Hales's machine, the late Dr. Arnott, F.R.S., invented a piston pump of simple construction (see Parkes's 'Practical Hygiene,' p. 172, fig. 23), in which, by a suitable arrangement of valves of oiled silk, air is received and expelled on both sides of the piston alternately. The great length of the piston-rod, and the physical difficulty of working it, would seem to be the chief objections to this apparatus, which would also apply to pumps on the gasometer principle. One of these latter was fitted up by Dr. Arnott in the York County Hospital, and another, with a double set of tubes, the invention of M. Peyre, is figured and described in Dr. Foussagrives's work on Naval Hygiene, together with the ventilator of M. Simon, which is a combination of pump and bellows.

(*b*) EXPANSION BY HEAT ARTIFICIALLY APPLIED.

Steam.—As a part of the ventilating system of Dr. Edmonds, R.N., a powerful upcast current is developed by steam-jets issuing from a circular perforated ring included in the ventilating shafts ; and being in communication with the auxiliary and main boiler of the engines, when the steam is turned on, it escapes with great force through the apertures of the jet ring. A strong current of air is thus carried up from all the ramifications of the longitudinal air-shafts and deck air channels with which the main ventilators are connected. This action, moreover, is favoured by the outer cowls being turned to leeward. The effect may be observed by holding the flame of a candle to any of the openings.

As, owing to the length of the steam pipes connecting the ventilators with the boiler, some steam must be condensed before it escapes upwards, the steam should be first turned into the pipes alone for a few minutes, and the condensed water blown through the extreme end before turning the cock which admits it into each ventilator.

Flame.—A circle of small lamps may be used with excellent effect instead of the steam jets just described. This principle was practically carried out in H.M.S. 'Zealous,' with the view of sweetening the bilges, by Mr. J. Husbands, the chief engineer. A side door in the metal shaft afforded access to the lamps, which were thus regulated and kept in trim by a little attention.

Stoves.—Previously to Mr. Husbands' adoption of a circle of lights, Mr. Crump, an officer in the same department of the navy, suggested the introduction of a small stove into the horizontal portion of a metal shaft bent twice at right angles; and though his ostensible object was merely the correction or rather removal of bilge effluvia, it was obvious that he really intended it to answer the purpose of thoroughly ventilating the ship.

If this system of extraction by heat were applied on a larger scale, or in several shafts at stated intervals, there can be little doubt but the expectation of the inventor would be fully realised. Independently of the detail of the application of a stove for the purpose here spoken of, perfect safety or protection from fire must of course be the first desideratum, the next should be the economy of fuel and the conservation of the caloric developed.

Some little time ago the writer devised a small cylindrical stove, so constructed as to meet the above requirements, and admit of being placed with safety within a straight vertical shaft, sufficiently dilated in this locality to preserve its mean capacity. From the sides of the stove thus included a septum or plate extends to the corresponding sides of the shaft so as to cut off the fireplace from the clear space behind it. The ash-drawer beneath, being also inclosed in a case, insures perfect safety, while advantage is taken of a heating surface which would otherwise be unavailable.

The current of air supplying the fire must pass down in front of the vertical partitions to enter the ash-pit beneath the grating of the stove. Fuel is supplied through an ample door in the outer casing, and a second one in the stove itself.

For every pound of coal 250 cubic inches of air must pass in front of the septum to be consumed, but a much larger amount of expanded air will pass up through the funnel, and still more through the body of the shaft behind the stove.

Beneath the flat flooring of the shaft alley in some ships bilge air is led forwards to the ash-pits of the furnaces where it ascends with the draught; and as proving the necessity of confining currents of air to preserve their course in a definite direction, it has been observed that the removal of several of the limber plates will sensibly diminish the force of the current in question.

Though the furnaces generate an ascensional force in engine-rooms and stokeholds, it would still appear to be necessary to supply pure air from above through the medium of wind-sails and air-shafts. Otherwise, though an up-draught may be produced by the fires, the general radiation of heat going forward would convert the air furnished by ordinary diffusion into an oppressive atmosphere, forming as fast as it is carried off.

By an ingenious contrivance, in the 'Lord Warden' and some other ships, the heated air of the stokehold is carried up by a tube which ascends through the axis of each funnel, a powerful draught being generated by the surrounding heat in the materials of incomplete combustion. Since the introduction of this improvement the temperature of the stokehold under full steam has been lowered from 30° to 40° in certain places, or from 170° to 130° Fahr. The plan of investing the funnel, upper part of the boiler, and as much of the steam apparatus as possible, with an iron casing, was originally devised by Mr. Baker, and Admiral Fanshawe seems to have espoused it zealously when he was superintendent of Chatham Dockyard. The space between the heating surface and the casing in question is sufficiently large (4 feet) to admit of the almost continuous ascent of a great body of air.

Motion may be given to comparatively still air, though of high temperature, by the judicious arrangement of septa or curtains of sheet iron, so as to determine an up and down current on their opposite sides. Instructive examples of this principle may be seen in the engine-rooms of some ships.

Section D.—*Special Systems of Ventilation.*

In the description given of the structure of wooden ships, it was pointed out that the ribs or timbers do not lie quite in contact, but are separated by intervals of variable breadth named openings. Now these openings communicate freely with the bilges below, so that foul air from this source will readily permeate them.

The outer and inner skins, or planking of the ship, form the corresponding walls of the openings, which are abruptly cut off where they meet the port sills, and frequently also where chocks are introduced to succour the ring bolts used in working the guns. In some few instances they may ascend uninterruptedly to the rough tree rail which supports the hammock netting. It is clear, however, that a free circulation of air between the two layers of planking is stopped in the fore and aft direction by the frame timbers themselves, while its ascent between the latter is arrested by the port sills (each of which closes three openings) and the chocks already mentioned. On the contrary, the permanent lodgment of foul air would be the universal rule, were it not for the exposure of these openings just above the shelf piece and between the beam ends resting upon it. The spaces here indicated are usually covered in with ornamentally perforated zinc or wood, as though they were intended for the removal of the heated air from between decks, but this idea is precluded from the fact that there is no upward means of escape. It is probable, therefore, that the object of retaining them was to ventilate the bilges. But on this supposition it is difficult to say why they have been so long permitted to roll their offensive vapours into the cabins of officers and the living and sleeping places of the seamen.

As experience has so clearly proved the natural uptake function of the openings between the timbers, any system that would use them for down draught must be occasionally at least imperfect, namely, during any intermission of the drawing power. Provision should be made for the most complete intercommunication of these openings, the detail of which should form a part of the original design of the ship. Thus, by judiciously arranged anastomosing channels and conveniently planned apertures through the rough tree rail, or either layer of planking just below the hammock netting, a good vent would be obtained. In H.M.S. 'Topaze' and other vessels in which this idea has been imperfectly carried out (on account of the difficulty of finding patent channels communicating with the bilges), the vent-holes are made to open inboard on the upper deck. On one occasion in H.M.S. 'Racoon,' actual steam from the boilers found its way into the lining, and was in due time carried up by the openings and finally poured out through the gratings above the shelf piece, into the breathing zone of the men to a considerable depth beneath the beams (see Plate XVIII., fig. 30). How-

PLATE XVIII.—IMPROVEMENT IN THE VENTILATION OF H.M.S. 'RACOON.'

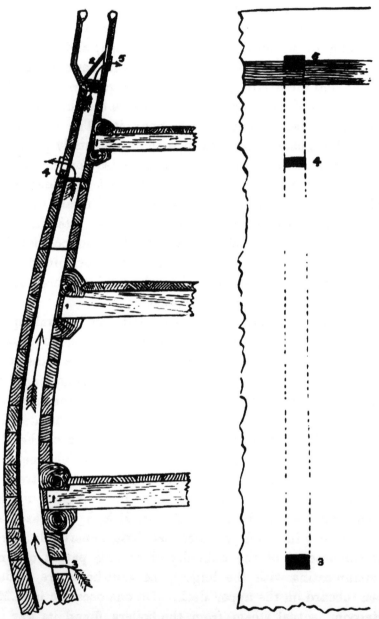

FIG. 30.—1, Chocks introduced between the beam-ends, waterways, and shelf piece to shut off all communication previously existing between the timber openings and the interior of the ship. 2, A piece of wood to cut off the foul air passing through an opening in the rough tree rail from the hammock berthing. 3, An opening for the escape of foul air made in the inner skin, below the shelf piece. 4, A louvre opening in the outer skin, below the hammock netting. 5, An opening through the inner wall of the hammock netting. A side elevation is shown in the drawing to the right, and a vertical section in that to the left.

ever accustomed the ship's company might have been to vitiated air, this was quite insupportable, and a remedy was sought for immediately. An assistant shipwright was sent off to investigate the matter, and the first thing that he did was to sound the patent openings with a *mouso*, so-called, namely, a piece of lead attached to a line, and when these were found the gratings (1 and 2) were closed, and vents were made in connection with them in the inner skin below the lower deck (3), while they led upwards to outlets in the external planking clear of the hammock netting (4 and 5). The result was a complete success, and the general ventilation of the ship was much improved. The condition of the ship just noticed reminded one of a washing day in a laundry, when the ceilings of all the passages are clouded with steam, and those who are employed in it lower their heads to breathe pure air. A similar state of things obtains naturally in the caverns of Nero's baths, near Naples. But whether it be steam or foul air, it is sure to accumulate under the beams of a ship where the hammocks of the seamen are slung in the most unsuitable position for their health and comfort.

It is quite certain that the whole power of a perfectly uninterrupted circulation between the skins with proper outlets has never been tried. We have, however, sufficient knowledge of the probable effect to see that it cannot altogether supersede the use of wind-sails or other available means of ventilation in ordinary use.

In the system of Dr. Reid, F.R.S., as applied to H.M.S. 'Minden' and other ships, more especially those of the celebrated Niger Expedition, although he was fully aware of the importance of a free circulation of air between the timbers, he kept the ordinary gratings open, and determined a down-draught throughout the openings, as it would appear, contrary to the nature of the case, by establishing an up-draught through a large median shaft furnished with an internal rotatory fan or Archimedean screw.

Her Majesty's Indian troopships are ventilated on the

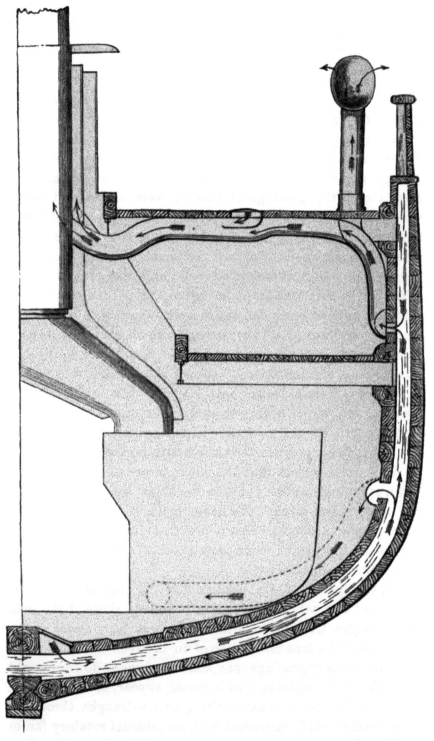

Fig. 31.—In this drawing it will be seen that two aspiratory fences are in operation, viz. first, the ordinary cowls turned away from the wind, by which, as shown by the

system patented by the late Dr. Edmonds, R.N., which is in many respects similar to that of Dr. Reid, already referred to (see Plate XIX.).

Ordinary tube and cowl ventilators are placed wherever their action is thought to be desirable and space will permit. They are five in number.

The first and second pass up from the lower deck through the forecastle near the side of the ship. The ventilating shafts with which they are in communication are placed on each side in the angle formed by the lower deck and the ship's side. One branch passes forwards as far as the prisons; the other extends aft along the fore troop deck, ventilating these parts by the air-shoots which join them, and terminate in the perforated zinc openings close under the beams, and of which so much has been already said. These two varieties are also connected with the 'deck air channels' over the women's compartment, the heated air from which will pass into them and up the ventilators through the circular apertures overhead.

The third and fourth main ventilators are also lateral, and pass up near the commencement of the poop. They pass down into the after cockpit to assist in its ventilation and that of the cabins which are on each side.

The fifth main ventilator is central, placed a short distance before the mizenmast, and passes through one of the ventilating hatches. Its action is distributed to the lower cabins, and it is also connected with the after 'deck air channels' which ventilate the central cabins of the lower saloon. These channels, which may be described as a substitution of a lon-

---

(*Continuation of Description of Plate XIX.*)

direction of the arrows, the air is extracted from the openings between the timbers; and secondly, the funnel, and funnel casing, and the furnaces in steamers. A large trunk is seen leading upwards and then inwards, beneath the deck, receiving the air from a deck air-channel in its course, and terminating either in the funnel casing or the funnel itself by a simple arrangement for the purpose. Another air trunk is seen descending from an opening in the inner skin to the furnaces.

gitudinal air-space for the width of about a foot of the deck planks, covered in above with thick plate-iron, and below with thin sheet-iron, in which circular apertures are cut in suitable localities. They act directly on the foul air which tends to collect between the beams, and which is heated by the lights, respiration, &c.

All the main ventilators are designed to act by the wind alone when this is sufficient. By turning the cowls to windward fresh air will be diffused equally through their branch air-shoots, and even in calms, when the ship is going rapidly through the water, much air will be forced below by their action; but in hot, close weather, when a more powerful ventilation is necessary, provision is made for it by means of steam-jets, already referred to (p. 87).

The supplemental means of ventilation on Dr. Edmonds's plan are, first, double-acting ventilating shafts, and second, the gunwale ventilators.

The double ventilating shafts are divided vertically into four or six divisions leading down to the lower deck. These divisions open outwardly above the deck, and one or more of them will face the wind from whatever quarter it blows, and will introduce fresh air, while the remainder will be to leeward, and by the exhaustive action of the wind, added to the upward tendency of the foul air below, its escape will be aided by them. Thus, they have a double ventilating action, and will exert a powerful effect in removing and purifying the atmosphere of the lower deck. The outlets below are so arranged that the influx and efflux currents will not interfere with one another. Covering doors are provided to close the windward openings in wet and stormy weather. A half round canvas screen may be substituted should these be carried away. The revolving gunwale ventilators placed at short intervals along each side of the ship for the whole length of the gunwale are designed to ventilate the frame of the ship, and the parts with which they communicate by the before-mentioned grated openings along the side of the main deck cabins. Each water-closet has one of these over it, which must be used to draw up foul air, *i.e.* with the open part of the tube above the gunwale turned from the wind. The others may be used either as uptakes or downtakes, whichever may be required, but they act more powerfully with the open part turned to the wind for forcing air downwards.

'As a general rule,' says Dr. Edmonds, 'the cowls of all ventilators should be turned from the wind in wet, cold, or stormy weather, using them as uptakes. In hot weather, on the contrary, every means of introducing fresh air should be made available, and their cowls should be turned to the wind; the heated air below will then be forced up the hatchways. In calms or very light winds, when the steam-jet is used, all the cowls of the other ventilators should be turned to windward, and all ports or scuttles for the admission of external air should be open.'

This system is, no doubt, very excellent; but it is defective in the attempt to ventilate the officers' cabins and the main deck through openings which must inevitably also permit the escape of bilge effluvia into the same space.

The accompanying drawing (Pl. XIX., fig. 31) exhibits the application of this system either to sailing vessels or steamers, the upper conduit leading to the funnel casing on the one hand, and into an uptake cowl on the other. The references to the several parts will afford all the explanation necessary. The arrows show the direction of the air-currents.

The Ventilation of H.M.S. 'Undaunted.'—Three important purposes are carried out in the ventilation of this ship. 1st, The supply of ample air-shafts to certain localities hitherto proverbially deficient of ventilation. 2nd, The adoption of deck air-channels, but with considerable improvement in their construction for the ventilation of the lower deck. 3rd, The shutting off all communication of the openings between the timbers with the body of the vessel above the orlop deck, while the escape of the foul air contained in them is provided for by louvres fitted in the topside.

1. Amongst the parts of a vessel usually requiring more efficient ventilation may be mentioned the after-part of the ward-room, the after cock-pit, the fore-part of the lower deck, the fore store-rooms (carpenter's), the prison-cells, and lastly, the gunner's store-room, holding a still lower position. In the 'Undaunted' the after-part of the ward-room is furnished with a poop skylight, and there is one of similar extent over the admiral's apartments; also, in connection with the after-part of both, a square glazed casement shaft extends downwards to the space between two of the beams in the ward-room. This affords not only a large supply of fresh air from without, but a considerable amount of light in an otherwise comparatively dark and confined locality.

A long vertical tube piercing through four decks in succession, and surmounted by a cowl on the poop, conveys fresh air to the bread-room, and a corresponding shaft answers the purpose of an uptake. A trunk of larger calibre, close abaft the after hatchway, supplies cool air from the upper deck, and a certain amount of light, though small, to the after cock-pit.

For the ventilation of the stoker's washing-place, a hatch opening through the lower deck has been fitted with great advantage. On the inner side of the bulwarks above are three louvre openings, in positions determined by such channels between the timbers as have been experimentally found to be patent throughout.

The outer portion of a double cowl and tube terminates at the upper deck, while the inner and longer one descends to the sail-room, and then turns backwards to the prison cells. From the fore-part of the hatch above the galley, an ample shaft extends to the lower deck, where its effect is sensibly felt.

2. The deck air-channels of Dr. Edmonds, already described, usually run along the main deck in the wake of the

guns, and owing to the convexity and slipperiness of the upper iron plate they prove a fruitful source of accidents, either when the ship is rolling at sea, or during the active movements of the men at gunnery drill. In H.M.S. 'Undaunted' these defects are remedied, and the upper plate rests laterally upon iron instead of wood, while additional support is given to it in the middle by a vertical piece secured by angle-irons to the beams. It is thus permitted to lie quite flush with the surface of the deck without impairing its capability of sustaining the weight of the guns. Each deck air-channel sends five conduits inwards, namely, one to each of the three masts, and two to the funnel.

3. We have yet to consider what may be regarded as the most important part of the ventilation of the ship, having for its object the protection of the middle and upper part of the body of the vessel from the invasion of foul air ascending between the timbers and planking of the hull, while provision is made for the outward escape of that air.

The drawing (Plate XX., fig. 32) represents an athwartship vertical section of the vessel showing the manner in which the above-mentioned purposes are effected. To the left is seen the funnel (F), with a transverse conduit (C), from one of the deck air-channels (D), opening into it. Louvres (L) are fitted in the topside to provide for the escape of foul air entering the channels between the timbers in the direction of the arrows, namely, from the bilge under the lining, and from the orlop over the shelf-piece of the lower deck. The openings that happen to be patent throughout are ascertained experimentally by a plummet for this purpose, named a *mouse*. Thus, while the bilge air is shut off from between decks, an external escape is provided for it, and the lower deck is ventilated by the deck air-channel or ventilating strake. Hitherto, while external vent has indeed been given to some of the foul air ascending beneath the lining, as in the 'Topaze,' and more lately in the hospital ship, 'Victor Emmanuel,' fitted out for the Ashantee war, the

PLATE XX.

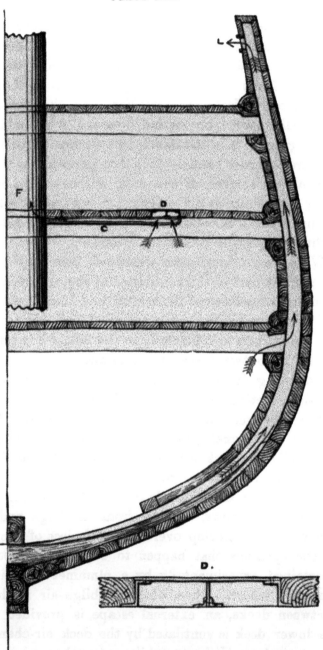

FIG. 32.—SYSTEM OF VENTILATION IN H.M.S. 'UNDAUNTED.'

F Funnel.   C Conduit to funnel.   D Deck air-channel, on a larger scale below.   L Louvre opening.   The air in the openings between the timbers ascends to the louvre openings.   Currents are seen passing from the bilge and over the shelf-piece of the lower deck.

intervals between the beam-ends with their perforated ornament have still remained open, so that the old standing evil has been only mitigated, not removed.

Proposed Scheme for the Ventilation of Ships of the Frigate Class.—Some years ago the writer had the honour of submitting a paper to the Admiralty on the substitution of tubular ventilating shelf-pieces for the existing solid ones, as shown in Plate XXI. fig. 33, with the view of providing for the removal of the foul air finding access to the openings between the timbers, and so frequently the source of ill-health and discomfort in wooden ships. The authorities to whom that paper was referred for judgment were good enough to say that 'the plan was well conceived, and very clearly described both in principle and detail,' but they could not recommend its adoption for several reasons, which, however, did not in any way challenge its practicability. Further study, moreover, has shown that the original design might be simplified for ships of the prevailing frigate type, in connection with ventilating strakes fitted to the upper instead of the main deck.

As before intimated, the provision for ample means of egress for vitiated air is the most important problem in connection with ship ventilation, and by what arrangement can this be most satisfactorily effected, should be our first question in contemplating the ventilation of a frigate, for example. The means of escape are usually very unsatisfactory on board ship, and are either permitted to remain so, or a compensation is attempted by introducing ventilating mechanism and appliances. Thus we seem as it were to distrust Nature, while we practically repudiate her own laws.

Experience has proved it to be desirable that at least the principal parts of a ship requiring ventilation should be furnished with separate outlets of their own. In a frigate the principal parts comprehended in this proposition are, 1st, The orlop and bilge, for the ventilation of which the shelf-piece supporting the main deck should be tubular, with its

102 CONSERVATIVE HYGIENE.

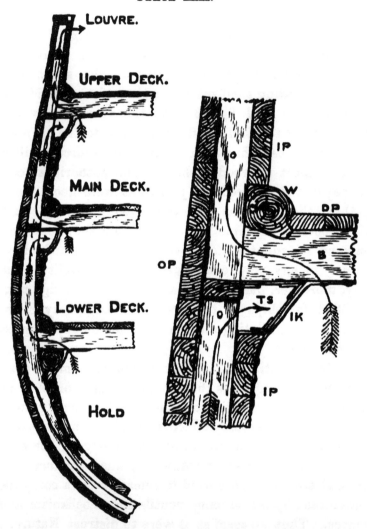

FIG. 83.—VENTILATING SYSTEM WITH TUBULAR SHELF-PIECES.

O P Outer planking. W Waterway. D P Deck planking. B Beam. C Chock of wood, interrupting the lower current in the opening and directing it into the tubular shelf, while an upper current ascends over the shelf-piece. In the text this principle is only mentioned in respect to the ventilation of frigates, but it is obvious that any number of decks might be ventilated in the same way, and quite independently of each other. A similar arrangement might be adopted with great advantage in the construction of hospitals on shore as well as hospital ships. I P Inner planking. T S Tubular shelf. I K Iron knee. O Opening.

conduits leading chiefly into the funnel or funnel casing. 2nd, The lower deck, which should be ventilated by the ship's side, with louvre openings above, as in the 'Undaunted.' 3rd, The main deck, which should be ventilated by means of deck air-channels fitted into the upper deck.

With the view of exhibiting the propriety of making the main-deck shelf-piece tubular, reference must be made to the leading particulars of the framing of a wooden ship. All the timbers here concerned are shown in their proper order in fig. 34 (Plate XXII.), which is a normal elevation of a portion of the side of a line-of-battle ship, consisting of the frames and portsills only, without the planking, beams, or decks. It will be seen, on inspecting this figure, that all the channels connected with the frames corresponding with the ports are effectually cut off or interrupted in their ascent. Next, if we look to the single frames, with their single openings between the ports, it would seem that these openings alone were patent from the keelson to the toprail. But when it is mentioned that they are themselves interrupted by chocks inserted to succour the fighting bolts at every port, it stands to reason that the great bulk of the bilge air, finding its way between the skins, must be delivered again to the body of the vessel over the shelf-piece next below the first tier of ports.

This simple representation of the fact will fully account for the evil so frequently associated with it. The figure also shows the position and connections of the proposed tubular shelf for frigates, and the arrangement of oblique and transverse intercommunicating strakes, so disposed as to link together and utilise a large number of uptake channels, which are, under existing circumstances, quite locked up, and worse than that, as being still permeable to subtle infection, though usually beyond the reach of ordinary fumigation.

By covering the vacant space of a single strake of the internal planking with thin sheet-iron, and by ventilating trusses, a free circulation would be established. Oblique bands or trusses of iron have long been in use, with the vie

PLATE XXII.

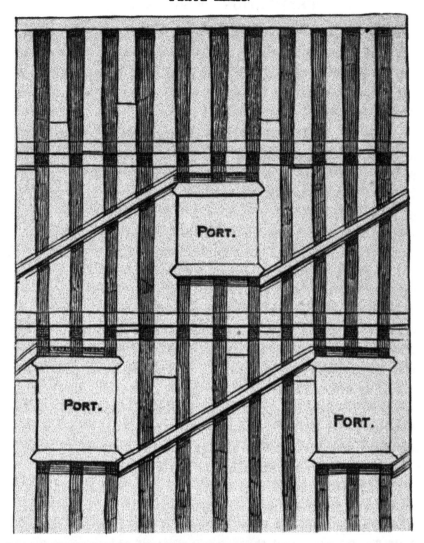

FIG. 34.—VENTILATING SYSTEM, WITH TUBULAR SHELF-PIECES, AND THE ADDITION OF VENTILATING TRUSSES.

The figure represents a portion of a ship's side, with the corresponding timbers and openings between them, and three ports. The transverse bands indicate the position of the tubular shelf-pieces, and the oblique ones the ventilating trusses. It will be seen that the upper and lower port-sills effectually shut off three openings; but they are brought into communication by transverse grooves above and below the ports, and, in addition to these, by the ventilating or hollow iron trusses passing from the groove below one lower port-sill to that above the next port-sill, a nearly complete patency will be effected in the whole ship's side. This arrangement, if thoroughly carried out in connection with tubular shelf-pieces and the extractive power available in all steamships, would it is presumed leave very little more to be desired in reference to the subject of ventilation, even in the case of merchant ships with a cargo of hides, bones, or guano.

of strengthening the ship's side and binding its parts more intimately together. Now, if such trusses were made tubular and so arranged (as in the figure) that the three openings below each port may be brought into communication with those above the port either to the right or left, a double purpose would be thus effected. This arrangement, however, would be better suited for ships in course of construction, though with a little trouble it might be easily adapted to those already built.

With the free circulation of air through the ship's side, secured by the means here suggested, a comprehensive louvre strake might be fitted in the topside instead of the few and circumscribed openings at present possible, even where the most favourable conditions exist with wide intervals between the ports.

It may be remarked, in passing, that not only in the 'Undaunted,' but in other cases where ventilating conduits enter the funnel or the hollow masts at right angles, with the delivering orifices unprotected from the lateral pressure of the ascending column of air, the whole effect of the aspiratory power of this movement can scarcely be secured. Indeed, it is quite possible to conceive that, in some instances, it might be nearly or altogether arrested or reversed. As the aperture of the conduit is exposed to the lateral pressure of the ascending air, the effect would obviously be to retard the movement in the conduit; and that movement would be altogether arrested or reversed if the aperture were directed slightly downwards.

Some extracts from the journal of Surgeon Levinge, M.B., R.N., may be worthy of insertion here, suggesting the utilisation of the caloric constantly wasted in the condensation of steam for ships' use. According to his experience, all ships appear to be constructed for one kind of weather, namely, fine, open, weather, without rain, and having a temperature of 65° to 75°. Any other combination of conditions will render them one and all uncomfortable. He adduces the case of H.M.S. 'Egeria' to illustrate the imperfections of the present system.

The 'Egeria' is a modern composite sloop divided into three water-tight compartments, the first including the captain's cabin, ward-room and steerage, the second the engine-room, and the third the lower deck.

The sum of all the openings of the captain's cabin, ward-room and steerage, gives an area of 52·8 square feet, but rain will reduce this to 18 square feet, while rain with wind or swell will bring it down to 12 square feet.

On the lower deck the openings give an area of 60·2 square feet. Rain will reduce this to 40·8 square feet, while rain with wind or swell will bring it down to 37·5 square feet.

Matters look better on the forecastle on account of a sort of flying deck (gallows), although, no doubt, at all times it must retard the escape of heated air. The defects of the present system appear to be threefold, namely:—

1. Inability to separate air from moisture.
2. No method of heating delivered air in cold weather.
3. Too slow movement, namely, in calms, cabins with scuttles in, &c.

The times and causes of failure in the several factors of ventilation will be seen in the following table, where the plus sign $+=$ working or effective, and the minus sign $-=$ not working or ineffective.

Weather	Wind-sails	Ports	Scuttles	Hatches
Wet	−	+	+	often −
Cold (below 60°)	−	often −	+	often −
Wind (fresh)	+	+	−	+
Gale	+	−	−	+
Calm	−	+	+	+

The result of a gale with rain may be easily seen, while a calm with swell and rain would be equally bad.

The scheme which Dr. Levinge recommends, and every

step of which he states he has proved with a working model, would involve no permanent expense, for the motor principle is the latent heat of evaporation, which steam must give up before turning into drinking water.

It would be continuous in its action, unaffected by heat, cold, gale, or calm, and obviate a very great nuisance in bad weather, namely, throwing tons of steaming hot water (often 130°) into the lowest part of a ship.

Wind-sails disappear at 60°, because people will not tolerate a draught at that temperature. A stove cannot well diffuse its heat unless openings are closed, and air must be changed too rapidly in an overcrowded space like a ship (if we would preserve even a tolerable degree of purity) to allow the effect of a stove to be felt at a distance. The side facing a stove is usually hot, while the other is chilled by the cold, incoming currents.

If we cannot hold the air when it is heated, why not heat it while it is entering? Heat, we are told, means motion, and it is a very great waste to allow all the heat which is produced in forming 60 tons of water (10 days' allowance for 500 men), and which represents an expenditure of from 3 to 6 tons of coal, while the crew may be either shivering in cold weather, or half suffocated in hot calms.

On board the 'Egeria' all the cooking was performed on the lower deck, which was scarcely habitable in warm weather from sunrise to sunset. The men accordingly slept on the upper deck. In the annexed table the temperature of the lower deck is contrasted with that of the ward-room, the daily average being taken for 23 days from November 16.

TEMPERATURES TAKEN AT

The Galley			Bows			Ward-room	
9 A.M.	1 P.M.	9 P.M.	9 A.M.	1 P.M.	9 P.M.	Min.	Max.
94	94	89	88	89	89	79	82

The great advantage to be gained by making the air distil the drinking water, Surgeon Levinge thinks must be apparent to every one acquainted with the internal economy of a ship. The principle of the scheme suggested by him is the following:—

The steam being delivered by a pipe from the boiler into a closed chamber through which an air-shaft passes, the air in the shaft which is surmounted by a cowl is immediately heated, say 40° or 50° higher than the temperature of the external air. The heated and expanded air must rise, while the steam which has thus imparted its heat will fall down as drops of drinking water, which will accumulate in the lower part of the condensing chamber and may be drawn off by a pipe. When the mouth of the cowl is turned away from the wind a very strong ascensional current, no doubt, would be caused by this arrangement, and, on the contrary, if turned towards the wind, a volume of warm air would be forced downwards into the body of the vessel.

Perkins' Automatic Ventilator.—In the early part of the present century an ingenious contrivance for the ventilation of ships was invented by Mr. Perkins, an excellent account of which is given in a little work by Dr. Finlayson, R.N., on the baneful effects of too frequently washing ships' decks, with a plate of the ventilator as a frontispiece.

Fig. 27 (Plate XV.) represents this arrangement, in which the following parts will be recognised:—

1. Tanks or water butts.
2. Hose for conducting foul air into the tanks.
3. Hose for the escape of the foul air from the tanks.
4. A pipe connecting the tanks inferiorly.
5. Valves for admitting the foul air into the tanks.
6. Valves for allowing the foul air to escape.

'The operation of this self-acting ventilator,' says Dr. Finlayson, 'is as follows:—Each tank or butt is half filled with water, which flows from one to the other through a connecting pipe.

PERKINS' AUTOMATIC VENTILATOR.   109

'The quantity of water running alternately from each depends upon the motion of the ship. When one of the tanks is elevated by the ship's motion, the water will run through the pipe and into the depressed tank, and thereby discharge as much foul air as the additional water displaces. The elevated tank at the same time is receiving the foul air through a pipe, from the hold of the ship to supply the vacuum that would otherwise be made by the escape of the water. (See the course of the arrows in the figure.)

'If the tanks are fixed at right angles with the keel of the ship, the ventilator will operate only with the roll of it; but if placed diagonally, both the pitch and the roll of the vessel will discharge the foul air. It would be most economical to fill the tanks at the beginning of the voyage. The first water for the ship's use should be taken from the ventilating tanks, leaving, however, half of it behind for operation. If the remaining water should ever be wanted for the ship's use, it can be drawn off and replaced by salt water.

'It will be seen that, by this mode of ventilating, nothing but the hose and valves are to be added to what must necessarily be on board every ship.

'Any improvement in the arts generally becomes valuable in exact proportion to its strength and simplicity, for when an improvement is complicated or easily deranged, it is only useful in the hands of the inventor and the scientific.

'Mr. Perkins' not only combines those properties in a most eminent degree, but from its principle works hardest when most wanted.

'In a gale of wind when the hatches are on, and when there is much straining and rolling in a ship, the noxious gases are then generated to the greatest extent, then also the operations of the ventilator become most powerful, both in admitting fresh and expelling foul air.'

This principle, so lucidly described by Finlayson, has lately been made the subject of a patent under the name of 'Thier's Automatic Bilge-pump and Fog-horn' (see fig. 35, Plate

PLATE XXIII.

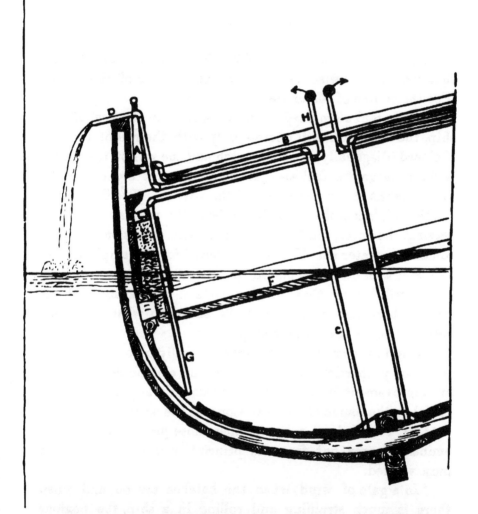

FIG. 35.—THIER'S AUTOMATIC SHIP VENTILATOR, BILGE-PUMP, AND FOG-HORN.

It has been already stated that Mr. Thier's patent very much resembles Mr. Perkins' scheme shown in Plate XV., fig. 27. A, The port mercurial cylinder. B, The intercommunicating pipe between it and the starboard one. C, The bilge-water pipe; and D, The discharge pipe. This part of the apparatus constitutes the 'bilge-pump,' but the means at present available would appear to answer the requirement sufficiently well. E is the water cylinder of the port side, F the intercommunicating pipe, G the air conduit from the bilge, &c., and H the vent-pipe, to which a fog-horn may be attached when the motion is considerable, but this is seldom the case in a fog.

XXIII.). This apparatus has been furnished to the 'Thetis' and several other ships; but although the first reports as to its efficiency were quite satisfactory, it does not appear to have kept up its credit on more extended trial.

The principle is the same as that of Perkins, but with this difference that Perkins seems to have taken advantage of the pitch as well as the roll. In Thier's plan the motion is purely lateral, the rolling only being taken into consideration. Perkins placed his tanks obliquely so that a partial effect might attend the pitch as well as the roll. The following concise account of Thier's invention is taken from the 'Times' of November 9, 1872:—

'Thier's Ship-ventilating Bilge-pump has been fitted to H.M.S. "Vigilant."

'The ventilator and the pump are identical in principle, but one acts upon air and the other upon water, and either may be separately used.

'Each consists of two vertical cylinders (A and E) placed one on either side of the ship, and connected together by a horizontal tube (B and F) of smaller calibre than themselves. From each cylinder a pipe (C and G) descends to the place from which air or water is to be drawn, and another pipe ascends as a channel of exit (D and H), both being provided with ordinary check valves.

'For the air-pump, the horizontal tube and cylinders are partially filled with water; for the water-pump, with quicksilver. As the vessel rolls to starboard, the water or quicksilver ascends in the starboard cylinder, and descends in the port cylinder, thereby causing a vacuum in the latter, which is immediately supplied by the ascent of air or water from below. As the vessel rights herself, the valves close, to prevent the air or the water from returning, and, as she rolls to port, the water or quicksilver rising in the cylinder on the port side not only expels through the eject-pipe whatever has been drawn up, but also causes a vacuum on the starboard side by which the foregoing process is repeated.'

Staff-Surgeon Martin Magill, M.D., of H.M.S. 'Thetis,' gives the following account of the ventilator from his own experience of it at sea. 'The action of the system is very simple, and the theory very plausible, but the actual work done is small indeed, and on occasions when ventilation is most required it is altogether inactive.

Height of each cylinder	4 feet 6 inches.
Diameter ,, ,,	1 foot 6 ,,
,, of connecting pipe	0 ,, $3\frac{3}{8}$,,

'If the ship were to be constantly rolling so as to fill each cylinder completely in rapid succession, the displacement of air thus caused might be perceptible, but a ship does not usually roll to such an extent, and the utmost practicable result is an occasional puff, and this puff will only be given when the ship rolls over three degrees, when ordinary ventilation is effective enough. When a ship is at anchor, perhaps in a close tropical harbour where a current of air would be a boon, the patent system is idle. To have it in full work the ship must be going before a gale of wind, rolling to both sides, and on such occasions the currents of wind on board are generally quite enough, and often more than is comfortable.

'I may only mention that its practical value in this ship was so little thought of, that when one side ceased to send out any air at all by its eject-tube soon after we left England, it was not considered worth the trouble to investigate the cause till we arrived at Hong Kong, although I need not say what a favourite it would have been if it could have sensibly increased the circulation of air through the ship when in the Red Sea.

'If a man had suggested that the feed pipe to a blacksmith's bellows on deck should be fitted so as to draw its supply of air from the bilge he would probably have been laughed at. Or if he had suggested that a small charcoal stove be placed in the bilge with a funnel $3\frac{3}{8}$ inches in diameter, its pigmy efforts to ventilate a ship 220 feet long would have been apparent, although either of these suggestions, and especially the latter, would have decided advantages over the patent system.'

The Ventilation of the French Ship 'L'Annamite,' a published account of which has been given by M. L. E. Bertin, naval engineer.—Notwithstanding the high authorities quoted by M. Bertin in reference to the principle on which the 'Annamite' is ventilated (and the detail as to the area of openings and the calibre of tubes required for the transmission of a given amount of air, in a given time, and at a certain degree of velocity to obviate draught, &c.), there would seem to be a radical defect in the system arising from the mode in which the principle is applied.

Thus, a downward current is established in the openings between the timbers, which will at any time be reversed when there happens to be a remission of the extractive force. For in the normal state of the case, where no such force is in operation, vitiated air will take an upward course in the openings in question.

The system of drawing vitiated air in a downward direction to give it egress has often been tried, but it should be much modified, or abandoned, as it is in opposition to natural law, instead of turning it to proper account.

In commenting upon the scheme of ventilation adopted in the case of the 'Annamite,' it should be premised, 1st, that the more nearly the ventilation of enclosed spaces is made to imitate open air conditions the more perfect it is. 2ndly, that to effect this purpose efficiently, ingress and egress must be so provided for as to insure insensible interchange without draught. We may now inquire as to how the latter conditions are fulfilled in the ventilation of this vessel.

1. *Provision for Ingress.*—Besides the openings of hatches and ports when their closure is not necessitated, downcast cowls and shafts are made to communicate below with horizontal tubes perforated as in the scheme of Dr. Arnott, which

is by no means new to us, as it has been already adopted in several of our ships, e.g. 'Lord Warden' and 'Royal Oak.'

2. *Provision for Egress.*—As in the system patented by the late Dr. Edmonds, R.N., and more recently by Mr. Stott of Halifax, advantage is taken of the funnel casing and the ascensional force of the heated air contained within it for extraction. Now, though it is by no means certain, in ordinary cases, that this ascensional tendency is always persistent or permanent, provision is made to insure it by supplementary extractive furnaces, when the ship is at anchor or under sail.

With the provision just mentioned it will be seen that the objection raised as to the manner in which the vitiated air is drawn downwards in other cases is here so well met that it would be quite worthy of a trial.

Ventilation of the 'Victor Emanuel,' Hospital Ship.— The following extracts in relation to the ventilation of the 'Victor Emanuel,' which was fitted up as a hospital ship for service on the West Coast of Africa during the Ashantee war, are taken from the Report of Surgeon-Major T. M. Bleckley, M.D., C.B., Senior Medical Officer on board :—

'Extending on either side amidships from the break of the poop as far forward as the fore side of the funnel, a ridge-covered projection is noticed rising above the planking. This is 80 feet in length (there being a break of 12 feet on either side to admit of passage to and from the galleys) by 2 feet 5 inches in breadth and 10 inches in height of combing. This is a trunk ventilating shaft, with a sloping roof, capable of being raised to a height of 8 inches by means of a butterfly-nut screw worked from below ; and its object is to act as an upcast and outlet for the foul air of the hospital deck. The lower ridge on either side is subdivided into four parts, each with its own screw, so as to admit of the degree of ventilation being regulated to different sections of the hospital deck, should such an expedient be at any time desirable. This is an admirable arrangement, simple, and at the same time perfectly effective.

'There are three small goose-neck pipes, opening above the bulwarks on either side of the upper deck, which communicate with the water-closets on the hospital deck, and thus serve as upcasts for foul air. Direct downcast ventilation is effected by means of cowled tubes, of which five are to be observed opening above the poop, and nine some feet above the level of the bulwarks on the upper deck. Of these, seven open below on the hospital deck, eight inches above the floor, two on convalescent decks, two on orlop deck, these latter communicating by means of an opening that can be closed by a shutter with the convalescent deck, and the remaining two open on the part of the lower or gun deck which is occupied by the ship's company.

'For the purpose of light and ventilation there are sixty-six ports $3\frac{1}{2}$ feet in height by 3 feet wide, and five scuttles, each 8 inches in diameter. The ports are fitted with sashes and jalousies, the latter of which can be shipped or unshipped at pleasure.

'The use of jalousies is known to all who have lived in the tropics, and their value in this ship was recognised both when stationary at Cape Coast and on the homeward voyage, as they kept out the sun, and at the same time admitted fresh air. General ventilation is also promoted by the hatchways, and by the three large stern ports. Direct downcast ventilation is effected by seven cowled tubes.

'The upcast ventilation is carried out by the ridge-covered projections in the floor of the upper deck, and by a perforated zinc shaft,[1] 5 inches in breadth, extending along the entire side wall of this deck, 6 feet 2 inches above the floor. This communicates with the external air through the hollow sides of the ship by louvred openings, and also with the bilges underneath. The expediency of this contrivance appears to

[1] This, no doubt, means the perforated zinc plates between the beam-ends taken collectively, which are a permanent nuisance in every wooden ship as originally fitted.

be, to say the least, very doubtful, as, however essential purification of the lower parts of the ship may be, this might be attained without the attendant evil of disagreeable smells from the bilges, which now and then pass inward through the perforated zinc plates, instead of outwards through the louvred openings in the ship's side.

'Extending all the way between the inner and middle row of cots is an iron shaft and ventilator in the flooring of the deck 21 inches broad, which serves as an upcast for the convalescent deck, and which communicates, by airtight boxes, with the hollow iron masts.' (This description applies to the deck air channels of the late Dr. Edmonds, R.N., which were supplied to the main and lower decks of the 'Victor Emanuel.')

Suggestions of Dr. F. Eklund, of Stockholm.

This section, though already of considerable length, would be incomplete without a notice of the valuable pamphlet of Dr. Eklund of Stockholm, amongst other things advocating the use of super-heated steam for drying and disinfecting not only the bilges, but the openings between the timbers.

It would, indeed, be very important if the drying, disinfooting, and extractive power of heat could be brought to bear upon bilge moisture and contagia in a practical way without involving much apparent outlay or inconvenience.

Hygienic measures, like many others, often become simple questions of expediency; even admitting that certain sanitary conditions can be effected at a definite cost, it is only fair to ask, would the benefit to be derived so far exceed the necessary expenditure as to render the proposals feasible or expedient? Dr. Eklund has given no figure or fairly descriptive outline of his plan, but the principle, no doubt, might be practically applied by any person sufficiently acquainted with the structure and economy of ships, and the benefit to be derived would certainly justify the small outlay required.

The difficulty of cleaning out the bilges on board ship is quite proverbial, arising from the usually narrow means of access to them, and the faulty construction of the floors in particular. The accumulation of water in the bilges takes place either by leakage or drainage, or both. In steamers, oil and grease, cotton waste, and filth of various kinds, add to the general effect; and in wooden ships, chips and shavings, remaining after dressing the timbers, undergo decomposition, and assist in setting up putrefactive changes in the bilges.

Dr. Eklund very properly advocates such an enlargement of the bilge areas as would be sufficient to permit a middle-sized man to enter them, that they might thus be easily and perfectly cleaned and dried. He also alludes to the usual flatness of the bilges through so considerable an extent of the square body in modern ships, as being favourable to the permanent accumulation of water in certain parts beyond the influence of the pump-suckers.

In the attempt to cut off the ascent of bilge air, which has been suggested by some, a difficulty at once arises as to how the descent or the percolation of drainage from above can still be permitted to take place. It might be easy enough to do the former by sealing up the channels which are normally subservient to both functions, but a vicarious bilge accumulation is sure to take place if such a proceeding is carried out. We should, therefore, endeavour, 1st, to favour the ascent of the bilge air between the timbers, with the view of conducting it safely into the outer air; or, 2ndly, divert it into some reservoir, from which it could be conveniently extracted without permitting it to diffuse itself between decks. The former of these indications has already been sufficiently enlarged upon; but the trial of the latter might be suggested as perhaps affording a better promise. It is only reasonable to suppose that a reservoir for bilge air, laid fore and aft upon the keelson, would take it up as fast as it is formed, and thus not only confine it within definite limits, but permit of its speedy removal by extractive means, such as conduits leading to the furnaces or funnel casing, to the hollow iron masts, or to air drums with coils of steam pipe, fans, respiratory cowls, &c. Steam pipes could also be introduced into this bilge reservoir, so as to rarefy the air and favour its removal and ascent in drying up the moisture, while by using super-heated steam any existing contagia might be more satisfactorily sterilised than by any other system of disinfection.

It has been already intimated that although the bilges form part of a drainage system, the physical requirements for such a system are but imperfectly met.

The bilge floors on either side of the keelson should be made perfectly smooth, cemented, lacquered, or tiled, so as to protect the wood from decay on the one hand, and permit of being wiped dry on the other.

It is, moreover, a matter of the greatest importance that a sufficient fall should be given from both ends of the vessel to the pump-well to ensure the complete removal of the water, and obviate any lodgment requiring the use of a hand-pump or any special mode of treatment.

Ventilation of Ships of the 'Monitor' Class.—The peculiar construction of low free-board vessels, in which all communication with the outer air is reduced to a minimum, seems to have suggested the necessity of introducing air by mechanical means to compensate for that which, under ordinary circumstances, would be permitted to enter without obstruction.

The *plenum* principle has without exception been adopted in the ventilation of those ships. A short general account of the ventilation of H.M.S. 'Glatton' and 'Devastation' is given in the April number of 'Naval Science' for 1873. Of the former vessel it is stated that 'a shaft 5 feet 6 inches by 6 feet 4 inches is sent from the top of the upper deck to the level of the main deck just abaft the smoke stack, and is continued above the upper deck to a height of 12 feet, the walls being rifle-proof and furnished with doors leading to the upper and first decks, both of which must, however, always be closed in rough weather.

'At the bottom of the shaft are four fans connected with two transverse tubes, the upper of which is 16 inches by 12 inches, and the lower 16 inches square. The fans propelled by the engine collect fresh air from the shaft and send it into the tubes, from which latter it is conveyed by means of pipes to every cabin and compartment of the ship, fore and aft, by goose-necked funnel ends, that open a few inches from the floor of the deck, and are each supplied with a screw valve. There are in the " Glatton " 133 of these outlets.'

'The principle adopted in the " Devastation " is pretty much the same, but the arrangements are different in many respects. Thus there are in this ship three shafts and five fans. One shaft is fixed just abaft the mainmast, and has two fans. The other shafts are placed just abaft the foremast, and are close to each other but distinct, the smaller enclosing one, and the longer two fans. All these fans are provided with distinct sets of engines and work independently; but it is an important arrangement, and one that contrasts favourably with the system adopted in the "Glatton," that if one or two shafts are blocked, or otherwise rendered useless, the third can by intercommunication supply air to all the compartments.'

Dr. James McCarthy, late Surgeon, R.N., on his appointment to the 'Devastation' studied experimentally the practical working of this system of ventilation. The more important results obtained will be found in the following remarks and tables selected from his journal, for the perusal of which the writer is indebted to Sir Alex. Armstrong, K.C.B., late Medical Director-General :—

Description of the Apparatus as originally fitted, and General Remarks thereon.

On the compartment, or lower deck, are three air shafts communicating with the outer air through the flying deck, and named respectively the *fore, main,* and *after* air shafts.

They are all placed over the stoke-hole; the fore immediately behind the fore funnel casing. Contiguous to this is the main, and five feet abaft the after funnel casing stands the after shaft. The dimensions of each are as follows:—

The fore shaft, length in feet 33, sectional area 37·78
„ main shaft „ „ 33 „ „ 21·78
And after shaft „ „ 38 „ „ 21·78

Reference to the table of observations will show the respective and aggregate hourly and daily cubic delivery of air through these shafts, as registered by Cassella's pocket anemometer.

The annexed diagram (Plate XXIV. fig. 36, B) is a horizontal section of the ship at the compartment deck.

The square spaces in the middle show the relative position of the shafts on this deck.

The fans, recognised by their form, are placed within the fore, but without and below the level of the after shaft.

The main trunks, 2·25 square feet sectional area, give off round pipes of ·5 square foot sectional area, and from these again arise the inlet or distribution tubes of ·0341 square foot sectional area, which are led into the various compartments. These latter may not inaptly be termed the capillary system of the apparatus.

The starboard fan boxes of the fore and after shafts furnish two trunks running horizontally, and two vertically: the latter go to supply the stoke-hole, the air travelling through them into the central trunk being distributed by eight T-shaped inlets.

Communication can be cut off from each fan box and its trunk by sluice valves. Valves are also placed at certain distances along the trunks to cut off, if required, the air from any single compartment. The inlet tubes may now be traced into the three principal sleeping-places, namely, the cabins, belt deck, and lower deck.

In the cabins the inlet tubes open about a foot from the

PLATE XXIV.

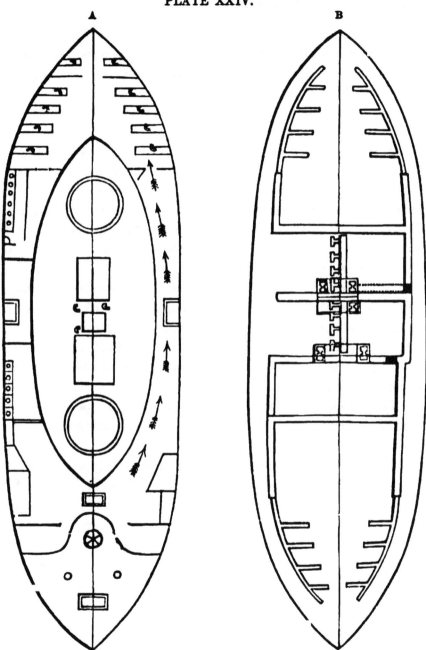

FIG. 36.—VENTILATION OF H.M.S. 'DEVASTATION.'

A and B are simply hand sketches of the system adopted, without claiming great accuracy. In B the central position of the five fans will be readily recognised, as well as the general distribution of the air-shafts, and the eight T-shaped inlets to the engine-room. In A three curved inlets are seen near the end of the hatchway in the middle, and five on each side under the mess tables of the men. The arrows show a prevailing current of air alluded to in the text.

floor of each, the consequence of which is that the air as it issues from the tube escapes into the passage outside, and is carried along to the stoke-hole by the extractive force of the furnaces. The cubic delivery of these tubes is about 1,000 feet per hour, which would be ample if it were more effectively confined to the space to be ventilated.

In the belt deck, which contains an available air space of 32,580 cubic feet, and sleeping billets for 136 men, there are three inlet tubes; two placed at the combing of the main hatchway, and one near the windows of the funnel casing. The result of this malposition is that as the air issues from the tubes it escapes up through the hatchway and casing, and the primary object must thus be largely defeated. Fortunately, owing to its direct communication with the pilot deck through the main hatchway and funnel casings, this deck is, even in rough weather, independent of mechanical ventilation. So effective, indeed, are these two means of ventilation, that under the very worst circumstances the CO_2 has never been found to exceed 1 per thousand volumes.

The lower or forecastle deck (fig. 36, A) possesses an available air space of 16,063 cubic feet, and sleeping billets for 120 men.

The aggregate sectional area of the hatchways, cowled ventilators, and side ports opening into this deck is about 67 square feet. When in harbour, however, the CO_2 in the air was seldom found below 1·5 per 1,000 volumes.

One would imagine that the above-mentioned immense area would supply enough air to keep the CO_2 considerably below the amount stated. The fact, however, is that in harbour both watches sleep below, and the deck is overcrowded, 120 men occupying a space of 16,063 cubic feet. This would be equivalent to but 133 cubic feet per man, and in each case would require 3,000 cubic feet of air to keep the CO_2 down to the standard of practicable purity, and 3,000 multiplied by $120 = 360,000$ cubic feet per hour, which it would be quite impossible to supply under the circumstances.

At sea in rough weather this deck is converted into an hermetically sealed box, and is then, with the exception of the air flowing through the starboard wing passage, into which the starboard upper deck hatchway opens, entirely dependent on its artificial supply, which is quite inadequate.

There are ten inlets in this deck opening beneath the mess tables, five on either side. The average aggregate cubic delivery from these tubes is about 10,000 feet per hour, which for 60 men, allowing the other 60 to be on watch, is 166 cubic feet per head per hour.

On four occasions, when battened down, the air of this deck was examined, and on each occasion the CO_2 was found to be within a decimal of 2·75 per 1,000 volumes. On one night, August 20, it reached 3·14. This was owing, however, to the upper deck hatches being closed all that night, the deck being thus deprived of the air flowing through the wing passage into which these hatches open. The above figures represent the maximum impurity of the air in this deck; for it was always collected between 3 and 4 A.M., and on a level with the hammocks.

Besides the method of distribution, the position chosen for the shafts, the abrupt diminution in calibre of the transit media, and their frequent angularity might deserve comment. Dr. McCarthy next goes on to describe the adoption of a suggestion of his own to mitigate the stuffiness complained of in the cabins and elsewhere. He says, 'in the absence of an extracting shaft the only means left was to distribute the air supplied in such a manner as to insure its diffusion. I, therefore, proposed the following alteration in the position of the inlets:—To continue the tubing up over the foot of the bed close to the beams, stop up the end, and perforate the sides with a series of half-inch holes. The air thus delivered would be thrown immediately over the bed, and in falling mix with and dilute the respiratory impurities as they arise.'

This was done in the staff surgeon's, the master's, and his

own cabin, and on a comparative analysis of the air in these and other cabins whose inlets were still *in statu quo*, he found the CO_2 in the former never much above 9, while in the air of the latter always above 1 per 1,000 volumes. This, he admits, is a small difference, but it is sufficient to show that the air was more efficiently distributed by the latter than by the former plan. But, apart from this, the pleasant feeling experienced by the person in bed as the cool air was thrown over his face rendered the alteration a success. The method was not carried out in all the cabins until the ship was docked in October, when somewhat similar alterations to the above were also made in the distribution tubes of the lower deck.

As previously stated, the cubic delivery of these ten tubes was for 60 men, only 166 feet per head per hour. It was imperatively necessary to increase that, and give at least 500 cubic feet per head per hour, and at the same time to alter the position of the inlets. 'I therefore proposed,' he says, 'to treble the number of inlets, lead them from their present position under the tables, up by the ship's side along the beams and over the hammocks, the horizontal portion of the tubes being perforated on both sides and closed at the end. The current of air thus delivered would be distributed equably, and prove, as in the cabins, an effective diluent of the respiratory impurities and also, especially in summer, agreeably cooling to men in passing over them at night.'

Twenty-nine analyses of the air given in Table I. were made in the three principal sleeping-places of H.M.S. 'Devastation' during her trial trips in 1873, carbonic acid being taken as the index of impurity. From the following observations, however, it will be seen that the results contrast favourably with those obtained in other ships. Thus in H.M.S. 'Doris' between decks the CO_2 was found to be 3·21 (Dr. Hayne, R.N.); in the 'Alert's' wardroom reached 4·82 (Dr. Moss, R.N.); and in the 'Discovery's' lower deck 5·57 (Dr. Ninnis, R.N.).

Table I.—Twenty-nine determinations of CO_2.

Date	Conditions under which the observations were made	Belt deck air-space 3,258 cub. ft. 136 men	
		Port side	Starboard
April 30	In harbour, fans going, hatches and turrets open	·87	·9
May 9	Ditto	·93	·98
,, 16	Ditto	·95	·979
,, 20	At sea, battened down turrets, ports closed, fans going	1·03	1·
,, 29	Same as April 30	·9	·89
June 3	Ditto	·99	·97
,, 9	Ditto	·9	·9
,, 13	Ditto	·098	·967
		·946 av. (Per 1,000 vols.)	·948 av. (Per 1,000 vols.)
		Lower deck air-space 16,063 cub. ft. 120 men	
May 3	In harbour, with hatches and ports open, fans not going	1·20	1·23
,, 5	Same, but fans going	1·15	1·10
,, 7	As May 3; still night	1·33	1·40
,, 22	Ditto; ports closed	1·45	1·48
,, 26	Ditto; fans going	1·17	1·21
,, 30	Ditto; windy night	1·13	1·09
June 1	At sea, not battened down	1·04	1·1
,, 6	As May 3	1·30	1·34
Aug. 13	Battened down, fans going	2·65	2·29
,, 14	Ditto	2·70	2·55
,, 30	Ditto; upper-side hatches closed	3·05	3·10*
Sept. 1	Ditto; fans going	2·51	2·20
		1·723 av. (Per 1,000 vols.)	1·647 av. (Per 1,000 vols.)
		Port cabins	Starboard cabins
May 13	Harbour, fans going, after hatches and W.R. skylight open, good wind	·91	·97
,, 15	Ditto	·93	·91
,, 25	Ditto; no fans, still night	1·15	1·23
,, 28	Ditto	1·20	1·17
June 4	Ditto; good wind down skylights and hatches	·960	·981
,, 16	Ditto; calm night	1·21	1·29
Aug. 15	Battened down, at sea, fans going	·987*	1·55
,, 31	Ditto	1·5	·99*
Sept. 1	Ditto	1·0*	1·42
		1·089 av. (Per 1,000 vols.)	1·167 av. (Per 1,000 vols.)

* Denotes those cabins in which the inlet tubes were altered in the manner alluded to in the text.

Table II.

Cubic delivery of the three shafts per hour.[1] Thirty-two observations.
Average velocity of fans, 160 revolutions per minute.

Date	Fore shaft		
April 12	330026·4	298430·6	
,, 12	294436·0	277625·8	469872·1
,, 15	310940·3	362989·0	490876·6
,, 15	220410·9	324321·6	479987·5
,, 21	314684·7	351248·4	567532·8
,, 21	298297·2	300987·0	547280·7
,, 23	297998·6	292438·6	440801·6
,, 23	Irregular movement	347891·4	483242·3
,, 23	261172·8	Irregular movement	469873·0
,, 30	No movement	291134·2	520401·2
,, 30	Irregular movement	351762·3	547340·0
,, 30	270069·1	310420·1	407112·3
May 5	359676·7	363423·2	
,, 5	280579·6	310107·0	487239·6
,, 9	291874·3	Irregular movement	433160·6
,, 9	170498·7	Not working	431003·0
,, 15	359700·2	276984·3	369009·2
,, 15	Irregular movement	212398·0	526201·5
,, 16	369874·0	349195·3	487321·6
,, 16	309998·6	270403·0	444397·6
,, 18	Not working	Not working	460711·7
,, 22	Irregular movement	Irregular movement	310914·4
,, 26	Ditto	210694·3	510911·6
,, 26	Not working	Not working	530731·2
,, 27	279876·3	340691·3	311389·4
,, 27	321443·2	319455·8	476214·0
June 1	277691·4	276731·1	468401·7
,, 1	Not working	185627·1	534658·5
,, 2	Ditto	190876·3	500337·0
,, 2	225365·7	364454·5	492346·0
,, 2	313344·3	389548·5	497201·0
Mean hourly delivery	283631·9	302627·9	479466·0
Mean daily delivery	6807165·6	7263067·6	10786200·8
Aggregate total daily delivery		24,856,434 cubic feet.	

[1] The late Professor Parkes kindly lent the anemometers used in these experiments.

VENTILATION OF THE MAGAZINES. 127

Ventilation of the Magazines.—From the very nature of the case the magazines are excluded as much as possible from all external communication, and it will be easily understood how defective the ventilation must be under such circumstances. Indeed, it was long a desideratum how this could be improved

PLATE XXV.

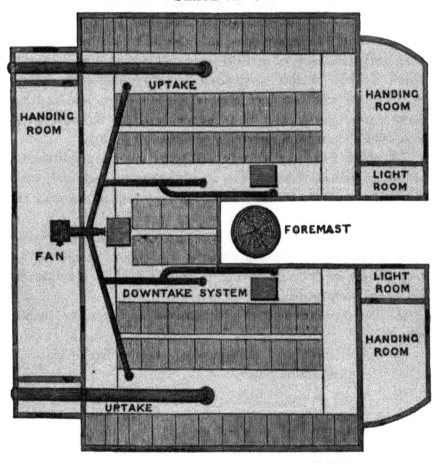

FIG. 37.—THE VENTILATION OF THE FORE MAGAZINE, H.M.S. 'DUNCAN.'
This figure will be sufficiently understood without further description.

with safety, until a plan was suggested by Captain Jerningham, R.N., the leading features of which are shown in fig. 37, Plate XXV.

From a Desagulier's fan, usually worked by hand, a main

shaft leads downwards to the floor of the magazine, where it divides symmetrically into several branches, each of which communicates with the interior, having the opening protected by a little copper grating. To complete the system an uptake shaft is provided on either side. This scheme would appear to have given the initiative to the *plenum* system of ventilation, which has since been so generally adopted. When the fan is in full play, the displacement of dust from the floor of the magazine often becomes quite as serious an evil as the temporary inhalation of a little more carbonic acid than usual. There is good reason to believe, however, that this defect would be remedied and a better result, generally, obtained by using extraction rather than propulsion, the inferiority of which latter has been elsewhere sufficiently shown.

To what has been already said in relation to ventilation, ventilating tubes, relative size of main trunks and offshoots, bending at angles and subdivision, some practical remarks on the following important topics should be added :—

1. The vitiation of air by a single individual in a given air-space per hour, and the amount of fresh air required to keep the air of such space up to the standard of practicable purity for respiration.

2. The measurement of cubic space available for respiration.

3. The chemical and microscopical examination of air.

4. The purification of air.

---

1. The amount of carbonic acid in the external air may be taken as ·4 per 1,000 vols., and it will be at once admitted that it would be quite impracticable to renew the air of any circumscribed space so frequently as to keep the CO_2 down to that proportion. Since, therefore, a certain amount of vitiation is inevitable, the question arises how much should be admitted as the standard of practicable purity? It has been shown by Pettenkofer that a single individual

will evolve by respiration ·6 of a cubic foot of CO_2 in an hour, which amount will of course be doubled at the end of the second hour should no interchange have taken place. Thus, if the air-space = 1,000 cubic feet, the CO_2 will be ·6 per 1,000 in the first hour, which would require 2,000 cubic feet of fresh air to dilute it to ·2 per 1,000, or ·6 if we also take into account the initial amount in the air, namely ·4 per 1,000 vols. We see, then, that, as a rule, each individual should be supplied with 3,000 cubic feet of air per hour, to maintain the air of any breathing space in the purest condition which is practically attainable.

2. In the measurement of cubic space available for respiration, three simple rules must be observed:—

1st. To take the largest measurements of length, breadth, and height that the space will admit of for the main cubic capacity.

2nd. To take the capacity of all irregular spaces and recesses in communication with the principal space, to which the sum should be added.

3rd. To take the measurement of all obstructive bodies, projections, and everything that would impinge upon the available air space, and subtract the sum from the gross cubic capacity already obtained.

It will greatly facilitate calculation to take the measurements in feet and decimals rather than feet and inches, and for this purpose the following table will be useful, copied on a slip of paper to assist the memory:—

ONE FOOT.

Inches	1	2	3	4	5	6	7	8	9	10	11	12
Decimal parts of a foot	0·08	0·17	0·25	0·33	0·42	0·50	0·58	0·67	0·75	0·83	0·92	1·00

Naval architects use Sterling's rules in the measurement of areas bounded by a straight line as a base, and a curve line.

If, however, every such area be regarded as the segment of a circle, a simpler method is the following, taken from Professor Parkes's 'Manual.' Thus, the area of the segment of a circle = ⅔ of the product of the chord and height *plus* the cube of the height divided by twice the chord: $(Ch \times H \times \frac{2}{3}) + \frac{H^3}{2Ch}$.

Next in importance in a practical sense is the measurement of triangular spaces, which is very simple. Thus, the area of a triangle = the base × ½ the height, or conversely the height by ½ the base, and it will be observed that areas of the most irregular kind will admit of being divided into triangles, so that the measurement of all may be added together.

When the measurement of the whole cubic space has been ascertained, and then divided by the number of individuals occupying it, the result will give the cubic space per head available for respiration.

3. In the chemical and microscopical examination of air many of the processes exactly resemble those employed in the case of drinking-water. Thus, by employing a measured aspirator and drawing a definite quantity of the air to be tested through a series of wash-bottles, each charged with 100 c.c. of pure distilled water, all soluble matters will be arrested in the water, which may then be submitted, as such, to chemical examination.

The ammonia should be tested with Nessler's fluid, the oxidisable organic matters with the permanganate of potassium, after the manner described under the head of the 'Chemical Examination of Water.'

On the other hand, all the suspended matters, which will form a settlement at the bottom of the bottles, should be collected in conical glasses, taken up with a pipette, and examined under the microscope.

As the proportion of carbonic acid may be taken as the most reliable index of the whole organic impurity present in any air-space, the method of determining it should be simple, efficient, and thoroughly understood by the operator. Petten-

CHEMICAL AND MICROSCOPICAL EXAMINATION. 131

kofer's method, so clearly stated with all the necessary precautions in Parkes's 'Practical Hygiene,' should be chosen for this purpose. The materials required are comparatively inexpensive, and when once obtained will be always ready for use. They are the following:—

1. A glass jar of about the capacity of a gallon or $4\frac{1}{2}$ litres, with a wide mouth fitted with an india-rubber cap.

2. A bottle of clean lime or baryta water.

3. A solution of crystallised oxalic acid, 2·25 grammes to a litre of distilled water, 1 c.c. of which is equivalent to a milligramme of lime.

4. A wooden stand with a small burette carrying 10 c.c., with an india-rubber pipe, glass nozzle and pinch-cock.

5. Any small glass vessel that will hold 30 c.c. and a glass stirring rod.

6. An ordinary pair of bellows with about a yard of india-rubber tubing to fit on the nozzle.

Thus provided with apparatus, the operation is simple enough.

First ascertain the critical capacity of the jar in cubic centimetres by filling it with water and then measuring off the water. When the capacity of the jar is determined, it should be thoroughly dried for use. Next introduce the india-rubber tube attached to the bellows, which is to be blown energetically for a few minutes to dislodge the air contained in the jar. The air of the locality to be experimented upon will replace the air so expelled, and should be immediately shut in with the india-rubber cap, having previously introduced 60 c.c. of the alkaline solution.

If lime water is used, its alkalinity should be ascertained by placing 30 c.c. in the glass vessel, and then dropping in the acid solution from the burette until it becomes neutral to test-paper (litmus and turmeric). The number of c.c. used should be noted as the *first alkalinity*.

The lime water in the jar should be shaken about and then allowed to stand for eight hours, when 30 c.c. should be taken out and tested as before, the number of c.c. used being noted as the *second alkalinity*. The latter amount should be taken from the former, and the difference multiplied by the factor ·795, which by converting weight into volume will give the number of c.c. of CO_2 contained in the jar. This amount being then divided by the capacity of the jar, *minus* 60, to allow for the quantity of lime water originally introduced, will give the CO_2 in volumes per 1,000 which we desire to determine.

As air expands in the proportion of ·2 per cent. for every degree of Fahr., the standard being 32°, a correction must be made for temperature. Thus, if the temperature is 60°, $60 - 32 = 28 \times ·2 = 5·6$ per cent. to be added to the result. Or the latter may be multiplied by 1·056. $\therefore 1·103 \times 1·056 = 1·164$ per 1,000, the corrected result. If the temperature is below 32°, say 27°, deduct this from 32°, and multiply the difference $= 5$ by $·2 = 1·0$ per cent. to be subtracted; or multiply the result by $1·00 - ·010 = ·990$. $\therefore 1·103 \times ·990 = 1·092$. (Parkes.)

The relative humidity of the atmosphere should be determined by consulting the wet and dry thermometer, with which the humidity of the enclosed air-space should be compared.

In relation to iron ships it is provided by Article 1227, page 395, 'Queen's Regulations and Admiralty Instructions,' that 'when it is impossible to dry out completely any of the compartments, bilges, or wings of an iron or composite ship, in order to coat them with composition, paint, or cement, lime slaked thoroughly to prevent injury to the composition is to be placed in the water contained in such places.' (The addition of carbolic acid would no doubt be an improvement.)

Also, by Article 1229, 'the following precautions are to be observed while men are engaged in cleaning and coating the double bottoms of an iron ship:'—

'(a) The air-fan with hose is to be freely used for pumping in fresh air before the men are sent down, and while they are at work.

'(b) A leading stoker is to be responsible under the engineer in charge of the party, that no man enters a compartment unless a light has been held in and left at the bottom of the compartment for at least five minutes, to ascertain the purity of the air.

'(c) Still greater caution is required when the compartment has only one exit.

'(d) Communication is always to be kept up between the men in the inner compartment and those who have access to the outer air; and

'(e) The men are to be warned that they should leave a compartment immediately the light begins to burn dimly; a candle is to be supplied to each party, as a surer test than a lamp, since it might be thought that a lamp burnt dimly for want of trimming.

'(f) The same precautions are to be taken when examining boilers and bunkers, in accordance with Article 913, which provides that the engineer "will take care that whenever boilers are opened up sufficient time is given to allow any foul air to escape, and that before any one is allowed to enter the boilers or bunkers the purity of the air is ascertained as directed by Article 1229."'

CHAPTER III.

WATER SUPPLY.

Section 1.—*General Remarks.*

The importance of a good supply of wholesome water for ship's use must be evident to everybody, though it is more particularly felt by those who have at any time experienced the discomfort of short allowance at sea, or the issue of bad water under circumstances permitting of no remedy.

As a rule, in every ship a drinking tank is fixed in a convenient place near the main hatchway on the main deck, and it is only on extraordinary occasions that it becomes necessary to place it under restrictions. There is also, very frequently, a similar tank on the lower deck free at all times.

The usually athletic duties of the sailor, whether stationed on deck or aloft, lead him to draw very largely upon the water tank, and with this is inseparably coupled the responsibility of those whose duty it is to see that the water is of good quality. Moreover, as this article is, in ordinary, so freely consumed by the seamen, we can readily understand how it is that evils traceable to this source should spread so rapidly through a ship as they are too frequently known to do.

The origin and spread of a certain class of diseases, due to the contamination of the drinking water, was long known to the Government of India, until it was decided in 1866 that competent analysts should visit the various military stations and draw up accurate reports as to the condition of the water in use. This duty at first devolved upon civil officers, but of late years it has been conducted by military surgeons instructed in the laboratory of the Netley Medical School.

It is very satisfactory also to know that the chemical and microscopical examination of water to which any suspicion might be attached can now be made by naval medical officers on their own responsibility, instead of seeking the necessary information from without as in former years.

While bad water cannot be deprecated too much, good water cannot be too highly extolled; more especially if we share in the views of Pliny, who could not understand why men went to so much trouble and expense to manufacture drinks of various kinds while nature had furnished them so abundantly with the best of all beverages without cost.

Water is the grand vehicle of all the nutritious materials which are applied to the support and growth of organic beings, and hence arises the question as to its comparative utility in chemical purity, or while holding in solution the various constituents normally present in it as drinking-water. However this may be, it is probable that, whether such constituents are primarily combined with it or subsequently taken up by it on entering the system, the result would be practically the same.

In the ordinary sense good potable water may be said to be that which contains no deleterious materials, nor excess of those which are admissible from their more constant presence; and although our knowledge is yet very imperfect in relation to this subject, useful tables have been made to show what maximum proportion of each substance may be present without exerting a prejudicial influence on the health.

With the exception of carbonic acid and perhaps iron, the gaseous, saline or other constituents should not be in such quantity as sensibly to affect the taste or smell of the water.

The absence of all colour and suspended matters gives brilliant transparency to water, and evidence of the complete solution of the several substances contained in it, though no guarantee of its intrinsic purity. However repugnant to the convictions of practical men this simple lesson may be, they had better accept it at once than wait for its more general adoption at some future time.

Section 2.—*Natural Waters.*

Evaporation, condensation, and fall, are the three great processes by which a continual circulation of the watery element is maintained in nature. Of the total amount of rain falling upon the surface of the earth, a certain portion, varying in different localities with the permeability of the soil, will penetrate downwards, until it reaches a less penetrable stratum, above which it will accumulate and take a further underground course, determined by the inclination of that bed towards some point where it may cross out at a lower level, and the water will reappear as a dripping spring. If, on the other hand, the strata do not become superficial, but continue to slope downwards, the water may be thus conducted to a very great depth, whence it cannot ascend, except there be some defect or fissure in the beds, either occurring naturally or made by human skill, as in boring for an artesian well.

Springs situated in the high lands give rise to streamlets, which, after a longer or shorter course, run together, and the common bulk being augmented by tributaries as it descends towards the sea, may finally roll as a mighty river.

From the foregoing remarks it will be seen that besides the water of lakes, ponds, and brooks, the three principal descriptions of so-called natural waters are—(1) rain, (2) spring or well, and (3) river water, upon each of which some few observations may be made.

1. Rain water is, perhaps, the purest natural water. Ammonia, nitrous and nitric acids are the only substances which pure atmospheric air can impart to it. Chlorine, chloride of sodium, and the small trace of iodine said to be present in rain water, are probably derived from the sea. Principles resulting from the combustion of coal, and the sul-

phurous acid given off in manufacturing districts, may be classed with any others having a purely terrestrial or local origin.

Rain water from its solvent property is well fitted for various uses to which it is applied by man, and the numerous purposes which it serves in the economy of nature. Its primitive purity, however, favours its dangerous contamination with lead when conveyed by leaden pipes or received into cisterns lined with that material. When collected in the neighbourhood of towns, it should be boiled and strained to fit it for use.

Dew differs from rain water chiefly in containing more atmospheric air; and ice water, when first obtained, differs from both in being destitute of air. It is for the same reason mawkish and insipid, and no fish can survive long in it. Snow water is similar in this respect.

2. Spring water of course will vary as to the nature and amount of the materials which it holds in solution, in accordance with the conditions of its source and the composition of the strata through which it has passed. It contains most of the matters found in rain water with the addition of others, such as the salts of lime and magnesia, and when these are abundant the water is proportionately hard,—though this hardness, as indicated by the soap test, is often also due to free carbonic acid, as well as the carbonate of lime present in the water.

Dr. Paris states that large springs are in general purer than small ones, and those which occur in primitive countries and in silicious rocks or beds of gravel necessarily contain the smallest amount of impurities.

When particular constituents greatly predominate, their therapeutic properties are often highly extolled.[1]

3. River water mostly originates in springs, as before

---

[1] The study of composition of mineral waters in relation to the rock formations through which they flow has been taken up very satisfactorily by Dr. Gairdner.

mentioned, and is commonly augmented by rain water. If it flows over sand or granite it is found to be comparatively pure, depositing in its course many earthy salts, especially those of lime from the escape of carbonic acid.

The unicellular plants and animals are in much greater abundance in river than in spring water.

When lakes have an outlet, the properties of the water correspond mainly with those of river water; but if there is no outlet, there is more scope for the development of animal and vegetable life, and for the decomposition of organic remains. Or the water may contain the same ingredients as the ocean, but in a more concentrated state. These salt lakes are highly interesting in a geological sense, for there is indubitable evidence of their having been uplifted from the sea, beneath which the surrounding land was once submerged.

The constant evaporation going forward, and by which they occasionally become so concentrated, is compensated for by rainfalls and diluting streams of fresh water. Should a lake of this kind suffer an inundation of fresh water at any time sufficient to break down the barrier and make an outlet for the water charged with its salts, though as old as a geological epoch, it might be swept away in a week (*e.g.*, American lakes).

Little need be said of marsh water, which is usually in a stagnant state, charged with decaying organic matters, and exhaling noxious principles. It should be remarked, however, that the brownish tint often occurring in waters flowing through bog lands is not found to be associated with any definitely unwholesome effect.

The waters of sluggish streams moving through flat country should always be avoided in watering ship. On the other hand, when the land is diversified by hill and dale, any spring discoverable will be likely to furnish good water. The general features of the country will afford the means of judging where water would probably be found were it necessary to dig for it.

On the shores of a continent or island with a mountainous interior, the reservoir of fresh water usually reaches close to the beach, as at King George's Sound, where excellent water may be obtained by digging within a few feet of the ripple. In Western Australia, however, round the whole coast line of Shark Bay, at least 300 miles where the country is flat and monotonous, not a single streamlet was encountered by the surveying officers of H.M.S. 'Herald.' Exploring parties were sent in different directions to dig for water, but without success; and when some of the miserable aborigines of the district came on board they only begged for water. In one place a deep but dry pit was observed in the sand, with a large melo or melon shell at the bottom of it, evidently the instrument with which the pit had been dug in search for water.

If the bed of a brook be of pebbles and sand, and the banks sloping or abrupt, and its course rapid, there need not be much further question as to the good quality of the water, though it is always well to follow the banks of the stream for a little distance towards its source, to see there are no stagnant pools or other causes of pollution in communication with it.

In high winds the specific gravity of the surface water is above the average.

Section 3.—*Condensed Water.*

The credit of having been the first to suggest and carry out the distillation of fresh water from the sea is claimed for several individuals, who all nevertheless considered that it was necessary to mix particular substances with the water in order to obtain a satisfactory result. In the year 1761, however, Dr. Lind was fortunate enough to discover that sea water simply distilled, without the addition of any ingredient, afforded a water as pure and wholesome as that obtained from the best springs.

Rude methods of distillation, using the ship's coppers with still-heads and worm tubs, inverted tea-kettles, or the hand pump with gun-barrel condensers, &c., were carried into practice from time to time as suggested by Dr. Lind.

Lord Verulam says (Bacon's 'Nat. Phil.,' art. 9, ex. 881), 'It hath been observed by the ancients that salt water boiled, or boiled and cooled again, is more potable than of itself raw, and yet the taste of salt in distillations by fire riseth not, for the distilled waters will be fresh. The cause may be that the salt part of the water doth partly rise into a scum on the top, and partly goeth into a sediment in the bottom, and so is rather a separation than evaporation; but it is too gross to rise into vapour, and so is a bitter taste likewise; for simple distilled waters of wormwood and the like are not bitter.' However, it was not the salt itself nor the bitter taste which was supposed to rise in the distillation of sea water, but a bituminous substance and a spirit of sea salt, which had been the unanimous and uncontroverted opinion of chemists up to the date of Dr. Lind's discovery.

Sir Richard Hawkins, with four billets, was represented to have distilled a hogshead of water wholesome and nourishing; and Dr. Lind reasoned, that the billets were used for making wood ashes is apparent from a letter written by Captain Chapman to Dr. Fothergill ('Lond. Mag.' for August 1753), where the captain gives an account of his distilling fresh water from the sea, first with the assistance of soap, then of wood ashes, having lost most of his water in a hard gale of wind.

Not many years after the death of Lord Verulam several experiments were made on board ships at Spithead by Sir Theophilus Oglethorpe and others, who had obtained a patent for distilling from the sea a water fresh and potable by means of additional ingredients. In 1739 Dr. Hales proposed another method, but that which was devised by Mr. Appleby in 1753 attracted the attention of all Europe. The following announcement is extracted from the 'London Gazette' of January 22,

1754:—'Mr. Joshua Appleby, of Durham, chemist, having discovered an easy and expeditious method of rendering sea water fresh and wholesome at sea, and the same on a reference to the Admiralty having been thoroughly examined and approved by the College of Physicians and the Commissioners of the Victualling, the Lords Commissioners for executing the Office of Lord High Admiral of Great Britain and Ireland have published the process used by the said Joshua Appleby in the "London Gazette," that so useful a discovery may be universally known. It is as follows:—Put 20 gallons of sea water into a still, together with six ounces of lapis infernalis and six ounces of bones calcined to whiteness and finely powdered. From this 15 gallons of fresh and wholesome water may be extracted in two hours and a half, at the expense of little more than a peck of coals.' This proportion of ingredients will answer very well in these northern seas, but in some parts of the Mediterranean or Indian seas, where the water is more salt and bituminous, the quantity must be increased to nine ounces of each. The ship's boiler should not be used for this process, what remains being very noxious. To remedy this latter difficulty, Dr. Butter suggested the use of capital soap leys, Dr. Alston limestone, and Dr. Hales powdered chalk.

These facts speak for themselves, and incontestably show that the credit of having discovered that no ingredient whatever is necessary for the distillation of fresh water from the sea is due to Dr. Lind.

The distilling apparatus in former use is now quite superseded, since the introduction of steam power has been so general in the navy. The quantity of water condensed while under steam in vessels of war is usually so ample that it is rarely necessary to supply them with water in any other way. In the ordinary process of condensation the water passes over quite devoid of air, and is too often conveyed to the tanks at a high temperature, evolving steam, and precluding the absorption of air, which is always present in good tasting and wholesome water. To meet this deficiency Dr. Normandy has devised a patented apparatus, which is not only economical, but an invaluable resource in a hygienic sense. The water condensed and aërated in this way is perfectly wholesome, and we have the satisfaction of knowing that it may be freely drawn from the tank without producing disease, which can only spring from the causes already alluded to.

In this connection it will be important to bear the following facts in mind :—

1. Both sea and fresh waters contain air with a larger proportion of oxygen and carbonic acid than exists in the same amount of atmospheric air.

Thus: 100 volumes of atmospheric air contains—

Oxygen, 24; and carbonic acid, $\frac{1}{4000}$.

100 volumes of air in solution in water contain—

Oxygen, 32—33; carbonic acid, 40—42.

2. Rain water contains 15 cubic inches of oxygenated air per gallon of the following composition :—

Nitrogen	.	.	.	.	.	3·20
Oxygen	.	.	.	.	.	5·04
Carbonic acid	.	.	.	.	.	6·26

3. Sea water contains two-thirds less of oxygenated air than rain water, i.e., only 5 cubic inches, the larger half of which is composed of carbonic acid.[1]

---

[1] The total quantity of dissolved gases in sea water were found by Mr. Wm. Lant Carpenter to average 2·8 volumes in 100 volumes of water.
Average of thirty analyses of surface water:—

	Per-centage	Proportion
Oxygen . . .	25·046	100
Nitrogen . . .	54·211	216
Carbonic acid . .	20·243	80
	100·000	

As a general rule, the proportion of oxygen was found to diminish, and that of carbonic acid to increase, with the depth, as also with the ratio of the development of animal life; the latter particular was so frequently

Dr. Normandy's apparatus (fig. 38, Plate XXVI.) consists mainly of three parts, viz.: 1, an evaporator; 2, a condenser; and 3, a filter. The first takes advantage of the heat derived from the steam in the fasciculus of tubes of the evaporator A to drive off the oxygenated air contained in the sea water surrounding those tubes. In the next place, this air is conducted by air pipes into the condenser B, where it commingles with the water as it is condensed. Finally the condensed aërated water is conveyed into the filter C, from whence it is conveyed by a pipe and hose into the tanks to be stored for use. The air-pipe is of such considerable length, and the flow of salt water through the apparatus so constant, that the water is quite fit for consumption soon after it leaves the filter. Thus far a general idea may be formed of the process which must now be more particularly described.

1. The steam-pipe a leads into the cap b connecting the upper ends of a sheaf of pipe c, through which it passes to the cap d, connecting their lower ends. From the latter a pipe e leads to a steam box or trap f, with a ball-cock which only allows the distilled water to pass by the pipe g to the cap h, surmounting the lower sheaf of pipes i in the condenser B. Having descended through these tubes to the lower cap k, it thence flows into the filter C, from whence it is drawn off by the cock l.

2. The filter is divided by a vertical septum incomplete below, so that the water must descend through the charcoal of the first chamber, and ascend through that of the second, affording ample provision for its purification.

3. Sea water is introduced into the apparatus by the feed-pipe m, fills the condenser and the lower end of the air-pipe n, communicating with it. Passing along the pipe o, it fills the

observed by Mr. Carpenter that he would predict a good or bad haul of the dredge in a given locality from the relative proportion of the gaseous elements in the bottom water.

The total solids in solution in sea water may range between 3,920 and 4,132 grammes per 100,000 c.c. (Frankland).

144 CONSERVATIVE HYGIENE.

PLATE XXVI.

Fig. 38. Dr. Normandy's Condensing, Aërating, and Filtering Apparatus.

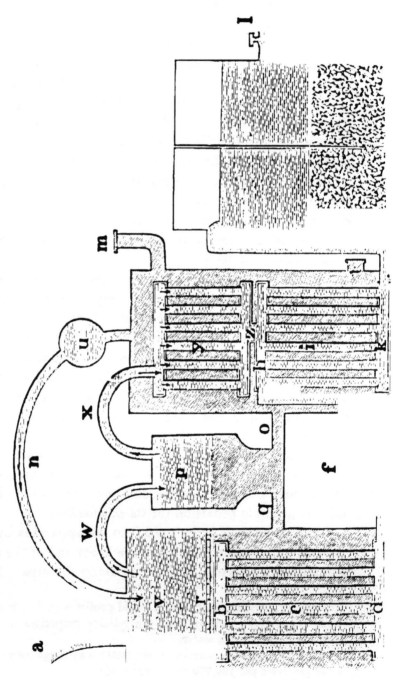

floor of the priming-box p, and is conducted by the pipe q into the evaporator A, which it fills up to the perforated plate r, an air-space remaining above that level being indicated externally by the gauge s. The waste sea water escapes by the pipe t.

4. The air contained in the sea water is driven off by the heat of the steam and hot water in the two first bundles of pipes; passes into the long air-pipe at u from the water in the condenser, and into the air-space v from the water in the evaporator, as well as from the water in the priming box to the air-space above it. The mixed vapour and air therefore passes in the direction of the arrows from the air-pipe n, furnished with a bulb to prevent priming into the air-space of the condenser. From the latter space it enters the priming-box by the pipe w, and from thence it traverses the pipe x to enter the cap of the upper sheaf of pipes, y, in the condenser, and then trickling down joins the condensed water in the lower sheaf of pipes by the short conduit, z, when the process of aëration is complete.

There are, of course, in the actual apparatus numerous cocks and appliances required for the efficient working of the whole, but these have been purposely omitted in the diagram so as to simplify it as much as possible.

(*Description of Plate XXVI.*)

FIG. 38.—A, The evaporator. B, The condenser. C, The filter. a, Steam-pipe entering b, a cap or chamber in communication with c, a sheaf of steam-pipes opening below into d, a receiver, with which the pipe e is connected. This leads to f, a steambox or trap. g, A pipe leading from f to h, a cap surmounting i, the lower sheaf of pipes of B. k, A receiver from which the distilled flows into filter C, and is drawn off by l, the water-cock, with which the hose leading to the tanks is connected. m, The feed-pipe for sea water to fill the condenser and the lower end of n, the air-pipe. o, A pipe for the passage of sea water to the floor of p, the priming-box, from which it is conducted by q, a pipe, to the evaporator A. r, A perforated plate for the passage of disengaged air. s, A gauge for the level of the sea water. t, The waste sea-water pipe. u, An expansion of the tube n, receiving the disengaged air from the water of the condenser. v, Air chamber of evaporator above the plate r. w, A pipe connecting v with p. x, A pipe connecting p with y, the upper sheaf of pipes in the condenser. z, A short conduit, by which the mixed vapours and air blend with the condensed steam in h, but still more perfectly in i and k.

L

It is important to observe that for every gallon of fresh water produced, about six gallons of sea water pass through the apparatus. Thus, though, as before mentioned, sea water contains two-thirds less oxygenated air than fresh, it follows that double the quantity of air capable of being taken up by fresh water is furnished to the pipes of the condenser. The air begins to be expelled from water at a temperature of 130° Fahr., and is quite dissipated at 212°. Recently distilled water, therefore, contains no air.

From $3\frac{1}{2}$ to 4 per cent. of salines, and much organic matter, render sea water unfit for domestic purposes, much less for drinking. Now, though the salts are left behind in the mother liquor, the organic matter is carried over in the process of distillation, having also undergone a certain change by previous contact with the heating surface. This change will be more perceptible in the flat and disagreeable taste of the water when the heat is intense, and, as a consequence, the process is more rapidly conducted. It has, moreover, been abundantly proved that re-distillation does not quite free the water from these subtle organic matters, so that the more effective process of filtration is now very generally adopted.

SECTION 4.—*Storage of Water, and Watering Ship.*

In former times water was stored in casks on board ship, and the evils connected with this system were both many and great. Of late years, however, casks have been superseded by iron tanks, with many resulting advantages.[1]

In a newly-commissioned ship the holds should be carefully swept out, and every strip or shaving of wood remaining in the limbers and lower openings between the floors and timbers removed, so that no particle susceptible of decomposition may be overlooked. The limber passages in particular should be searched with a rod to see that they are clear, so as

---

[1] Iron tanks appear to have been first brought into use about the year 1815, from which time their adoption became gradually more general.

to allow all water from leakages to find its way to the pump-well. As much moisture as possible should be taken up by hand, and the limbers dried as far as practicable. The hold and store room should next be carefully whitewashed, the whitewash being mixed in the proportion of 1 to 80 with carbolic acid. This done, the plan of the stowage of the hold supplied from the dockyard will point out how the ballast should be laid, as a foundation for the water tanks to rest upon. The pigs of ballast, so-called, are elongated square blocks of iron, having a hole at each end for the convenience of transporting them with chain hooks, and they vary in weight from 1 to 3 cwts. each. Upon this foundation the ground, or lower tier of tanks, is laid, and upon these, again, the riders, or tanks, of the upper tier are placed.

The tanks are sent down the main hatchway by a strop and toggle in the man-hole, and transported to their places by luff-tackles. As soon as they are placed *in situ*, the lids are screwed on, that no filth of any kind should enter them, and the space between the tanks is immediately filled up with battens and chintzed.

In stowing the tanks, when practicable, the corners with keyholes should come together for convenience in starting, and the lower keyhole should be clear to allow the water to run out freely.

By using iron stays for supporting the upper tier of tanks, the ground tier can be made available without disturbing the upper, which is a great improvement where space may be required for other purposes. Some tanks contain as much as 600 gallons of water; the smallest are supplied for oil, holding about 20 gallons.

A line-of-battle ship would take in between 200 and 300 tons of water, and a frigate about 180 tons. Therefore, when the trouble of obtaining the water in the first instance, and of pumping it into the ship, is taken into account, the importance of making a selection of wholesome water at the outset must be doubly apparent.

At all home ports and British stations abroad, as at Malta, Gibraltar, Bermuda, and Halifax, ships are supplied directly with water from tank vessels, which are brought alongside so that the water may be pumped into the ship by leather or canvas hose conveniently laid through one of the ports. In other cases, however, it may be necessary to take the water from rivers, streamlets, or springs opening near the beach, when it is either brought off in casks or baricoes and started into the tanks, or in the ships' boats themselves, for which purpose they must be thoroughly cleaned out beforehand. This is what is termed 'watering ship in bulk.' In some instances the water is received into a canvas lining accurately fitted to the boat, so as to form a clean collapsible reservoir, calculated to do away with many of the disagreeables associated with the reception of drinking-water into an open boat.

Section 5.—*Filtration.*

For many years back drip-stones and filters of various descriptions have been in use in the officers' messes on board ship, but it is only very recently that any provision of this kind has been attempted for the benefit of the ship's company at large. The excellent filters devised and patented by Major Crease, however, are now in general use in the service, and duly appreciated by the sailors.

The whole subject of filtration is one of great interest, and many particulars connected with it are even at present but imperfectly understood. Some very practical and important experiments with various filtering materials have lately been conducted in the laboratory of the Army Medical School, Netley, by Surgeon-Major J. Lane Notter, B.A., M.D., F.C.S., who obtained the following results, as published in the 'British Medical Journal' for October 12, 1878.

Filtration through finely-granulated animal charcoal.—The albuminoid ammonia is diminished 100 per cent., the whole being removed. The free ammonia is not increased (none in original). The organic oxygen is diminished 71 per cent., the volatile solids 33 per cent. One of these filters experimented on was a metallic one. The water was allowed to remain in it for three weeks, when it was examined and found to contain zinc in large quantity, evidently dislodged from the galvanised coating of the iron. The total solids were more than doubled. On testing for free and albuminoid ammonia, the following results were found:—

	Original water. Parts per 1,000,000	After filtration	After three weeks in filter
Free ammonia	Nil	Nil	1·3824
Albuminoid ammonia	0·2152	Nil	0·1440

The water had thus taken back from the charcoal about two-thirds of the albuminoid ammonia, and had also absorbed a large amount of free ammonia.

Filtration through a silicated carbon.—Treated in the same manner as the granular charcoal, the results were:—

	Original water. Parts per 1,000,000	After filtration. Parts per 1,000,000	After three weeks in filter. Parts per 1,000,000
Free ammonia	Nil	Nil	1·0800
Albuminoid ammonia	0·2152	0·2023	0·1420

The water had taken up a small quantity of free ammonia, but appears to have diminished its albuminoid by longer contact with the filtering media.

Spongy iron filter.—This, treated similarly, gives the following results:—

	Original water. Parts per 1,000,000	After filtration. Parts per 1,000,000	After three weeks in filter. Parts per 1,000,000
Free ammonia	Nil	Nil	Nil
Albuminoid ammonia	0·2152	0·0720	Nil

The water has taken up nothing from the filtering materials, but has got entirely rid of its albuminoid ammonia by prolonged exposure to the filtering medium.

A further series of experiments to test the keeping power of water passed through various filtering media. A sample was placed in a stoppered bottle and in a bottle unstoppered. After a considerable number of days had elapsed they were carefully examined. The original water contained very little sediment, and showed none on being kept.

1. *Granular charcoal filter.*—In both the stoppered and unstoppered bottles a reddish-yellow deposit showed itself, which, under the microscope, appeared to be granular, with numbers of moving particles—the sphærobacteria of Cöhn.

2. *Silicated carbon filter.*—No trace of sediment in stoppered bottle; a little in the open sample, containing a few micrococci and one or two infusoria.

3. *Spongy iron filter.*—There is no trace of sediment or organisms of any kind. With reference to spongy iron as a filtering medium, we found that its action on hard water was much more satisfactory than on soft waters. Iron is exceedingly soluble in soft water, and the action of the prepared sand in removing the iron is not nearly so effective as when hard waters were used, as these latter take up a smaller percentage of iron.

From the foregoing experiments we may, I think, adduce the following facts:—

I. Filtration through sand is simply mechanical for the most part, and not to be depended on as a purifier.

2. Water may be purified by animal charcoal to a large extent; that its action is extremely rapid on decomposing organic matters; that fresh organic matter passes through unchanged; and that water should on no account be stored after filtration, as this matter subsequently decomposes, giving rise to low organisms. It is advisable not to leave the water in contact with the animal charcoal for a lengthened period, as it again takes up impurities from the medium.

'3. That spongy iron is undoubtedly the *best* filtering material; its action is not so rapid as charcoal, but there is no danger in prolonging the contact with the water. As far as my experiments go, it is the only *safe* filtering medium we have at present. It appears to act on all organic matter, whether fresh or decomposed, whereas charcoal acts more as a dialyser when colloidal substances are fresh and in a state of extreme dilution, and are certain to decompose after filtration.

'One feature of filtering through charcoal must not be lost sight of—that charcoal becomes exhausted of its oxygen, and that foul gases held in solution by the water may replace it; its action is limited, and it requires constant attention.'

Though much has been said above in favour of spongy iron as a filtering medium, the *carferal* of Major Crease, R.M.A., which has been generally adopted in the naval service, is certainly its greatest rival, having a lasting-power equal almost to all other filtering materials.

Physical, Chemical, and Microscopical Examination of Water.

It is of great importance that the medical officer should be able to give a decisive answer as to the hygienic properties of any sample of water that may be submitted to him for judgment; and although he may not always be furnished with the means of making an exhaustive analysis, he may, with a very trifling addition to the usual apparatus supplied to him, obtain such qualitative results as shall afford him, in general, very valuable information.

1. *Physical Examination.*

The sample should be placed in a tall cylindrical glass vessel, if such is available, and inspected by holding it up to the light, and observing the nature of any suspended matter that may be present; and in particular, if any spontaneous movement is exhibited. Note the transparency, lustre, shade of colour, smell, or turbidity, if any. The transparency and colour are best observed by looking down through a considerable stratum on a white ground. A slight bluish tint augurs more favourably than yellow or brown, however faint.

There should be no odour, nor any peculiar taste in good water, though, from the experiments of Professor de Chaumont, it would appear that, with the exception of iron, a very considerable amount of any or all the dissolved solids usually occurring in water may exist without materially affecting the sense of taste. Sometimes the hardness of water may be estimated by rubbing it between the fingers.

2. *Chemical Examination.*

This subject can only be treated in a very general way in the present work. Indeed, qualitative results are all that will in general be needed; and if ever a more complete analysis is required, it will be easy to consult Parkes's 'Practical Hygiene,' which will afford all the information necessary for this purpose.

A stand of ordinary test tubes should be at hand, with the several re-agents specified in the following experiments.

First observe the reaction of the water to test-paper (litmus and turmeric) and then proceed as follows:—

(a) *Water Unconcentrated.*

For chlorine.—Acidulate with dilute nitric acid and add nitrate of silver solution.

Effect.—An opalescence passing on to a white precipitate, growing darker by the action of light.

Note.—In this case, as in the others following, the amount of the substance present will be indicated by the intensity of the precipitate, and a little experience will enable the operator to estimate it approximately.

For lime.—Add oxalate of ammonium.

Effect.—A white turbidity and precipitate of oxalate of lime.

For sulphuric acid.—Acidulate with dilute hydrochloric acid and add solution of barium chloride.

Effect.—A white turbidity or precipitate.

For free carbonic acid.—Lime water will give a white

precipitate of carbonate of lime, more or less evanescent in its character.

For ammonia.—Add Nessler's fluid.

Effect.—A yellow or amber tinted precipitate.

For nitrous acid.—Solution of iodide of potassium and starch, after the addition of a little dilute sulphuric acid, will strike a beautiful blue in the presence of nitrous acid. The value of this test depends upon the promptness of the reaction, for under any circumstances a blue colour will be developed in the lapse of time.

For nitric acid.—Mix two or three drachms of the water to be tested with the same quantity of brucine solution in a test tube, then add a little concentrated sulphuric acid, the tube being slightly inclined so as to allow the acid to pass to the bottom without mixing with the fluids.

Effect.—A beautiful pink ring, passing into yellow beneath, will be formed at the junction of the fluids with the acid. This appearance is evanescent, but by gently shaking the tube it will brighten up, and wane again for some little time.

For organic matter.—Take six or eight ounces of the water and boil it in a flask with a few drops of solution of chloride of gold for twenty minutes.

Effect.—If organic matter is present, the gold will be reduced with the development of a violet tint, passing to purple and an olivaceous hue when the contamination is large.

For alkaline sulphides.—The nitroprusside of sodium will develop a beautiful purple colour with the sulphides, though not with sulphuretted hydrogen.

For sulphuretted hydrogen.—The addition of a salt of lead to water impregnated with sulphuretted hydrogen throws down a black precipitate of the sulphide of lead, or if ammonia be added to the water, and the nitroprusside of sodium be employed, as in the last experiment, the characteristic purple colour will be produced.

For iron.—Ferrous salts are tested with the red prussiate

of potash, and ferric salts with the yellow. A mixture of the two will be most convenient for use.

Effect.—A deep green, passing to a more intense blue.

(b) *Water concentrated to One-third or more.*

For phosphoric acid.—Place some of the concentrated water in a test tube, add a little dilute nitric acid first, and then some solution of molybdate of ammonium. Boil for a minute or two in the flame of a spirit-lamp.

Effect.—A rich yellow colour, with a precipitate on standing.

For magnesia.—Add a little oxalate of ammonium to precipitate any lime that may be present. Filter into another test tube. With this should be mixed a few drops of phosphate of sodium, chloride of ammonium, and liquor ammoniæ, and the tube set aside for twenty-four hours to permit the formation of the triple phosphate, which usually assumes the feathery form, and may be examined under the microscope.

For silica.—A portion of the water should be evaporated to dryness, and the residue treated with strong hydrochloric acid and then washed with boiling distilled water and ignited. This process should be once more repeated, when only pure silica or silicate of aluminium will remain behind.

The more important indications afforded by the qualitative examination of water are the following:—

1. *Chlorine in excess.*

(a) This may indicate that the water is derived from strata containing chloride of sodium or calcium. Such water may be alkaline from the presence of carbonate of soda, and show little evidence of organic matter.

(b) It may arise from contamination with sea water, in which case there may also be much magnesia but little organic matter.

(c) Contamination with liquid excreta may be indicated if also ammonia, nitrous, and nitric acid, organic matter, and phosphoric acid are present in notable amount.

2. *Lime in large quantity.*

(a) If thrown down by boiling, is in the form of carbonate.
(b) If little affected by boiling, sulphate or chloride.

3. *Sulphuric Acid in excess.*

Is probably in combination with sodium when lime is in small amount, under which circumstances there may also be much chloride and carbonate of sodium present.

4. *Carbonic Acid large.*

As ground air is highly charged with carbonic acid, increasing with the depth, waters from deep sources are often strongly impregnated with it.

Bubbles of the gas may be seen adhering to the sides of the glass containing such water. So-called sparkling waters, though agreeable to the taste, may nevertheless be very impure.

5. *Ammonia large.*

(a) Without nitric or nitrous acid, probably of vegetable origin.
(b) With nitric and nitrous acids, of animal origin.

6. *Nitrous Acid.*

Without oxidisable matter, recent contamination.

7. *Nitric Acid.*

Without oxidisable matter, previous contamination.

8. *Phosphoric Acid in large amount.*

(a) From phosphatic strata (rare).
(b) Sewage impregnation very probable.

3. *Microscopical Examination.*

The microscopical examination of water may often supersede the necessity of anything more than the use of a few qualitative tests; but the subject is one requiring not only a competent knowledge of the lower forms of animal and vegetable life, but sufficient experience to discover the import of their presence after their identification.

We must not forget that living things as naturally abound in fresh and salt water as they do upon the surface of the earth immersed in the ocean of air; and consequently the mere discovery of living plants or animals in a sample of water could afford no necessary indication of its impurity. If, however, we study the natural history of the forms in question, we shall find that the conditions of their existence will vary so considerably as to inspire a hope that when we are better acquainted with them, we shall be able to draw more definite inferences on the whole. As to habitat, we find that some forms chiefly occur in lakes and ponds, some in streamlets, some in rivers, some in cisterns fed by river or rain-water, and others in wells. Some, again, rest in pure, but constantly changing water, while others are only found in stagnant water, or where organic matter is undergoing decomposition.

As a rule, it may be said that bright green algals, unicellular or filamentous, afford a much better indication than either dead or colourless forms, the latter being often parasitic, and flourishing more usually amidst death and decay.

When the suspended matters, and consequently the deposit, is large, there can be no difficulty in taking up a portion with a pipette for microscopical observation; but, if the water is lustrous and without apparent matters in suspension, it will be necessary to set aside a sufficiently large quantity in a tall glass for twenty-four or forty-eight hours, to permit the formation of a sediment, however small it may be.

An ordinary watch-glass, or a simple disc of glass resting on a loop of aluminium wire may be lowered to the bottom of the vessel, and again removed with the deposit for examination when a sufficient quantity of the clear water above it has been removed with a siphon. Or the clear water may be drawn off to within two or three ounces, which should be well shaken up and transferred to a conical glass for secondary subsidence and examination, as in the case of urinary deposits.

For further information the reader is referred to the author's work on this subject, published by Messrs. J. & A. Churchill.

Chemical Tests and Volumetric Solutions required for Hygienic Purposes.

A. *Ordinary Test Solutions.*

1 and 2. Sulphuric acid, strong and diluted
3 and 4. Nitric   „   „   „
5 and 6. Hydrochloric   „   „
} One part to ten.

7. Nitrate of silver, a strong solution.
8. Chloride of gold (for organic matter)
9. Brucine solution (for nitric acid)
} One gramme to the litre.
10. Phosphate of soda (for magnesia).
11. Oxalate of ammonium (for lime).
12. Mixed red and yellow prussiates of potash (for either ferrous or ferric salts of iron).
13. Molybdate of ammonium (for phosphoric acid).
14. Nitroprusside of sodium (for alkaline sulphides).
15. Chloride of barium (for sulphuric acid).
16. Acetate of lead (for sulphuretted hydrogen).
17. Ammonium, carbonate of (for recarbonating).
18. Ammonia, liquor of (for magnesia and other purposes.)

B. *Special Solutions.*

1. Iodide of potassium and starch (for nitrous acid).

Preparation: Iodide of potassium, 1 gramme; starch, 20

grammes; water, ½ litre. Make the iodide of potassium and the starch solution separately; filter the latter, and then mix the two together (for nitrous acid).

2. Alkaline permanganate (for albuminoid ammonia).

Preparation: 8 grammes of permanganate of potash and 200 grammes of solid caustic potash dissolved in 1 litre of water. The solution must be well boiled, to free it from all nitrogenous matters.

3. Nessler's solution (for ammonia).

Preparation: As directed by Professor Parkes, 'Practical Hygiene,' page 82.

C. *Standard Solutions.*

1. Permanganate of potassium. 0·395 grammes per litre, 1 c.c. of which = 0·10 milligrammes of oxygen.

„   „   oxidises 0·2875 milligrammes of nitrous acid.

2. Nitrate of silver. 17 grammes to the litre.

1 c.c. = 3·55 milligrammes of chlorine,

or 5·85 milligrammes of chloride of sodium.

3. Iodine. 6·35 grammes, with a little iodide of potassium to the litre (for sulphuretted hydrogen).

1 c.c. = 0·85 milligrammes of sulphuretted hydrogen. Multiplying the amount in a litre by the short factor 0·164 will give cubic inches per gallon.

4. Chloride of ammonium. 0·0315 grammes per litre. 1 c.c. = 0·01 milligramme of ammonia.

5. Soap solution. *Preparation*: Soft soap of the Pharmacopœia is mixed with spirit and water in equal parts. It must be so graduated by further solution that 2·2 c.c. will produce a beady lather lasting for five minutes in 50 c.c. of—

6. Barium nitrate solution. 0·26 grammes per litre.

7. Oxalic acid. Three solutions are employed, viz.:

1st. A strong solution = 6·3 grammes to the litre.

2nd. 100 c.c. of the strong solution mixed with 180 c.c. water.

3rd. 100 c.c. of the strong solution and 700 c.c. of water.

With the first the alkaline solution (8) is graduated, equal parts of each neutralising each other.

The second is used for determining the alkalinity of lime or baryta water, 1 c.c. = 1 milligramme of lime, or 2·73 of baryta.

The third is used for graduating the permanganate of potash solution, which will be decolorised by equal proportions of the acid solution in the presence of sulphuric acid.

8. Alkaline solution. Dilute the liquor sodæ or potassæ of the Pharmacopœia with 8 or 9 parts of water, and graduate with the strong oxalic solution.

1 c.c. of alkaline solution = 6·3 milligrammes of oxalic acid.

The above tests and solutions are in accordance with the system pursued in the 'Army Medical School'; but further detail in relation to their practical use in quantitative analysis would extend beyond the scope of the present work.

CHAPTER IV.

CLEANLINESS.

HAVING thus far considered the subject of water supply, can be no more befitting place for a section on personal cleanliness and the cleanliness of the ship respectively.

SECTION A.—*Personal Cleanliness.*

Sir Gilbert Blane quotes a passage from a letter of Erasmus to a physician in York, written over three hundred years ago, soon after his visit to England to show that the proverbially cleanly habits of the English are of more recent development. He noticed accumulations of filth in various places, and attributed the so-called plague, and especially the sweating sickness, of such frequent occurrence in England, to the almost total neglect of sanitary precautions or hygiene. But the Hollanders themselves being naturally a cleanly people, would be likely to pass rather a heavy censure upon any apparent neglect in this particular observable in others. Dr. Cullen, however, ascribes the low nervous fever (typhus) of Britain to an infection arising in the clothes and houses of the poor, who from sloth or indolence neglect to change their linen and ventilate their dwellings. It is only charitable, nevertheless, to remark that poverty, while it narrows the necessary means of attention to the person, carries with it an indisposition to use even those that are available in the estimation of others. How far this may be excusable or otherwise will, of course, depend upon the circumstances of the case. 'Nature has wisely so contrived our senses and instincts that the neglect of cleanliness renders a person loathsome and offensive to himself and others, thereby warning against those fatal diseases that arise from bodily filth.' Emanations from the human body imbuing the clothes too long in contact with it, and intensified by the products of respiration in crowded, close, and ill-ventilated localities, appear to be the specific source of jail, hospital, or ship fever, so-called. The often adduced case of the Black Assizes at the Old Bailey in 1750 proves that this cause is altogether independent of pre-existing fever, in which particular it differs from specific infection in its restricted sense. Without going to this extreme, however, inattention to personal cleanliness is the parent of evils which, although not so striking in their primary effect, yet are certain sooner or later to exert their prejudicial influence on the human constitution.

Every facility should be given the men for daily washing the body, and not to be satisfied with merely applying soap to the face, hands, and feet, which are ordinarily the only parts exposed, even to those who are responsible for the cleanliness of the division under their charge. Dr. Gihon, U.S.N., remarks that ninety per cent. of the men presenting themselves at the naval rendezvous are filthy in person, and ' every medical officer should refuse to examine them in such a condition.' He admits that ' some few men-of-war's men are exceptions, but the great majority of patients admitted into the naval hospitals, from before the mast, are shamefully unclean. Always the first, and sometimes the only prescription they require is a warm bath and a clean shift of clothing.' At the present day no difficulty can arise from lack of water, or the want of time or a suitable locality for ablution. Lord Dundonald's axiom was that ' anything can be done on board ship,' and it is astonishing what a cloud of obstacles break down with a simple word of command. In the morning watch, when the holystoning process is over, the head-pump would be brought into requisition with marine soap, and a canvas screen rigged in the top-gallant-forecastle, or round the manger, while a reasonable allowance of fresh water from the tanks, or even hot water, while under steam, would be furnished, and the 'service' so-called would be quite unconscious of the expenditure.

Before the year 1796 it is difficult to say how the seaman's ablutions were carried on. In that year, however, at the suggestion of Gilbert Blane, Lord St. Vincent, then Commander-in-Chief in the Mediterranean, made application to the Admiralty for the supply of soap, either gratuitously or by stoppage in the wages of the men, upon which better footing it has been ever since continued.

'If cleanliness, which may well be called physical chastity, is required by the laws of decency and health everywhere, on board ship it becomes a sacred duty which one owes to society under the penalty of endangering the health of oneself and others.'—(Fonssagrives.)

Section B.—*Cleanliness of the Ship—Humidity.*

Though fresh water is only used in cleaning paint-work, and for some few other purposes, the cleanliness of the ship itself, after that of the *personnel*, would naturally fall under consideration; and with this is inseparably connected the important question of humidity. *Ex aquâ oritur aër, ex aëre morbus.*

At a very early period, the evils arising from the permanent dampness or humidity of the air on board ship have been recognised by medical men; but, though warning voices have descended to us from the last century, those evils still continue to exist—happily, however, not to so great an extent as formerly. Having been found to be preventable, like many other things within the domain of hygiene, the drying up of all sources of moisture and cleansing the decks with as little water as possible, or by some other means, should be strictly attended to. The general flooding of the ship, which is, in some instances, supposed to be necessary every day in the week, should only take place at lengthened intervals, or when imperatively demanded.

The lieutenant of the morning watch usually superintends the washing of the decks in harbour. The watery operations commence about half-past four, or five o'clock A.M., and the main and quarter decks are generally finished a little before eight o'clock, or at breakfast time.

Cleaning the lower deck is performed in one of the three following ways, viz.: 1, By dry holystoning, *i.e.* using dry sand and rubbing it on the deck without water; 2, Washing the deck after the manner already described; and 3, By sprinkling and scrubbing, that is, watering the deck in a different way, either by throwing it out of a bucket with the hands, or applying it by means of wetted swabs to the whole surface of the deck. Afterwards dumb-scrapers are used, and when those implements cannot be applied, the seamen's knives are generally called into action for scraping the previously wetted tables and ladders, &c., and the second ablution is usually finished about half-past ten or eleven o'clock.

Thursdays and Sundays were the great cleaning days when sprinkling and scrubbing the lower deck were used so many times a week to do away with the name of washing decks.

It will appear from the foregoing statement that British seamen are in the habit of labouring in water at least three hours daily before breakfast, and nearly double that time (twice a week) in those ships where washing the lower deck is practised, and every morning after breakfast in other ships where sprinkling and scrubbing is deemed salutary (Finlayson).

The leading American writers on the subject of naval hygiene, namely Drs. Wilson Gihon and Hunter, have so thoroughly exposed the perniciousness of the system here detailed, that it would be merely repeating what they have already said, to enlarge much further upon it. The reader, however, might profitably peruse a little work by Dr. Finlayson,

R.N., 'On the Baneful Influence of so frequently Washing Decks,' published in 1823, and from which some of the above-mentioned particulars were derived, not because they were new or specially original, but because they were old, and in accordance with the writer's own experience, who cannot help also agreeing with Dr. Finlayson when he says that—
'No rule can be laid down for cleaning a ship's hold so good, as that it must be done as often as it becomes filthy; and it follows, as a consequence, that those ships which are most famed for having their lower deck washed, sooner acquire an accumulation of filth in their holds.' As a remedy for humidity, he suggests that 'any water that may have been accidentally spilt' on the lower deck 'should be carefully and speedily swabbed up, and afterwards dried by means of warm sand or sawdust, kept in a store in the galley for that purpose.' Further, as an interesting fact, the wet and dry thermometers are stated to have been recommended by Mr. Colebrook as a hygrometer indicating the amount of humidity in the atmosphere. Here it may be stated that the relative humidity of the air should range between 70 and 75, saturation being taken as 100, and this implies that the difference between the wet and the dry bulb should not be less than 3° or 4° Fahr. The range of comfort in the external temperature is between 58° and 68° Fahr. (Hunter).

SECTION C.—*Rendering the Deck Planking Impervious to Moisture to Facilitate Drying.*

While much may be said in reference to the baneful influence of too frequently washing or wetting the decks of a man-of-war, as commonly practised, it is certain that when large bodies of men are crowded together in a confined space— as, for instance, on the mess-deck of one of our Indian troopships—filth in a variety of forms is sure to accumulate rapidly and require expeditious removal. It is the absorbent power of the deck-planking which is the root of this evil; for even those who are scarcely able to suggest a remedy are obliged to admit that the cleansing of the decks is not more frequent than is actually required under the circumstances. Fleet-Surgeon Anderson, R.N., urges that the mess-decks, whether in troopships or men-of-war, should be tiled in cement on the planking at present in use; the decks could then be washed and dried in a very short space of time. In fact, the operation of cleaning decks would merely consist in sweeping off loose dust and refuse, wiping over the tiles with a wet swab or cloth, and then drying them up with a dry one. The vapour which is now constantly arising from wet and sodden planking would be obviated, and with it much of the present tendency to colds, lung disease, rheumatic affections, and other complaints of a serious nature.

The plan of tiling the washhouses, water-closets, bathrooms, and women and children's quarters might be first tried, and, if found to be satisfactory, it might be carried out on the mess-deck also.

Black and white glazed tiles, of from 6 to 8 inches square, would be very ornamental, and if crenated on the upper surface it would tend to prevent men from slipping when walking on them. It would be advisable to have a water-way, or shallow groove, all round the deck by the ship's side, so as to carry off the superfluous water used in washing, and any water that might be spilt during the day.

A deck of this description could be easily and expeditiously washed, and thoroughly dried, in the course of an hour or less; whereas troop and mess-decks, as they now are, seldom dry at all, even in fair weather, and never during damp weather or when the ports are closed. We might then dispense with those articles of ship furniture called 'bogies,' which are as inimical to health as they are dangerous to the safety of the ship; for although they help to dry portions of the decks, they, at the same time, consume and vitiate the air which the men have to breathe. One of the arguments adduced against the use of tiles for the above purpose is that they would feel cold to the men's feet. This, however, would only apply in very cold weather, and could then be obviated by laying a strip of cocoa-nut matting along the gangways fore and aft, while during warm weather, and in the tropics, the cool tiles would be rather an advantage than otherwise. These suggestions are not intended to include the gun or battery decks or the upper decks of ships.

Tiles have been in use in the 'Great Eastern,' in one of our turret ships, and on portions of the decks of H.M.S. 'Hecla'; so that some little experience must have been gained, as to their durability or otherwise, during the working of the decks at sea.

A layer of cement might be spread over an iron-plate deck, and fortified against the absorption of moisture by several applications of linseed oil, and subsequent coatings of silicated paint.

In the American navy, decks are sometimes lacquered, as it is termed; but while this will unquestionably repel moisture, the surface would appear to be slippery. Very little information is contained in the passing references made to it. Professor de Chaumont, F.R.S., suggests that a solution of silk in ammonio-sulphate of copper, or Scoffern's patent, might be tried with advantage. One of the purposes to which this preparation is applied by the patentee is to render ships' bottoms water-tight, and to this might be added also, to make the deck-planking of ships impervious to moisture.

The Admiralty instructions are clear enough in reference to cleanliness and dryness, however the law may be neglected, on the one hand, or too rigidly enforced on the other. Take, for example, Article 40 in the 'Instructions for Captains,' which runs thus:—

'As cleanliness, dryness, and pure air are essentially necessary to health, the captain is to use his utmost endeavours to obtain these comforts for the ship's company in as great a degree as possible. The ship is always to be pumped dry; the pump-well is frequently to be swabbed, and a fire let down to dry it (proper precautions being taken to guard against accidents). He is to take care that there is a free passage fore and aft for the water; and those places where, from the trim of the ship, there may be a lodgment, are to be baled out and dried. In steamships, especially, he is to take care that every possible means be taken to insure that the air may circulate freely, and that room be left for a man to get down upon the keelson to clear the limbers of all offensive matter that may accumulate. He is, as frequently as he may deem requisite, to examine, himself, the state of the holds and the lower parts of the ship, in company with the surgeon; and if he should not find them perfectly clean and free from obnoxious smells, he is to cause a thorough examination to be made, with a view to detect and remove whatever may be likely to engender disease.

'He is to cause an officer to inspect the holds and all parts of the ship below, every morning, and to report to him whether they are in a clean and well-ventilated state, or otherwise.

'The holds are to be whitewashed every six months, or oftener if necessary.

'In line-of-battle ships and frigates, if the weather should prevent the ports from being opened for a considerable time, fires are to be made in the stoves; and by means of them, and of wind-sails, the lower decks are to be kept as well ventilated as possible.

'He is to see that the men are properly clothed in the established uniform, according to the nature of the climate in which they may be serving; that their hair is properly cut, and clean; and that they are generally cleanly in their person and dress. They are never to be suffered to remain in wet clothes, or sleep in wet bedding, when it can possibly be avoided.

'The ship's company's bedding is to be aired once a week, when the weather will permit, each article being exposed separately to the air by being tied up in the rigging, or upon girt-lines. Twice in every year their blankets are to be washed with soap in warm water; and once a year the bed-tickings are to be washed, and the hair beaten and teased before it is replaced.'

CHAPTER V.

DIET.

SECTION 1.—*Historical Retrospect, and Present Scale of Diet.*

It has been already intimated that faulty ventilation, defective appetite, and a corresponding scale of diet, go together in the past history of our navy. It will be well, therefore, first to take a retrospective view of the systems of victualling in use up to the latter part of the last century, and then notice the several important changes that have been introduced, from time to time, towards the adoption of the present more liberal scale.

The weekly scheme of diet in use in 1720, and probably for many years previous to this, is given in the following table, the particulars of which were taken from a rare book, called the 'Mariner's Jewel,' quoted by Staff-Surgeon John M. Hunter, M.D., R.N., in an excellent paper on the subject of 'Naval Dietaries.' [1]

Besides this, each man was allowed a gallon of beer per diem, and oatmeal for burgoo when the store of dried fish was exhausted.

From each article in the table the purser deducted one-eighth as his allowance, to make up his salary; but, although his nominal pay was very small, his income was often very large. It was one of the complaints made by the men at the Nore, in the mutiny of 1797, that the sailor's pound was only 14 ounces.

[1] See *Health of the Navy*, for 1871 (Appendix).

Weekly Rations of the British Navy in 1720.

The nutritive value or composition of the articles is shown in the six latter columns of the table.

Species	Sun.	Mon.	Tu.	Wed.	Th.	Fr.	Sat.	Total	Alb., &c.	Starch	Fat	Salts	Nitrogen	Carbon
Biscuit	16	16	16	16	16	16	16	112	17·47	84·33	1·45	1·90	17·47	87·81
Salt beef	—	—	32	—	—	—	32	64	4·93	—	1·85	4·50	4·93	4·44
Salt pork	16	—	—	—	16	—	—	32	2·50	—	12·51	1·77	2·50	30·02
Peas	8	8	—	8	8	—	—	32	7·36	18·36	0·67	0·80	7·36	19·96
Dried fish	—	2	—	2	—	2	—	6	1·00	—	—	—	1·00	00·43
Butter	—	2	—	2	—	2	—	6	0·00	—	4·98	0·12	0·00	11·95
Cheese	—	4	—	4	—	4	—	12	3·40	—	3·73	0·54	3·40	8·95
Total dry food	40	32	48	32	40	24	48	264	36·66	102·69	25·19	9·63	36·66	163·56

This deduction reduced the weekly ration to the following proportions in ounces:—

        Albuminous principles . . . 32·09
        Starch . . . . . 89·85
        Fats . . . . . 22·04
        Salts . . . . . 8·42

'The following,' says Dr. Fletcher, R.N.,[1] writing in the year 1786, 'is the present scale of diet established for the use of British seamen, out of which the purser has his eighths:—

WEEKLY TABLE.

Days	1 lb.	½ pint	2 lbs.	Pint	2 oz.	4 oz.	Remarks
Sun.	Pork	Pease	—	—	—	—	They have also a lb. of biscuit every day and a gallon of small beer, or 1 pint of wine in warm countries, or ½ pint of spirits diluted.
Mon.	—	—	—	Oatmeal	Butter	Cheese	
Tu.	—	—	Beef	—	—	—	
Wed.	—	Pease	—	Oatmeal	Butter	Cheese	
Th.	Pork	Pease	—	—	—	—	
Fr.	—	Pease	—	Oatmeal	Butter	Cheese	
Sat.	—	—	Beef	—	—	—	

The simplest way to describe the table is to group the quantities of each article issued during the period of a week from Sunday to Saturday inclusive. Thus on Sunday and Thursday one pound of pork was served out to each individual; on Tuesdays and Saturdays, two pounds of beef; on Sunday, Wednesday, Thursday, and Friday, half pint of pease; and on Monday, Wednesday, and Friday, one pint of oatmeal, two ounces of butter, and four ounces of cheese. Or to put the quantities together, for seven days the whole amount of meat was six pounds; of pease, two pints; of oatmeal, three pints; of butter, six ounces; and of cheese, twelve ounces. But, to these must be added, one pound of biscuit daily, and

---

[1] A very intelligent naval surgeon, who wrote his own experience of naval hygienic matters about the time the celebrated Captain Cook was performing his circumnavigatory exploits.

one gallon of beer, one pint of wine, or half-a-pint of spirits diluted. Wheat was sometimes given in lieu of oatmeal. Flour, suet, and plums, instead of beef, oil instead of butter, and sugar in lieu of oil.

In commenting upon this scheme of diet, Dr. Fletcher says:—' They have a saying in Cornwall that, were it not for the peas and oatmeal, they wonder what would become of the pigs and sailors. So here we find pigs and sailors classed together as one species, whose food ought to be the same, of course, and it is, perhaps, from this idea that they have no more compassion for a sailor, when he happens to be wrecked upon their coast, than they would have upon a pig; at least, it was so formerly. But I beg here to ask whoever casts his eye over the above scheme of diet, and weighs it in the balance of justice and philosophy, whether it would not be found wanting? Whether the framers of it had not merely the same ideas of seamen as those of Cornwall?

'Oil! Oil instead of butter; what a palatable mess where such oil is an ingredient! The Russians, indeed, who refit in our ports, have often been seen dipping their coarse bread in the train oil used by the caulkers and eating it. Here, then, the Russian diet must have been at a very low ebb, and accordingly, we find that their fleets have been very unhealthy. Haslar Hospital has been filled with their infectious sick (400 at a time).'

Having descanted further upon the merits of the table, he contrasts the superior diet of an officer with that of a foremast man, mentioning the case of the Hon. Captain Ruthven, a man of perfect humanity, who, sensible of this matter, assigned, as a principal reason for his meat being carried aft in covered dishes, that he should not hurt the feelings of a foremast man viewing the diet of an officer. He would, of course, contrast his own with it; and if dejection of spirits or despondency be the first symptom of scurvy, perhaps that symptom will often be found to originate in this very idea. Dr. Fletcher then draws up a scheme of his own for the more effectual preservation of the health of seamen, of which the Table following is a copy. He makes no alteration in the issue of beef, pork, and cheese, but reduces the allowance of pease to one-half and expunges the oatmeal altogether. The butter is increased from six to ten ounces weekly, while the further additions to the table are four ounces of rice, four ounces of portable soup, and half-a-pound of sour-crout, each served twice a week with half-a-pound of flour, of suet, and of plums on Wednesday for a pudding.

TABLE FOR DINNER.

Days	Beef	Pork	Rice	Portable soup	Flour, suet, and plums	Butter	Cheese	Sour crout	Pease
Sun.	—	1 lb.	4 oz.	—	—	2 oz.	—	—	—
Mon.	—	—	—	4 oz.	—	2 oz.	4 oz.	—	½ pint
Tu.	2 lbs.	—	—	—	—	—	—	½ lb.	—
Wed.	—	—	—	—	{ ½ lb. of each }	2 oz.	4 oz.	—	—
Th.	—	1 lb.	4 oz.	—	—	2 oz.	—	—	—
Fr.	—	—	—	4 oz.	—	2 oz.	4 oz.	—	½ pint
Sat.	2 lbs.	—	—	—	—	—	—	½ lb.	—

'They are to have a sufficient quantity of spice powder with their rice, celery, thyme, and onions, or eschalots with their pease, and mustard and vinegar to be given liberally with their beef.'

Breakfast.

'Bread, one pound; butter, two ounces (as marked in the scale); tea, one pint; and sugar, two ounces. This for breakfast every day in the week except the beef days, Tuesday and Saturday; on which days I would have them get a breakfast of sowens, with small or spruce beer and sugar, or a gill of wine, with water and sugar, in countries where wine is served.

'They should likewise be served their daily allowance of

beer, wine, or grog as usual.' Seeing that this allowance was already injuriously large, it is rather extraordinary to find a medical man recommending any further addition of beer or wine as a matter of diet.

Dr. Fletcher dwells much upon the merits of tea and coffee, stating that 'the admiral, the captain, and other commissioned officers, the midshipmen and mates, and even the boatswain, gunner, and carpenter's mates, together with the quartermasters, all make use of tea. Yet, I appeal, from the robust appearance of these, most of them at the same time keeping watch and doing as arduous duty as the foremast man, and the health they enjoy out of all proportion superior to the others, whether tea can be supposed to injure them? whether it is not rather a service to them? Is the reigning disorder scurvy, these people either escape it, or are but slightly affected by it. Is the disease fever, or flux, the same may be said, and those of the foremast men who are provident, and possessed of a little stock of tea and sugar, are more healthy than others, as I have always observed.'

In the year 1797 the victualling of the Navy experienced a most salutary change, in connection with which the health of seamen improved very strikingly. Scurvy, typhoid fever, dysentery, and ulcer, which up to this period had produced great havoc, became comparatively rare in occurrence and light in impression. Some ships in particular circumstances suffered from one or more of those diseases, but the sweeping epidemics of former years, which often rendered individual ships and sometimes entire fleets totally ineffective, became unknown. Amongst the hygienic improvements introduced since the year 1797 may be mentioned the supply of cocoa in lieu of gruel (burgoo) for breakfast, issuing salt meat at a much earlier period after being cured, the selection of much better articles, and the substitution of tea for the afternoon allowance of spirits.

'The victualling of the Navy,' says Dr. Wilson,[1] 'is as

[1] *Health of the Navy*, for 1830–1836, Part I.

nearly uniform throughout the service as circumstances will permit. At sea it is almost entirely so; in harbour it varies more or less, according to the supplies of fresh provisions procurable in different places.' He thus alludes to a system of victualling which had been in operation since the year 1825, when further salutary changes were made, and the following conditions established in relation to the issue of provisions :—

'There shall be allowed to every person serving in His Majesty's ships the following daily quantities of provisions, viz. :—

Bread, 1 lb. Fresh meat, 1 lb.
Beer, 1 gal. Vegetables, ½ lb.
Cocoa, 1 oz. Tea, ¼ oz.
Sugar, 1½ oz.

'When fresh meat and vegetables are not issued there shall be allowed, in lieu thereof :—

Salt beef, ¾ lb. Salt pork, ¾ lb.
Flour, ¾ lb. Peas, ½ pint

and weekly, whether fresh or salt meat is issued, a quantity of oatmeal and vinegar not exceeding half-a-pint each for occasional use when required, but not to be considered as subject to be paid for when not used.

'On the days in which flour is ordered to be issued, suet and raisins or currants may be substituted for a portion of the flour.

1 lb. of raisins,
½ lb. of currants, or
¼ lb. of suet

being considered equivalent to 1 lb. of flour.' In case of substitution being necessary in regard to other articles a list of equivalent quantities was given, but the more frequent was that of spirits for wine or beer, and of tea and coffee for cocoa or chocolate.

Beer was supplied on the home station only while ships were in harbour, or during a short period after leaving the port, as it could not be conveniently stowed or kept for any length of time at sea. Wine and spirits mixed with water were consequently more frequently used. Before the year 1740 spirits were taken neat, or in the undiluted state. At that period, however, Admiral Vernon issued a most salutary order that they should be mixed with water, and the mixture has ever since borne the name of 'grog,' facetiously derived from 'Grogram' (apparently a kind of camlet) of which material the Admiral's boat-cloak was made. Wine was occasionally supplied, but spirits (generally rum) were gradually gaining the pre-eminence, until the year 1831, when the ration of beer was superseded altogether, and wine in lieu of spirits was finally only issued on the Cape station.

Previously to 1825 half-a-pint of spirits was allowed to every person above the rating of boy. At that date, however, a judicious change was effected by the reduction of the spirit ration to a quarter of a pint daily, and the allowance of tea and coffee instead. The practice formerly was to divide the half-pint of spirits into two equal parts, one of which was issued at dinner-time, and the other in the afternoon. When the change was first made, it was apprehended by some that the seamen, if they did not resist, would be greatly dissatisfied with it. It was, however, introduced without disturbance or general complaint, and, as might be expected, acted very beneficially, for it is unnecessary to state that one of the most fruitful sources of disease and insubordination is the immoderate use of spirituous liquors.

To give a lad of eighteen a half-pint of spirits daily, with the precepts and example of his seniors, was tantamount to teaching drunkenness; for if he abstained from the allowance of grog he was ridiculed as a milksop, but was praised for his manly and seamanlike qualifications if he drank it with avidity. The quantity allowed produced unhealthy excitement, if not intoxication, under the influence of which he neglected duty or committed acts of insubordination entailing punishment, followed sometimes by repentance and amendment, but, often by further indulgence, procuring spirits beyond his allowance by every means in his power, becoming reckless and a confirmed drunkard, and finally a pest and a burden to the service (Wilson).

The spirit ration was still further reduced in 1850, the quarter of a pint of rum formerly divided into two parts or half gills, one of which was taken at dinner-time, and the other in the afternoon. The effect of this was that every evening, in nearly every ship, the cook of each mess was found to be more or less under the influence of liquor, and at the evening exercise accidents from aloft were common enough. At the period mentioned, however, the evening grog was done away with, and the scale of diet ran thus:—Biscuit, 1 lb.; fresh meat, 1 lb.; vegetables, 1 lb.; spirits, $\frac{1}{2}$ gill; tea, $\frac{1}{4}$ oz.; chocolate, 1 oz.; sugar, $1\frac{1}{4}$ oz. daily. Oatmeal, $\frac{1}{4}$ pint; mustard, $\frac{1}{2}$ oz.; pepper, $\frac{1}{4}$ oz.; vinegar, $\frac{1}{4}$ pint weekly. When fresh meat cannot be procured, there shall be substituted salt pork, 1 lb.; pease, $\frac{1}{2}$ pint every alternate day; and salt beef, 1 lb., with flour, $\frac{3}{4}$ lb.; or preserved meat $\frac{3}{4}$ lb., and preserved potatoes or rice $\frac{1}{4}$ lb. on every alternate non-salt-pork day. Suet and raisins issued as before.

In 1856 the ration of pease was reduced to $\frac{1}{3}$ pint split pease being issued instead of whole pease as heretofore. In 1859 the daily allowance of biscuit was increased to $1\frac{1}{4}$ lb., and sugar to 2 ozs., and an extra occasional issue of an ounce of cocoa and $\frac{1}{2}$ oz. of sugar was provided for.

In 1865 preserved meat of superior quality was introduced, and the scale of diet at present in use was adopted by Admiralty Circular in 1867, ordering the issue of $\frac{3}{4}$ lb. of preserved meat to alternate with the salt beef every third day, with preserved potatoes or rice. In harbour salt meat is issued twice a week, viz., salt pork on Monday and salt beef on Thursday; while at sea, 9 ozs. of boiled beef are substituted for salt beef, as above stated, on every alternate third day, with 4 ozs. of preserved potato, or 2 of 3 ozs. of oatmeal are allowed weekly for thickening th soup, and after 9 days at sea ½ oz. of lime-juice with sugar daily.

The scale of victualling now in use in Her Majesty' is shown in the following Table (see Appendix xxvi m, Part I., Queen's Regulations, &c.) :—

1. Daily Issue.

		Nitrogen	Carbo
Biscuit	1¼ lb.	214·0 grs.	360·0
or Soft bread	1½ lb.	110·0 grs.	238·0
Spirit	⅛ pint	—	—
Sugar	2 oz.	—	374·0
Chocolate	1 oz.	—	—
Tea	¼ oz.	—	—

2. Weekly Issue.

		Nitrogen	Carbo
Oatmeal	3 oz.	26·1 grs.	516·0
Mustard	½ oz.	—	—
Pepper	¼ oz.	—	—
Vinegar	¼ pint	—	—

3. Issued Daily when Procurable.

		Nitrogen	Carbon
Fresh meat	1 lb.	304·0 grs.	1883·2
Vegetables	½ lb.	3·5 grs.	144·0

4. Issued when Fresh Provisions cannot be Procured.

A.—*Every other day.*

		Nitrogen	Carbon
Salt pork	1 lb.	288·0 grs.	1360·0
Split pease	⅓ lb.	799·5 grs.	858·1
Celery seed	½ oz. to every 8 lbs. split pease put into t coppers.		

B.—*On one alternate day.*

		Nitrogen	Carbon
Salt beef	. 1 lb.	. 326·4 grs.	. 1115·2 grs.
Flour	. 9 oz.	. 68·4 grs.	. 1521·0 grs.
Suet	. ¾ oz.	—	—
Raisins	. 1½ oz.	—	—

C.—*On the other alternate day.*

		Nitrogen	Carbon
Preserved meat with either	. ¾ lb.	. 331·2 grs.	. 185·4 grs.
Preserved potato *or*	. 4 oz.	. 6·0 grs.	. 4·0 grs.
Rice *or*	. 4 oz.	. 20·0 grs.	. 3·2 grs.
Preserved potato *and*	. 2 oz.	. 3·0 grs.	. 2·0 grs.
Rice *or*	. 2 oz.	. 10·0 grs.	. 1·6 grs.
Flour	. 9 oz.	. 68·4 grs	. 1521·0 grs.
Suet	. ¾ oz.	—	—
Raisins	. 1½ oz.	—	—

SECTION 2.—*Source and Mode of Preparation of some of the more Important Articles issued.*

1. *Lime-juice.*—The produce of the West Indies, obtained under contract. Average specific gravity, 1036. Percentage of citric acid, about 9 per cent. It is fortified before issue to the navy with 10 per cent. of rum, 40 per cent. over proof.

2. *Cocoa.*—Obtained under contract, principally from Trinidad, Grenada, and Guayaquil. The beans are roasted at a high temperature, and, after being crushed and shelled, are ground and mixed with a percentage of sugar, the process of grinding being repeated twice.

3. *Soluble Chocolate* is prepared in the same way, but has a proportion of sago-flour mixed with it, to render its preparation for use more easy. The husk being removed carefully before the bean is ground, there is nothing irritating or deleterious in the chocolate produced.

4. *Flour.*—The wheat is first kiln-dried, and subsequently

ground in steam flour-mills, producing about 82 per cent. of flour, 16 per cent. of offal, and 2 per cent. loss.

5. *Biscuit.*—Manufactured from a meal consisting of flour and middlings made from raw wheat. The dough is mixed, rolled, and kneaded, and biscuits stamped and cut by steam machinery, and after being baked, the biscuits are removed to drying lofts, where they are deprived of nearly all their moisture previous to being placed in store ready for issue.

6. *Ship's Beef.*—The beef is cut into 8-lb. pieces, rubbed with white salt, and stowed in a bin, with white salt also occasionally thrown between the layers. It remains there four days, when it is shifted into another bin, so that the meat at the top of the first bin shall be at the bottom of the second. The brine which runs from the bins is boiled and mixed with pickle; to the extent of one-half is thrown over the beef again at least twice a day, the top pieces each time being covered with white salt. The meat remains four days in the second bin, after which it is carefully packed in casks with bay-salt and saltpetre, mixed together and distributed between the layers of the meat as it is packed. The several casks are properly marked, and filled up with proof pickle. American corned beef of excellent quality is now also in general use.

7. *Pork* is not cured by the Government, but obtained under contract from Ireland, and also from the Continent. The large amount of fat in pork serves to preserve its nutritive value longer than is usually the case with beef by keeping. No change, therefore, appears to have been necessary in respect to it. Only that every precaution is taken to have both issued sooner after the curing process has been completed than was formerly practicable.

8. *Rum.*—Ship's rum is received from the West Indies as imported, subsequently vaulted, and before issue it is reduced to navy strength, viz., 4·5 under proof.

9. *Vinegar.*—Malt vinegar is obtained under contract, containing from $4\frac{1}{2}$ to 5 per cent. of acetic acid.

Section 3.—*Adaptation of Diet to Climate.*

Though much has been said, from time to time, as to the necessity of establishing a change in the scheme of diet to suit tropical, subtropical, and temperate climates, but little has been practically effected in relation to it. In some instances great stress has been laid on suggestions of comparatively little importance, while existing institutions are perhaps too heavily censured. Sufficient attention has not been paid to the difference usually existing between the nominal and actual value, at least, of some of the rations.

In commenting upon the assumed necessity for three scales of diet, Mr. H. Leach says: 'We take it that two scales would fulfil any ordinary requirements, and that in framing them the following rules should be adhered to—1. To give salt meat not oftener than three times a week in cold and temperate, and twice a week in tropical latitudes; 2. To give soup and bouilli in lieu of solid meat in tropical latitudes; 3. To give no grog in the tropics; 4. To make the water supply practically unlimited, or at all events not less than a gallon a day. We have been told by some authorities that sailors will not eat preserved provisions, and that shipowners are compelled to adhere to the old scales, even though they are, in many cases, more costly than those which contain a varied diet. But the argument,' he thinks, 'is not supported by facts.'

There is, however, but too good reason to believe that Jack is averse to any innovation, however salutary it may be, from the chronic feeling or apprehension he has of being 'done,' so that he would rather have his beef and pork to the end of the chapter, than vary his diet with the best mutton that ever was cooked, if it were once known to be a halfpenny a pound cheaper to the Government.

There is a singular disparity between the weekly meat ration of the man-of-war's man and that of the merchant

seaman; thus, in the former case, we have 6 lbs.
against 9 lbs. 12 ounces in the latter, the difference
3 lbs. 4 ounces per week in favour of the merchant sea
Here, though little attention has apparently been paid
we have range enough for the ingenious to devise
schemes of diet.

SECTION 4.—*The Nutritive Value of Food.*

It is all important in a theoretical way to determine
actual quantity and character of the waste taking plac
the human system, in ordinary daily work for example;
to calculate the amount of the different kinds of food requ
to supply that waste; but we must take into account
there is not only a difference in the digestibility of
article as compared with another, but also in the diges
powers of different individuals. Taking the case of rice,
instance, 4 ounces will contain: albuminates, ·25; fats,
carbohydrates, 3·18; salts, ·02; but, if it is desirable t
this specific amount of constituents should be assimila
the gross amount of the rice itself must be considera
increased. Rice is admitted to be so easy of digestion t
it is supposed to leave the stomach in a single hour; but
large amount of it that passes away without yielding one-h
of its nutritive constituents, must be apparent to all w
have had any experience in India or China, or any coun
in which it is largely consumed. The benignity, so to spe
of the grains, would seem to put the pylorus off its guard, a
so obtain a passport for them even before they are complet
digested. It is certain, however, that although there m
be some percentage of loss in this way, the addition of a f
ounces of rice to the daily allowance of persons living alm
exclusively on this article of diet, will very soon manifest
effect in the greater plumpness of their face and figure.
good diet must, therefore, not only contain all the cons
tuents required for the repair of the body, but these cons

tuents must be in good relative proportion,[1] and in proper quantity.

It is customary now to estimate the different kinds of food in ordinary use as the supporters of potential energy, rather than solely as flesh-formers or heat-producers, in accordance with the views of Liebig. The bare maintenance of the internal work of the body, the supply of the waste of the frame which is constantly going forward, even during rest, the increased amount of waste occurring in moderate exercise, in an ordinary day's work, and in hard labour, have all been considered in reference to the food required in each case for the production of force.

Professor De Chaumont, F.R.S., has taken the mean of Moleschott's and Pettenkofer's estimation of the albuminates, fats, carbohydrates, and salts, demanded for the ordinary daily work of an adult (equivalent to from 250 to 300 foot-tons per diem), which is made up by additions to the diet of rest as shown in the annexed Table.

	Diet for Ordinary Work. oz.	Diet of Rest. oz.	Difference. oz.
Albuminates	4·70	2·50	2·20
Fats	3·54	1·00	2·54
Carbohydrates	13·40	12·00	1·40
Salts	1·06	0·50	0·56
Totals	22·70	16·00	6·66

Potential Energy of the Above in Foot-Tons.

Albuminates	816·80	435·00	382·80
Fats	1338·12	378·00	960·12
Carbohydrates	1795·60	1608·00	187·60
Totals	3952·42	2421·00	1530·52

Looking upon the first column here as a standard, the naval dietary may be compared with it:—

[1] Viz.—Albuminates, 1; Fats, 6; Carbohydrates, 3.

	Standard.	Naval Dietary.	Dr
	oz.		
Albuminates	4·70	5·51	
Fats	3·54	5·47	
Carbohydrates	13·40	21·39	
Salts	1·06	1·30	
Totals	22·70	33·67	1

Potential Energy of the Above in Foot-Tons.

Albuminates	817·80	958·74	14(
Fats	1308·12	2117·66	72!
Carbohydrates	1795·60	2852·86	105?
Totals	3921·52	5929·26	192?

The difference is all in favour of the naval dietary; fats are considerably higher, but the chief excess occ the carbohydrates. Even the naval dietary of 1720, gi page 170, contained—

Albuminates . . 5·24 = 911·76 ⎫
Fats . . . . 3·60 = 1360·80 ⎬ 4238·34 foot-t(
Carbohydrates . . 14·67 = 1965·78 ⎭
and salts . . 1·30

Section 5.—*Inspection of the more important Article the Seaman's Diet.*

1. *Biscuit.*—Ship's biscuits are hexagonal in form, to o] the waste that would occur by cutting the dough into c The baking should be so conducted as to give them a un dingy yellowish white, without any obvious browning or ing. When the gluten is in large amount, or unequall! tributed, and the baking long continued, though gentl(biscuit is flinty, so called, and must be kept a long tir the mouth before it can be properly masticated. On the hand, when biscuit is too friable, great waste is inevitabl

Captain Cook had his biscuit packed in casks, and it kept in excellent condition; indeed, there appears to been no complaint made in relation to it. Biscuit stowed in bags is too much exposed to the invasion of insects. These are more commonly the Weevil (*Calandra granaria*) and other small coleoptera, as the genus *Ptinus*, distinguished from the weevils by their lighter colour and having no curved proboscis. The larva of *Ephestia elutella*, or the 'Chocolate moth,' often renders large quantities of biscuit unfit for use. This insect is found to migrate from the cocoa stores to the biscuit. Professor Huxley makes the following suggestions in relation to it. 1. To have no cocoa stored in any place in which biscuits are manufactured. 2. To head up all biscuit puncheons as soon as they are full of the freshly baked biscuit. 3. Coat puncheons with tar after they are headed up, or at least work lime-wash well into all the joints and crevices. 4. Line the bread-rooms of ships with tin, so that if the *ephestia* has got into a puncheon it may not get into the rest of the ship. 5. If other means fail, expose woodwork of puncheons to a heat of 200° F. for two hours.

The usual method resorted to on board ship to free biscuit from weevils is to spread it on a tarpaulin or oil-cloth in the sun, when the insects will be seen to creep out from their concealment in large numbers; and the sound biscuit is hand-picked and returned into store. An 'old sailor,' so called, almost intuitively taps his biscuit on the table to dislodge any weevils that may be present.

Microscopical Examination.—Several small particles selected from different parts of the biscuit, moistened and spread thinly on a glass slide, may be examined under the microscope, to see if any impurity or adulteration with other starches can be detected. The wheaten starch grains usually retain their characters sufficiently well to be distinctly recognised as such. Fungi are readily distinguished by their branched mycelium. Mineral grit often occurs in large amount in foreign biscuit, from the rude methods adopted both in the removal of the chaff and grinding of the grain.

2. *Soft Bread.*—The crust and crumb of good bread should

be in the proportion of 3 to 7 respectively, the baking even and general, without burning. Much bran, or the addition of pea and bean flour, will give it a brownish colour; otherwise the bread should be white. It is commonly believed that alum is added to bread to whiten it, but this is not the fact. It has really a different effect, and is rather employed to assist the manipulation of mouldy flour. Acidity to a marked extent indicates bad flour, or the use of leaven. More than 45 per cent. of water is not allowable; such bread is liable to spoil and become mouldy.

The *chemical examination* of bread, in ordinary, need only be confined to the following particulars, viz.: 1. the determination of the *percentage of moisture* by drying a weighed portion of crumb, and then weighing it again. 2. *The amount of acidity*, by making an infusion of a weighed portion of the bread, and testing with a standard alkaline solution, as in the case of lime-juice (which see). 3. *The addition of alum*, by soaking a sample of the bread in cold distilled water, filtering well, and testing for sulphuric acid with hydrochloric acid and chloride of barium, as in the case of drinking-water. Unless the white precipitate is large, there will be no need of conducting the examination further. Sulphates may exist in the salt as in the water used in making the bread, as well as in the grain itself.

Microscopical Examination.—The starch grains of wheaten flour in bread suffer rather more change than they do in the manufacture of biscuit. By the dough-making and baking the grains are enlarged, doubled up, and more or less distorted, and lose much of their refracting property. The smaller ones exhibit an angularity resembling detached grains of rice-starch.

Stringy gluten from the walls of the air-cells may be seen entangling the structural elements of the wheaten grain as they occur in the flour.

Wheaten Flour.—Flour should be of a uniform whitish tint to the eye and almost impalpable to the touch. A portion taken between the fingers should have sufficient cohesion to be retained in great part when thrown with some force against a wall. Should any mineral matters be mixed with it, they will fall to the bottom, when a sample is shaken up with chloroform. There should be no apparent acidity in good flour, and it will readily permit of being worked up into dough. The gluten may be estimated by gradually mixing a weighed portion of the flour with water, giving time for the gluten to set or become plastic, and then working it with a glass rod and more water, to wash out all the starch. The gluten thus obtained should be dried and weighed, or, taken as moist gluten, one-third of its weight may be assumed to be the amount of dry gluten (from 8 to 10 per cent.). If the process is carefully conducted, all the starch so separated may be collected, dried, and weighed to determine its percentage.

Flour may contain from 10 to 18 per cent. of water. Weigh a small quantity and spread it out in a watch-glass or small dish, and dry at a temperature not exceeding 200° F.; the difference in weight will give the percentage of moisture.

Microscopical Character of the Cereal and other Starch Grains in relation to Wheaten Flour.

To form a right judgment as to the purity or adulteration of wheaten flour, by means of the microscope, implies at least a knowledge of the characters of all the other cereals also. For, without this, the determination of the particular nature or amount of any admixture or adulteration with other grains would be quite impossible. By way of introduction to this subject, the following particulars should be borne in mind:—

1. A grain of wheat or barley, for example, is not a simple seed, as many suppose; but, botanically speaking, a one-celled, one-seeded fruit, the seed being adherent to the pericarp

throughout, and thus constituting what has been named a *caryopsis*.

2. Just as the typical leaf, which by metamorphosis is converted into the pericarp of a fruit (say the *caryopsis*), presents an upper and an under surface, and an intervening substance, so, in the envelope of the cereal grain, we find, 1st, an outer coat, or epicarp; 2nd, a middle coat, or mesocarp; and, 3rd, an inner coat, or endocarp. This latter corresponds with the upper layer of the leaf, which is folded upon itself longitudinally, the infolded margins constituting the characteristic hilum. A fourth coat is usually described in the wheat grain, but this should be regarded as the testa of the seed, and is quite characteristic.

Intimate Structure of Wheat.—1. *The outer coat* consists of elongated cells disposed longitudinally and interspersed with smooth, sharp-pointed hairs, which become more closely set at the summit of the fruit. A thin and interrupted deposit of sclerogen on the walls of the cells gives them a delicately beaded outline. 2. *The midde coat* is made up of much shorter cells, arranged transversely and in columnar series, with the beaded outline more sharply defined than in the cells of the outer coat. 3. *The inner coat* is minutely laminated, corneous, and transparent, recognised more frequently when its broken border may happen to project beyond the outer coats. It is always, however, well seen in vertical sections, which will also show its intimate connection with the fourth coat, or the testa of the seed. Very delicate markings upon its surface would indicate a compressed cell-structure, quite distinct from the impressions made upon it by the cells of the middle coat. 4. The cells of the fourth coat form a beautiful single or double gravement; the walls are much thickened by deposit and highly refracting, contrasting remarkably with their dark granular contents (gluten and salts). Within this coat the cells gradually increase in size, while their walls become thinner, more like simple cellulose. It is within these cells the true starch granules are developed.

With certain differences that will be recognised by a little comparative study, the above description will be applicable to the other cereals, and when thoroughly understood the particular structures will be readily distinguished even when minutely broken up in the flour.

To economise space, the characters of the more ordinary starch-grains in use are given in the following Table, to which reference may be made. It will be seen that, as the starch-grains are always found within the cells, their form and appearance will much depend upon the conditions under which they are developed. If they remain separate and distinct, and free to move, the surface will be smooth and unbroken; but if they tend to unite in little glomeruli and still free to move, the compound grains will be either rounded as a whole, with all the granules facetted (oats), or mulberry-like, *i. e.* facetted within, but smooth and rounded when they project from the surface (Rio arrow-root).

In other cases the cellulose is accurately filled in, and the granules are tightly packed together, so that they will naturally break up into angular or irregular masses (maize and rice).

CLASSIFICATION OF STARCHES.

I. *Grains all smooth.*

General form	Hilum	Special characters	Name
Oval	At the small end	Continuous rings including less than half the grain	Tous les mois (Canna arrow-root)
		Continuous rings including more than half the grain	Potato (British arrow-root)
	At the large end	Often with a beak-like projection	Bermuda arrow-root
Elliptical	Longitudinal linear lateral	Often kidney-shaped. Hilum puckered	Bean starch
		More regular. Hilum simple	Pea starch
Lenticular	Central	Convex at the hilum	Wheaten starch
		Concave at the hilum	Barley starch
		Often with stellate fissure at the hilum	Rye starch

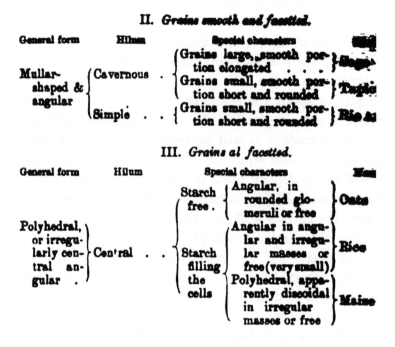

3. *Inspection of Fresh Meat.*

Though the paymaster and others, concerned in t[he] [selec]tion and supply of fresh meat to the ship's company, [may have] acquired good empyrical ideas to guide their judgm[ent of] its quality and fitness for issue, or otherwise, there c[an be no] doubt that a little more scientific supervision of so i[mportant] an article of diet would in many cases be desirable.

The particulars of importance to be attended to [are the] following:—

1. In relation to the flesh or muscular part, it s[hould be] remembered that in young animals the fibres are of a [pale] colour, which become darker as they grow older; [as] might be expected, the flesh of animals that have died [without] having the blood drawn in the ordinary process of sl[aughter]ing is of a deep purple tint. The colour of meat begi[ns to] turn by keeping grows paler at first, and then pas[ses to a] greenish hue. This latter will be distinctly seen thr[ough]

skin and fascia. Coincidental with this change, the characteristic odour of fresh meat gradually gives place to that of incipient decomposition, until finally, with the further development of bacteria, the putrefactive odour is fully established. Just as by heating drinking-water any bad odour that may be present will become more apparent, so by cutting and stirring up some of the suspected meat in hot water any existing taint will be readily detected.

2. A marbled appearance of the flesh, due to the interlacement of fatty veins in streaks, is said to be indicative of good meat; but, just as too much fat is surfeiting to most persons, and must relatively diminish the amount of nitrogenous matter, so very lean meat is harsh and indigestible, and the fat is not in sufficient quantity to represent that amount which should always be present in a well-proportioned diet.

The fat should not be too white and glairy, on the one hand, nor too rich and yellow, on the other. This latter effect is known to be produced by some kinds of food, oilcake for example.

It is a remarkable fact that very soon after an ox is killed the marrow in the bones of the hinder limbs coagulates, while that in the fore limbs remains like honey, both in consistency and appearance. This point should be attended to, as the arrest of coagulation in the marrow would be indicative of some pre-existing disease. The proportion of bone should not exceed 20 per cent.

Fresh meet should be examined for parasites—trichinæ and cysticerci in particular. Indeed this precaution would also apply to salt meat, since it has been found that salting will not always kill any parasites that may be present.

4. *Inspection of Salt Meat.*

To what has been already said in relation to the salting of meat (p. 180), the following remarks may be added. When the salt and brine are good, our judgment will be confined to the character and quality of the meat. The parts may be good, when a favourable opinion must be given; if the parts are inferior, the meat may be objected to on this ground alone, or if it is old, which will be indicated by toughness and a shrivelled appearance. If the meat is originally bad, salting will not completely arrest the changes going forward.

The pickle or brine may be originally too weak, or become so by continued use. It is known also to acquire poisonous properties under certain conditions that have not been thoroughly investigated.

CHAPTER VI.

EXERCISE, FOR RECREATION, HYGIENIC PURPOSES, AND IN CONNECTION WITH DUTY.

The old adage of 'all work and no play,' &c., is just as applicable to the sailor as it is to the schoolboy, and, even after very trying labours of necessity, when the hands are piped to 'dance and skylark' Jack is very soon ready for a hornpipe, highcockalorum, or any other fun that may be suggested, whether athletic or otherwise. When it is otherwise, of course the otium might be enjoyed without further testing the powers of the system, even with the solace of being under no restraint. Civilisation and moral influences have produced their effect upon sailors as well as upon the other ramifications of society, and the old coarse sea song, or fore-bitter of the past, has been replaced by less objectionable sentiments, and often even by part singing which would horrify the spirit of 'Benbow,' if it could be summoned to the forecastle of a modern ship of war on a summer's evening.

Indeed, it has been said by admirals of bygone days that they have never seen a sailor since the toke was cut off, but more modern experience has given us full confidence in making the assertion that the sailor of the present day will fight as manfully for the honour of his country as any toked sailor that ever existed is known to have done in days of yore. By this digression we have just lightly touched the subject of rest, the value of which would demand a section to itself.

If the use of gymnastics can be of benefit to anyone, it must surely be to the sailor, whose ordinary avocations on board ship often call for more activity and physical exertion than is perhaps brought into exercise in any other calling whatever. In recognition of this fact, a certain number of sailors of the French navy are sent every year to the gymnasium of Joinville-le-Pont, and in their turn these men become first-rate instructors to the men afloat (De Méricourt).

The amount of exercise falling to the lot of some men is much greater than that required from others. Thus some have possibly too much, while others have positively too little. Such men as the yeomen of stores, and those whose occupation confines them a great deal to the lower parts of the ship, should be assigned some light periodical work on deck for the preservation of their health under circumstances so inimical to it. It must be remembered, however, that while this is recommended with the view of benefiting the persons concerned, and aërating their blood even against their own inclinations, it would be injudicious to submit stokers, just off the fires, to sudden cold and exposure on deck until the system were permitted to rest for some little time and adapt itself to the change. Indeed, it would be much better to give these men the benefit of all the rest the interval between their watches will admit of.

Dr. Hunter, of the U.S. Navy, who supports his position by the most cogent reasoning, says, speaking of stokers in this connection, 'As these men are enrolled under special provisions, they should not be called upon for any duty outside their vocation. There is a physiological, and consequently a hygienic, necessity for this. It is no uncommon thing in vessels propelled by sail and steam to have all the engineer's force not on watch engaged pulling and hauling on sheets and halyards on deck, only to go below and take up their work in the engine and fire room when the watch is changed. It is all wrong, from whatever standpoint it may be viewed. After a watch they should not be disturbed except in cases of great emergency.' It will be scarcely a digression here to speak of the drink required by stokers to satisfy their thirst, arising from the peculiar nature of their toil. 'It is impossible to realise,' says Dr. Bourel Roniere, 'the enormous quantity of plain or acidulated water consumed by a stoker in the course of a watch, more especially in hot countries. In Europe it amounts on an average to three or four quarts, and is at least doubled in the tropics. The health soon suffers from this excess and over-excitement of the secretory functions of the skin. The immediate results are profuse sweats, insatiable thirst, and subsequently atony of the digestive organs, colic, diarrhœa, a feeling of heaviness and sinking in the epigastrium, a flabby and inert condition of the muscles, absence of colour in the skin and mucous membrane. This over-indulgence in drinking water is certainly most injurious to the stoker's health, and the injury is all the greater as there is no restriction to the quantity consumed.' As early as 1853 the same authority recommended the issue of what he considered to be a more wholesome beverage than the regulation acidulated mixture. He then proposed a weak solution of coffee with the sugar and brandy already allowed ; and in this he has received the support of M. Fonssagrives and many other naval surgeons.

By an order of July 1880 men employed in the French West Indian colonies and the tropics are allowed daily a small quantity of sugar, brandy, and vinegar, or, instead of the latter, as occasion may serve, fresh limes or oranges.

In the Royal Navy, stokers are commonly in the habit of mixing oatmeal with the water used for drinking during the watch, or, at the recommendation of the medical officer, an additional allowance of lime juice may be issued to them. It must, however, be admitted, as Dr. Leroy de Méricourt remarks, that 'it is difficult to fix upon a good wholesome beverage suitable to the stokers when employed on the fires.'

CHAPTER VII.

CLOTHING.

The subject of clothing is one of great importance, and would naturally follow that of exercise. Many things in relation to the characteristic dress of the sailor are so time-hallowed that it would be difficult to effect a change in them, even if such change were clearly shown to be a hygienic necessity. Thus, there can be no doubt that the needless exposure of the upper part of the chest is productive of much evil, and the health of many a fine young fellow has been sacrificed by bronchitis and other pulmonary affections arising from this cause alone. The use of navy-blue woollen comforters was intended to mitigate this evil; but any remittent article of this kind will often be either worn or discarded without sufficient judgment, and thus even favour the accession of a cold that may lead to something of a more serious nature.

Notwithstanding the great solicitude shown by the Admiralty for the health and comfort of the British sailor, provision for a change of clothing on exposure to wet in the ordinary discharge of duty would appear to be more carefully attended to in the American navy than in our own.

A list of the established articles constituting the outfit of the sailor will be found in the new Instructions; and, whatever may be said to the contrary, there can be no doubt that the attainment of neatness, tidiness, cleanliness, dryness, efficiency, and economy characterise all the rules relating to their nature, quality, and mode of issue, as well as their supervision by the lieutenant of divisions and periodical inspection.

Hygienic Notes and Particulars in relation to Clothing.

Many hygieists are of opinion that white clothing should be altogether done away with in the navy. 'Their chief use,' says Dr. Gihon, U.S N., 'is as a Sunday morning mustering-dress in the tropics; but in recent years the whim of the executive officer of the flag-ship, or, in its absence, of the vessel, determines whether the dress shall be white shirts and pants, blue shirts and white pants, white shirts and blue pants, or blue shirts and pants, apparently more for the sake of variety than anything else, straw hats and blue caps, with or without white covers, extending the number of permutations.' 'The absurdity of requiring a man to clothe his legs in flannel and his arms in white duck to-day, while to-morrow he is blue above and white below, ought to be evident to even the non-professional, as it is to the old quarter-master, whose "rheumatiz" is made to shift from his shoulders to his loins and back again.'[1]

On White Cap-Covers.—Dr. E. Payne, of the U.S. Navy, has made some interesting experiments in reference to the question of white cap-covers, so much in vogue in tropical climates; and he has clearly shown that when the ordinary service cap is covered with a white material of any kind, a thermometer placed within the cap and upon the head will record no diminution of temperature as effected by the white cover. A naval cap for officers, with ventilating eyelet-holes pierced through the top, was tested for ten minutes in the sun, and the thermometer registered 83° F. With the glazed cover, however, the temperature was raised to 104° F. On the other hand, under a white-duck cap of the same pattern the thermometer stood at 83°.

It would thus appear, 'first, that the glazed cover should not be worn except for protection against storms. Second, in comparing a cap with an air-chamber, and having holes for

[1] *Naval Hygiene*, p. 62.

ventilation, with one (as in the ordinary cap for sailors) which sits close to the head and has no ventilation, the difference in temperature is in favour of the former by 11° F. Third, in comparing a cap made of white duck and having an air-chamber, with a cloth one which sits close on the head (as the sailors') and is covered with white linen, the difference is in favour of the former by 21° F.; from which it would appear that caps should be made of white duck for warm weather, and that blue caps with white covers, as a substitute, should be discarded.'

Mr. Payne has also made some excellent remarks in relation to the manufacture of slop shoes for the navy, and demonstrated by practical experiment their inefficiency and radical defects in a hygienic point of view; but these evils could no doubt be easily remedied by simply enforcing the supply of more serviceable articles. He further deals with a most important subject, namely, the under-clothing of the sailors, suggesting that, as an interchange from blue to white in the outer garments has already been sanctioned by both experience and custom, the same provision should be made in reference to the under-clothing, though this has not hitherto been so cogently brought under the notice of the authorities. Referring to the cruise of the U.S. ship 'Jamestown' in the Pacific, he says, ' My frequent observation was that a large percentage of the men who applied for admission to the sick-list were either without proper under-clothing or neglected to wear it. Their neglect was usually the result of dislike to heavy articles served out during such periods of our cruise as were passed in the tropics. To such an extent was this dislike put in practise, by neglecting to wear such garments, that I made requests to have the men examined at morning quarters, thereby trying to detect the neglectful and force them to their use. This measure had the desired effect; and a good opportunity for comparing it with the one of allowing the men to follow their own inclinations was found at Panama in March 1871. At that time we were in company with a ship whose crew was but a little more in numbers than our own, and while our sick-list was only from six to ten, theirs was soon above thirty. The explanation was simple: our men wore under-clothing, and no special care was exercised to compel the men of the other ship to do so. And it is not surprising that when men are worked during the day in such a climate as exists at that place they perspire profusely, and on every opportunity throw themselves down for rest in the coolest spot they can find; neither is it surprising, when men are allowed to lie down on deck with no under-shirt on, and the outer one freely thrown open, and a smart breeze coming under the awning apron (as I have witnessed), that thirty men out of a crew of two hundred should soon be down with fever.'

The quality which is now in use (a heavy dark-blue material) seems to him to be all that could be desired for cold climates, but he believes that it would be a great advantage to have its place supplied, for use in warm climates, by a quality which would be both lighter in texture and lighter in colour. Then the men would be found to wear it more regularly, and would at all times be protected from sudden changes of temperature.

The ordinary flannel worn by British sailors is defective in several ways: thus (1), it is usually too loose, though not long enough; (2) it does not ascend sufficiently upon the upper part of the chest and root of the neck; and (3) it is totally without sleeves. A much more efficient article would be a kind of Guernsey frock, of some light material, as merino, which would be elastic and close-fitting, and at the same time permit of the transpiration of the skin, which it would thus supplement, taking up excessive moisture and obviating chill by its non-conducting property. Many sailors suppose that shifting into dry clothes when one gets wet is only necessary for delicate people, and they are rather disposed to let their clothes 'dry upon the same bush they got wet on;' and this mistake is further sustained by the common impression—in which there is, doubtless, some truth—that salt-water dampness is not so injurious as that of fresh. It is certain, however, that getting wet in flannel under-garments, whether the moisture be salt or fresh, is less to be feared than a similar exposure to wet and cold by evaporation without them.

Sailors are enjoined to put away every article in a clean and creditable state in their bags, and those that have been newly washed in particular should be thoroughly dry before they are put away. Moreover, on no account should articles of clothing be left about, whether wet or dry.

The ditty-box and bag of the seaman, the desk and sea-chest of the midshipman, and the cabin of the commissioned officer are but three grades of equivalent things, and it might be easily imagined how any infringement of justice in relation to any of them would give rise to discontent. In some ships clothes-lockers, answering also as seats between the mess-tables, are substituted for bags, and the bag-racks consequently abolished. There are, however, some disadvantages connected with the change; thus, the clothing is more likely to become damp, and the accumulation of filth is scarcely avoidable, the access to it is so easy. There is also some difficulty in removing the whole kit to the upper deck for inspection and periodical exposure to the sun.

DIVISION II.

PROPHYLACTIC HYGIENE.

CHAPTER I.

SECTION A.—*The Customary Issue of Lime-juice as an Antiscorbutic.*

AFTER having given a definition of scurvy, Professor Aitkin, M.D., F.R.S., observes that ' an altered state of the albumen of the blood is associated with this condition, and the phenomena are brought about by a deficient supply of the organic vegetable acids, or the salts of fresh vegetables.'[1] This simple statement, while it really expresses all that we are quite sure of as to the cause of the scorbutic condition, and affords us no explanation of the precise physiological effect, or *modus operandi*, of the vegetable acids in the healthy system, is nevertheless a practical guide to us; for experience has shown that, however defective our theory may be, the vegetable acids, and in particular lime-juice, are not only the best prophylactics in relation to scurvy, but also the most certain remedies when the malady has actually made its appearance.

When omnivorous capabilities are curbed by monotony of diet, necessitated or otherwise, it stands to reason that the blood, which should be renewed by the assimilation of diversified food, must suffer defect in some of its staminal elements,

[1] *Science and Practice of Medicine.*

either as to their quantity or quality, and it is to th[e] state of the vital fluid so induced that the train of sy[mptoms] known as scurvy is attributable.

The proximate organic principles of vegetables a[re] readily assimilable in the fresh or recent state th[an] drying or keeping, and even well-preserved vegeta[ble] stances cannot be supposed to make up altogether [the] absence of fresh vegetables in the ordinary diet [.] Moreover, the vegetable acids, malic, citric, &c., seem [to play] an important part in the human economy, as is demo[nstrated] in the important fact that the scorbutic diathesis, and [scurvy] itself, are brought immediately under control by t[heir] ministration.

The earlier writers attached much importance [to the] supposed influence of salt and other provisions dete[riorated] in quality in producing scorbutic disease. This view [in any] case, however, is quite erroneous, for there is a[n] instance on record where salt meat, having been alo[ne avail]able as a change of diet, produced a most salutar[y effect] upon existing scurvy. On the other hand, there can [be] little doubt that a salt meat diet would favour the d[evelop]ment of scurvy, from its natural tendency to lo[wer the] stamina of the system, reduce the weight of the bo[dy, and] induce a corresponding amount of debility. Thoug[h scor]butic patients living on salt provisions may still be c[ured by] the liberal use of antiscorbutics, it is certain that b[oth the] prevention and cure of scurvy would be much mor[e easily] effected when fresh meat can be supplied. Too great [confi]nence, however, cannot be given to fresh meat alone, [as it is] well known that a bad form of scurvy often occurs a[mongst] the Australian colonists who are not provident enough [to grow] vegetables, but who live almost exclusively on fresh [meat] of the best quality.

Just as scurvy itself must have long existed in th[e world] before it obtained a definite place amongst classified d[iseases,] so it is probable that its sovereign remedy, lime-jui[ce,] long known before it found its way into the recognised lists of therapeutic agents.

In the writings of Solomon Albertus (1573), Sir Richard Hawkins (1593), Sir James Lancaster (1600), and John Woodall (1617) we find, perhaps, the earliest records of the efficacy of lime-juice both as a prophylactic and cure for scurvy. It was not, however, until the year 1795 that the regular issue of lime-juice was introduced into the British navy, through the importunate solicitations of Sir Gilbert Blane, Bart. 'This fortunate circumstance,' says Sir Alexander Armstrong, 'was brought about in consequence of the alarm created by the prevalence of the disease in the fleet under the command of Lord Howe in the spring of 1795, the outbreak being traceable to causes entirely analogous to those which induced the epidemic on former occasions, namely, the deprivation of fresh vegetables. So prevalent was scurvy in this fleet, and so much enfeebled were the crews by its visitation, that the ships were rendered quite inefficient, and the safety of the empire became, in consequence, absolutely imperilled.'

Much inconvenience at first arose from the deterioration of the lime-juice on keeping. It was then suggested that pure citric acid should be substituted. Subsequently very extensive trial was made as to the relative value of the artificially prepared acid and lime-juice, in which, as a natural vehicle, it is contained, with a much smaller proportion of other vegetable acids, viz. malic and tartaric. The preference has been given to the lime-juice, just as quinine in the bark might be preferred to the alkaloid in the isolated state. It is remarkable, however, that what little is known of the separate use of citric acid is quite in its favour. After having noticed an excellent case by Thomas Watherston, of the 'Superb,' and stated the fact that Trotter gives reports from seven or eight naval surgeons, who all state that they found the citric acid more efficacious than lemon-juice, Dr. Parkes[1] remarks

---

[1] 'On the Pathology and Treatment of Scurvy,' *British and Foreign Medico-Chirurgical Review*, vol. ii. 1848.

that the disappearance of 'scurvy from the Royal Navy has not allowed any further experience of citric acid; but on board the Australian convict-ships the disease has occasionally appeared;' and he further says that 'Sir William Burnett, whose attention has been directed for many years to this subject, has been in the habit of supplying convict-ships with citric acid and nitrate of potash, as well as with lemon-juice, in order that comparative trials might be made of the relative value of these remedies.' The examination of all the documents bearing upon this point was liberally granted to Dr. Parkes, and his digest of the evidence will be found in the philosophical and exhaustive article already referred to, and his final remarks are of great importance.

'We cannot conceive that anything can be more convincing than the above evidence; the efficacy of citric acid is clearly proved, and the nitrate of potash is evidently inferior to it in power;' and further on, 'We know, on the other hand, that when lime-juice becomes musty, a mucilaginous principle is developed at the expense of the citric and malic acids. This is proved by several analyses, particularly by some which Sir William Burnett has had made, and which show very clearly the gradual decrease in the percentage of the citric acid.

'Everyone knows the immense difficulty of preserving lime-juice, and how often it becomes ineffectual at the time it is needed most. We need not wonder, then, if these circumstances are not properly estimated, that the reputation of lemon-juice as an antiscorbutic has at times suffered. In a document in Sir William Burnett's office it is stated that scurvy broke out on board a convict-ship. The lemon-juice was in casks and bottles. That in casks had fermented and become thick; it had more the appearance of pea-soup than lemon-juice. The patients "loathed it" instead of manifesting, as usual, the greatest avidity for it. It was, however, used, but was ineffectual. The lemon-juice in bottles was good, and was employed with the best effects in the worst cases.

'We may state here that we have no doubt that good lemon-juice is more effectual than pure citric acid; this may be from its containing malic and tartaric acids, besides citric, or, as is very probable, from the citric acid being in the form most easily absorbed or decomposed. The Materia Medica gives us many analogous examples of the superior efficacy of a medicine in its *natural combinations.*'

Notwithstanding the elaborateness of the report of the committee appointed to inquire into the causes of the outbreak of scurvy in the recent Arctic Expedition, very little more has been added to the facts and deductions contained in the masterly article from which the above quotations have been taken.

The navy allowance of lemon-juice is 1 oz., with the same amount of sugar, daily, after the men have been 9 days on salt provisions; but, as a discretionary power is vested in the medical officer in charge, it is now very usual for ships to issue lime-juice regularly during their whole period at sea, without waiting for the lapse of any specified time. It was the custom formerly to serve out the lime-juice and sugar to the several messes separately, and it was by no means certain that each man had taken his full allowance, or even any at all. 'When the lime-juice is taken into the different messes,' says Sir Alexander Armstrong,[1] 'many of the men are careless about it, and seldom or never take it; others will give it away, or, what is a common occurrence, will barter it with the few who are wise enough to prefer it to spirits, so that one-half of the crew may not, in all probability, take it. Thus there is no certainty whatever that it is taken by all with any degree of regularity, but there is positive evidence to the contrary.' With the view of testing the relative merits of lime-juice simply boiled and lime-juice fortified with spirits, it was necessary to adopt some plan that would ensure a fair trial. He therefore recommended 'that each half of the crew should partake of the different kinds of acid.

[1] *Naval Hygiene and Scurvy.* 1858.

In pursuance of this plan it was mixed in separate tubs, from which each man daily drank his allowance in presence of an officer. The adoption of this practice was attended with the happiest results. I had thus,' he says, 'the positive evidence afforded me that every man in the ship drank his allowance (1 oz.) daily, and was thus fortified with a regular daily quantity of a powerful antiscorbutic. To this circumstance, therefore, I unhesitatingly attribute not only the immunity we enjoyed from scurvy for a longer time than has ever been known before in the Polar Sea, but also our good fortune in maintaining an unprecedentedly high standard of health among our crew during the same period.' Further on the same authority remarks, 'I could wish that this plan was enforced in the navy, not only as regards lime-juice, but likewise spirits; for I am quite satisfied that by making the men drink their allowance of either at the tub, where it is mixed in presence of the officer who always superintends the "grog-tub," the most beneficial results would accrue, not only in a sanitary point of view, but in preventing the occurrence of drunkenness and its attendant evils on board ships of war.'

The late Dr. Alexander Eugene Mackay, D.I.G., R.N., used to say that 'the North Pole will never be reached without lime-juice.' Nevertheless some medical men affect to ignore the vegetable acids, and set up milk, meat-juice, alkaline salts, phosphoric acid, oils and fats as sufficiently prophylactic and curative in relation to scurvy. It is doubtful if ever the physical labour on any former occasion was so great as that which fell to the lot of the sledge-crews in the late Arctic Expedition; and there must have been a commensurate demand for wholesome food to repair the inordinate waste. Yet this was not all, for the effect of insufficiency of food, or starvation in the ordinary sense, and scurvy must not be confounded. The nutritive functions are in full action in the scorbutic condition, but held in abeyance in starvation. Indeed, one might die of scurvy without starvation, or die of starvation without scurvy. The secret of the matter was that lime-juice was withheld, which, however incredible it may seem to the uninitiated, would have preserved the necessary alkalinity of the blood, and thus furnish in a single article that essential part which was deficient in the rest of the daily food. Now, besides the inconvenience of carriage, one reason for omitting to send lime-juice with the sledging parties was, that by freezing the bottles would be broken and the lime-juice rendered unfit for use. It has since occurred to several persons, even simultaneously, including Sir George Nares himself, that if the lime-juice were sufficiently concentrated, mixed with sugar, and made into lozenges, this valuable agent might be carried without the feeling of encumbrance, but issued in a most simple and agreeable form. A sample of such a preparation, manufactured for the author by Mr. Cooper,[1] of Oxford Street, was exhibited to the members of the committee appointed to inquire into the outbreak of scurvy alluded to. Though citric acid is very deliquescent, Mr. Cooper showed the writer quite lately some of the original lozenges, which were still in excellent preservation, with all their agreeable odour, flavour, and other properties intact.

It was much to be desired that practical trial should be given them; but, as the Director-General of the Medical Department of the Navy did not sanction their use in the service, Mr. Harry Leach did not consider it advisable to employ them in the merchant marine. In favour of their efficiency it may be mentioned that lime-juice, reduced by evaporation almost to dryness, without charring, is still perfectly soluble, and when made up to the original strength with distilled water exhibits no diminution in the amount of acidity. Indeed, it has also been found that the acidity of lime-juice, taken both before and after submitting it to the freezing process, is quite the same. It may be said, however, that we are quite sure of the efficacy of lime-juice in its natural state, while we know nothing of its effect in the concentrated state.

Good lime-juice is of a rich or greenish yellow colour, quite

[1] The patentee of the effervescing lozenge.

transparent, and free from turbidity and stringiness. odour is fragrant, and the taste an agreeable acidity, ▇ bitterness, at least to any unpleasant extent. On ▇ testing the quality of a sample, take its specific gravity 1023), then evaporate to one-half to drive off the spirit take the specific gravity again (say 1035). Next determin amount of acidity with a standard alkaline solution (say grs. to the ounce). 1 cc. of the alkaline solution is equiv to ·0064 of citric acid. Now, if 10 cc. of lime-juice be ▇ with 90 cc. of water, 10 cc. of the mixture will contain of the original lime-juice. Let us now suppose that 9·5 ▇ the standard solution were required to neutralise the Multiply this by the coefficient ·0064, which will give ▇ grammes per cc. of lime-juice; then multiply by 1000 to ▇ up the litre, = 60·80 grammes per litre. This multipli 70 will express grains per gallon = 4256. There being ounces in a gallon, 4256 ÷ 160 = 26·6 grains per o This result may be at once arrived at by multiplying number of cc. used by the short factor 2·8. Thus 9·5 =26·60 grains per ounce, as before.

Sulphuric, hydrochloric, and nitric acids may be teste as in the case of drinking water. If tartaric acid is pre a white precipitate will fall in the course of twenty-four h after the addition of a little acetate of potash.

Finally, by evaporating a portion of the lime-juice to consistency of an extract, the relative amount of the l and the fragrant aroma evolved in the process will gre assist in forming an estimate of its quality.

SECTION B.—*Issue of Quinine in Malarious Districts.*

The benefit resulting from the use of Peruvian bark in fevers of the African coast having been represented to Admiralty by Mr. Robertson, of the 'Rainbow,' ships fitt out for that station were gratuitously supplied with it, and same boon was extended to the West Indies in the year 17

The great efficacy of this medicine was also attested by the fact that Count Bonneval and his suite through its means had escaped sickness in the camps in Hungary while half the army were cut off by fever. Subsequently the sulphate of quinine was used instead of bark. In Article 9, p. 11, of the 'Instructions for Medical Officers,' it is enjoined to be given in four-grain doses, morning and evening, to men when employed on shore to procure wood or water, or on other laborious duty; and the subsequent state of health of the men to whom quinine had been given is to be attentively observed and very fully reported to the Director-General. In obedience to these instructions, much important information has been received at the office, showing most clearly that in those cases in which the quinine had been duly administered an immunity was enjoyed, and conversely, where it had been neglected, either by carelessness or some unavoidable circumstance, malarious disease seems to have made its accession. This theme might be enlarged upon to almost any entent, but the simple notice of the fact must suffice for the present.

SECTION C.—*Vaccination or Re-vaccination as Prophylactic against Small-pox.*

In Article 33, p. 22, 'Surgeons' Instructions,' it is provided that, 'No person is to be admitted into Her Majesty's service unless he has had small-pox, or has been vaccinated; and should the vaccine cicatrix not be considered satisfactory, he is to be reported fit only on condition that he immediately submits to the operation.' An important circular has, however, since been issued on the subject of re-vaccination, March 7, 1871, running as follows:—

'*Re-vaccination.*—The Lords Commissioners of the Admiralty, having taken into consideration the severe epidemics of small-pox which have occasionally occurred in Her Majesty's Naval Service, the risks incurred by the crews of all vessels on foreign stations, especially in China and Japan, where that

disease is annually epidemic in the winter season, a
that the protective influence of vaccination per
childhood is liable to be much diminished, and i
stances altogether destroyed in the passage from
manhood, are pleased to direct—

'1. That all men and boys on entering into the
to be re-vaccinated.

'2. That all men who have not been re-vacci
tween their first entry in the service and the age o
be re-vaccinated as soon as possible, however, good
mary vaccination cicatrices may appear, or even sh
present unmistakable evidence of having suffered fr
pox previous to that age.

'The re-vaccination to be made with lymph eit
fresh from the arm of a child or from supplies to be
from the National Vaccine Institution.

'3. That no person shall be considered re-vaccin
has had the operation performed with lymph taken
arm of a re-vaccinated person, such an operation aff
protection from the poison of small-pox, and that all
so re-vaccinated shall again be vaccinated with lym
from the sources specified above.

'4. That a notation of the date of re-vaccination
on each certificate of service, specifying the result,
"a perfect vaccine vesicle," "modified vaccine ves
"no result."'

The terms of this circular are certainly on the sa
for although it may be difficult to prove that the 'o
performed with lymph taken from the arm of a re-va
person' affords 'no protection from the poison of sm
the efficiency of lymph taken from the arm of a c
scarcely be doubted.

Though the three sections briefly treated in the fo
remarks include the more important particulars co
with Prophylactic Hygiene, yet in practice we may a
with it also all that is anticipative of evil *and the most
protective measures.*

GENERAL ORDERS. 211

SECTION D.—*General Orders. Sanitary Regulations and Suggestions.*

(a) *Abstract of Admiral Sir M. Seymour's orders* (Hongkong, 1857):—

'5.30 A.M. Hands to be turned up.
6.0   ,,   Breakfast.
8.0   ,,   Decks to be finished and ready for any evolution.
9.0   ,,   Quarters for inspection.
Noon, P.M. Dinner.
4.30 ,,   Supper.
5.0   ,,   Work aloft as requisite.

'On Tuesdays and Fridays hands to be turned up at 5, and breakfast at 5.30.

'A cup of coffee, with a small portion of rum and biscuit, may be issued the first thing in the morning (by order of Admiralty).

'Monthly leave after October 15 to April 15 (forty-eight hours).

'Punishment cells not to be less than $6\frac{1}{2}$ feet long by 3 feet broad, with the full height between decks (Admiralty order).'

(b) *Sanitary Measures adopted during the visits of H.M.S. 'Investigator' to the Niger, and while stationed near Lagos Lagoon, which were so successful as to attract the attention of Commodore Hornby in 1866. (Medical Officer, R. G. Sweetman, R.N.)*

'1. It is of the utmost importance that men to accompany this expedition should not be taken indiscriminately, but the strongest, most healthy, and by all means temperate men available should be chosen for this purpose; and that there should be no boys, as they invariably suffer severely from the after effects of these expeditions.

'2. Each white man (including officers) to have 4 grs. of quinine in 1 oz. of sherry every P.M. after the day's work is done, commencing seven days previous to entering the river, and continuing the same for ten days after having returned from it.

'3. To have a cup of hot coffee before comi[ng]
every morning.

'4. To have one pint of porter at dinner, whic[h]
in addition to the service allowance of grog.

'5. Not to be allowed to drink the river wate[r]
other than condensed water.

'6. To be permitted to smoke when they please[,]
as much freedom generally as the service will admi[t.]

'7. Any exposure to the sun to be most careful[ly avoided]
by the use of proper awnings, and more especial[ly the]
man in the chains. It is most necessary to watch [and]
prevent unnecessary exposure.

'8. If men get wet, they should be seen to shi[ft]
clothes as quickly as possible.

'9. The bilges to be thoroughly cleaned and dried [every]
day, and chloride of zinc used if in the least foul.

'10. The lower deck should not be wetted more [than]
a week, and should invariably be dried up afterward[s.]

'11. It is most important that every man shoul[d be sup]
plied with mosquito curtains.

'12. The awning should be spread at least 9 feet [above the]
deck, and in fine weather furled at 5 P.M., every [day, and]
spread again at 6 P.M., before the dew begins to fall, [which]
does very early in the river.

'13 No white should be allowed to sleep on sho[re under]
any circumstances.

'14. It is well to anchor in mid-stream if possib[le, so as]
to avoid the closer proximity of the swamps; the[re]
mosquitoes give less annoyance, and there is general[cur]
rent of air, and however slight it may be it is most re[freshing]
and conducive to a good night's rest.

'15. Music, singing, or other harmless recreatio[n should]
be encouraged by all means. Indeed, every effort s[hould be]
made to render the time as little monotonous as possi[ble.]

'16. It is of great importance that the ship shou[ld leave]
the Niger sufficiently early to admit of the expeditio[n]

brought to a termination before the water has fallen to any extent.

'The intermittent fever of lagoons, no matter how slight, is almost invariably followed by some splenic affection'

(c) *Standing Order issued by Rear-Admiral Wyman, U.S.N., for the Guidance of Commanding Officers of Ships in the West Indies.*

'The crews will be exposed as little as possible to the heat of the sun. On calling all hands in the morning (in port), no work of any kind will be done until the men have had a meal of hot coffee and biscuit, and the market-boat will not be allowed to leave the ship until the officer of the watch has ascertained that each person in it has partaken of some food before leaving. The awnings, in port, will be triced up for a time in the morning and an hour before sunset, to ventilate the ship, and spread before nightfall, before the dew falls. If the weather be rainy, the awnings will be spread to keep the ship as dry as possible. The berth-deck will be kept clear of all articles that absorb moisture, and the deck will be sprinkled with dry sand. If the sand be damp, it can be heated at the galley and used and swept up carefully and removed every day. Water from the ship's distillers will alone be used for drinking or cooking purposes. The "bumboat" will be regularly inspected by a medical officer, to see that no unripe or improper fruits are sold to the ship's company, or in fact improper articles of diet of any kind. The authority of the medical officers in this matter is hereby made absolute. Officers going on leave will wear light clothing and straw or pith hats, observing, however, the spirit of the regulations touching uniform, so that they may be known as American officers. Liberty will not be granted to enlisted men, appointed men, or non-commissioned officers of the Marine Guard, without the express sanction of the commanding officer. Stewards and messmen will be cautioned not to visit the suburbs of towns where infection may linger, and will confine their visits to the shore strictly to the business upon which they are sent; as a rule, disease and infection are more to be apprehended in the crowded portion of a city than in the suburbs of a town. There is comparatively little danger in the suburbs or environs. When practicable, boats' crews, except the gig's crew, steam-launch, and dinghy's crew, will be sent in charge of a junior officer. When possible, coloured crews should be chosen for market and other boats in the sickliest islands of the West Indies. The men will wear flannel next to the skin, and at evening inspection divisional officers will see that this rule is observed. The ship's bilges will be thoroughly cleaned and disinfected not less than once a week, oftener if necessary. The bilges should be kept as dry as possible, but when even a small quantity of water stands in the bilges, fresh sea-water should be let in at least once a week, the bilges washed with the hose and steam-pump when practicable, and then pumped out, except in close harbours, where the water alongside, being in a measure stagnant, should not be used for any purpose. The exercises will be short, and not of an exhaustive or fatiguing nature. Instruction may take the place of actual manual labour at the guns. The "head" will be white-washed and disinfected daily; disinfectants to be procured from the Medical Department. The officers' water-closets will be thoroughly disinfected daily. The enlisted men will be cautioned by their divisional officers as to the absolute necessity of thorough personal cleanliness, as well as of the necessity of keeping the ship clean below, so as to avoid unnecessary scrubbing. If wet by rain on boat or other duty, they must shift in dry clothes as soon as possible, rubbing the person down well with coarse cloth or towel before putting on the dry suit. The men to be informed through their divisional officers that if they suffer from slight headache or diarrhœa, they are not to neglect it as a thing of no consequence, but apply to a medical officer at once for a remedy. It does not follow that a man need go on the sick-list, of which good sailors seem to have something of a dread. Commanding officers of vessels will promulgate this order, which is for the general benefit of all, and they will see that its provisions are rigidly adhered to.'

(d) *Secretary Preston's Regulations.*

Dr. Albert Leary Gihon, A.M., of the United States navy, states that the sanitary regulations of Secretary Preston, issued January 23, 1850, are still in operation, and should be enforced on all other stations where similar climatic conditions prevail, as in the East and West Indies, and on the coast of Central America. They are as follows:—

' 1. No officer or man will be permitted to be on shore before sunrise, or after sunset, or to sleep there at night; this rule to apply not only to the Continental coast, but to the Cape de Verde Islands.

' 2. No United States vessel will ascend or anchor in any of the African rivers except upon imperative public service.

' 3. Boat excursions up rivers or hunting parties on shore are forbidden.

' 4. Vessels, when possible, will anchor at a reasonable distance from shore; far enough not to be influenced by the malaria floated off by the land breeze.

' 5. Convalescents from fever and other diseases, when condemned by medical survey, are to be sent to the United States with the least possible delay.

' 6. When the general health of a ship's company shall be reported as impaired by cruising upon the southern or equatorial portion of the coast, the earliest possible opportunity will be given them to recruit by transferring the ship for a time to the Canaries or other windward islands of the station.

' 7. Boat and shore duty, involving exposure to the sun and rain, is to be performed, so far as the exigencies of the service will permit, by the Kroomen employed for that purpose.

' 8. All possible protection from like exposure is to be afforded to the ship's company on board; and the proper clothing and diet of the crew, as well as the ventilation and care of the decks, will be made a frequent subject for the inspection and advice of the medical officers.

'9. These regulations are to be considered as permanent, and each commanding officer of the squadron, on retiring from the station, will transfer them to his successor.'

(e) *Precautions to be taken where Malignant Cholera is prevalent.*

1. Check the slightest degree of looseness of the bowels.
2. Wear a flannel bandage round the belly.
3. Avoid protracted fasts by eating a little every five or six hours, and take the customary allowance of stimulants.
4. Change damp clothes, and keep the feet dry.
5. Do not take Seidlitz powders or Epsom salts, or any strong purgative dose.
6. Do not eat salads, melons, cucumber, shell-fish, pine-apples, plums, pork, oily fish, uncooked vegetables, cocoa-nuts, pastry, pickles, carrots, pease or beans, salted dry meats, geese or ducks, or any meat which is at all high.
7. Avoid excessive fatigue, damp and cold, especially at night or soon after meals.
8. Avoid exposure to extremes of heat and cold.
9. Keep all parts of the ship as dry as possible.
10. Air the bedding daily, and wash the clothing frequently.
11. Keep up fires during the night, as attacks most usually occur then.
12. Move from the locality where the disease is prevailing to some place which it appears to have passed by. If in a ship, shift the anchorage and get springs on the cable, to allow a free current of air to pass through her (Saunders).

(f) *Sanitary Precautions in regard to Cholera, issued by the Admiralty, August 3, 1866.*

1. The petty officers of messes are desired to exercise an unobtrusive watchfulness over the men complaining in their messes, and report to a medical officer any man whom they

may know, or have reason to suspect, to be labouring under diarrhœa, or who may appear to be in ill health, and that it be impressed upon them that by evincing an interest in this direction they will do much to prevent any outbreak of cholera on board.

2. Once daily at least, at a time when the majority of the men are in their messes, a medical officer shall go round the different mess-decks and ascertain from the petty officers of messes whether there is anyone requiring his attention.

3. The officers of divisions, when inspecting their men, shall take notice of any man who may appear to be in ill health, and shall cause him to be at once taken to the sick-bay and reported to the surgeon.

4. Twice daily at least the head-shoots, as well as the shoots of the different water-closets in the ship which are much used, shall be washed down with a solution of carbolic acid, or chloride of zinc, and instructions shall be given to the captain of the head to report to the surgeon any man who, from making frequent use of it, may be suspected to be labouring under diarrhœa.

5. Should cholera have established itself on board any ship, the utmost care is to be taken that the choleraic discharges, whether from the stomach or bowels, are largely mixed with the solution of the chloride of zinc, or other disinfectant, before they are thrown away, and that any clothing or bedding contaminated with the discharges be destroyed.

(g) *Aphorisms for Bathers* (R.H.S. Rules).

Avoid bathing within two hours after a meal.

Avoid bathing when exhausted by fatigue or from any other cause.

Avoid bathing when the body is cooling after perspiration; but—

Bathe when the body is warm, provided no time is lost in getting into the water.

Avoid chilling the body by sitting or standing naked on the banks or in boats after having been in the water.

Avoid remaining too long in the water; leave the water immediately there is the slightest feeling of chilliness.

Avoid bathing altogether in the open air, if after having been a short time in the water, there is a sense of chilliness, with numbness of the hands and feet.

The vigorous and strong may bathe early in the morning on an empty stomach.

The young, and those that are weak, had better bathe three hours after a meal. The best time for such is from two to three hours after breakfast.

Those who are subject to attacks of giddiness and faintness, and those who suffer from palpitation and other sense of discomfort at the heart, should not bathe without first consulting their medical adviser.

SECTION E.—*Hospital Ships* (' Victor Emanuel ').

When military operations are being conducted along a coast-line, the establishment of hospital-ships for the reception of sick and wounded is usually found to be expedient; and their organisation and fittings have frequently called forth much ingenuity and forethought to meet all portending emergencies and anticipate every possible requirement, even beyond the limits of probability.

Good accommodation and good ventilation are the first items of importance. The former implies sufficient cubic space for breathing, and the latter sufficient interchange of air, both of which, if essential, under ordinary circumstances, to health, are doubly so to the sick and hurt confined to bed.

Vessels of the frigate class have generally been employed as hospital-ships, though in some instances line-of-battle ships have been converted for this purpose and turned to very good account instead of lying up in ordinary.

It is commonly believed that a ship with two decks is

more salubrious than one with three, and that a one-decked ship would be still better, but for the corresponding want of

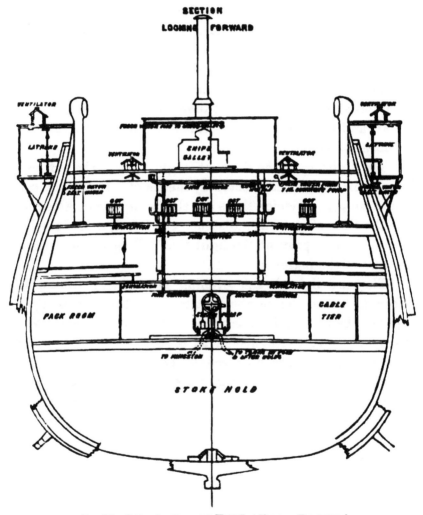

FIG. 39.—BODY SECTION OF H.M.S. 'VICTOR EMANUEL.'

This figure is very neatly executed, and speaks for itself. Reference, however, may be made to the text for more particular information.

accommodation. Perhaps the most complete and efficient hospital-ship of modern times was the 'Victor Emanuel,' for-

merly the 'Repulse,' a screw line-of-battle ship of 5,157
and 2,414 horse-power. This vessel was built in Pembr
Yard, and launched in September 1855.

Soon after the Crimean war she was laid up in hart
without further commission until the Ashantee war broke
when she was taken into dock at Portsmouth and fitted u
a cost of about 38,000*l.*, as a hospital-ship for service on
coast of Africa.

Allusion has already been made to the ventilation of
ship, nor is it intended to give here an exhaustive accoun
her internal arrangement, but there are many hygienic
ticulars and matters of detail worthy of notice in relatio
the hospital-deck.

'The lighting of the deck at night,' says Dr. Bleck
C.B., in his report, 'is effected by means of "Palmer's pa
candle-lamps," of which there are thirty arranged alterna
over the lines of cots, at a distance of 14 feet, and fitted w
shades, so as to prevent the light from falling too strongly
the eyes of the patients.

'They are lighted each evening at a quarter of an h
before dark, and the number left burning during the nigh
regulated by the requisitions of the prescribing medical offic
Other lights are extinguished at or before 9 P.M., by wh
hour all patients are required to be in bed. Any defe
during the evening in the lamps are at once brought to
notice of the master gunner in charge of the hospital-de
and defects in the same during the night are reported
the orderly of the Army Hospital Corps on duty, through
sentry at the hatchway, to the lamp-trimmer on night du
The arrangements for personal ablution on this deck cons
of a lavatory forward with eight washing basins, fitted
either side of the bowsprit, and supplied by taps with fr
and salt water. There are besides 14 basins with water-ts
screwed at intervals into the walls of the deck, for cases
emergency. There are six baths, provided with pipes to co
vey salt and fresh water from the large poop tanks abo

described, with steam jets connected with the engines, to heat the water, all the taps being clearly lettered and painted in different colours.

'There are two of Captain Crease's charcoal water-tank filters on the deck, each holding two tons of drinking water, and supplied from the large tanks in front of the poop. There is a smaller filter-tank, holding one ton of water for the use of the dispensary, which is situated forward, amidships. This is a commodious building, 18 feet 3 inches in length by 10 feet 6 inches in breadth and 6 feet 7 inches in height, lighted from above, and admirably fitted by Messrs. Savory and Moore, of London, with every requisite appliance.

'There are on the hospital-deck 18 water-closets for the men, arranged in three sets on each side. They are fitted up after Stone's patent, and with Baker's disinfectant, i.e. permanganate of potash, in solution, in a reservoir connected with the pan, and a jet of which is, by a simple arrangement, thrown into the pan after it has been washed out by ordinary water. This principle has been found to answer well. Close stools were in very little request, and, as Stone's closet also forms a urinal, chamber utensils were at no period kept on the hospital-deck.

'Before leaving England the floor and sides of the hospital-deck were coated with white zinc paint, with a view to admit of their being kept clean by ordinary scrubbing; a very good arrangement and one that experience has shown to answer well. On getting to sea it was found that, as the painting had been done in damp weather, the deck had almost to be scraped bare in order to get a smooth and dry surface. It was, therefore, proposed by Captain Parkin, R.N., that the deck should be repainted, and this was accordingly done under the superintendence of the first lieutenant, Mr. Hutton, to whose energy and good taste in the selection of colours I would here express my obligations. The floor of the deck, which was unoccupied on the outward voyage, had two fresh coats of white paint, slightly tinged with chrome-yellow, the bulwarks being painted white, with a relieving line of cobalt-blue. The ventilating shafts and fresh-water filter-tanks were painted a warm French grey, the bands of the tanks being left zinc white, relieved by a fine vermilion line. The four cable-bits and two of the centre ventilating shafts were painted a grey granite, and the buckets a zinc white, with chrome-yellow hoops. The two capstans received the same shade of French grey in use elsewhere, relieved by zinc white panels, rope mouldings, and gilt beading. The numerous pipes of different classes on this deck were distinguished by painting the joints of steam fire-mains vermilion, those of fresh-water taps blue, and those of salt-water green. By this arrangement the extensive white surface was toned down and the eye relieved, while the colouring of the taps was turned to practical account.

'A special feature in the arrangement of the hospital-deck is the erection at each side, about the centre of the ship, of a large outside platform, 26 feet 8 inches in length by 3 feet in breadth, on which such of the sick as are able to leave their cots may lounge or walk about. These platforms, furnished with easy chairs, and protected against the chance of accident by a strong wire netting, 6 feet in height, were a great boon to the poor fellows in hospital while on the West Coast. Here they lounged, read, or talked, and enjoyed what little breeze there was. Here, too, permission was given, on the certificate of the prescribing medical officer (to such men as were too weakly to go above for the purpose), to smoke between the hours of 8.30 and 9.0 A.M., 12 noon, and 2 P.M., and 6 and 8 P.M. When the number of convalescents increased towards the end of our stay at Cape Coast Castle, and on the homeward voyage, Captain Parkin was good enough to sanction the use of the port side of the poop by the sick and wounded soldiers, and to provide benches and chairs for their use. Here also smoking was allowed on the same condition as on the promenades. Before quitting the platforms I may mention that through them, and the gangways leading therefrom, all the severe cases requiring to be slung up in cots were taken on board and conveyed to the hospital-deck. The arrangements for the reception of such helpless cases will be considered at a subsequent part of this report. For the accommodation of sick officers there are six cabins at the stern of the hospital-deck, comfortably furnished, opening off an airy and commodious saloon, 32 feet in length by 19 feet in breadth and 6 feet 4 inches in height, in which those who were able to be up had their meals served. This compartment has a special gangway and accommodation ladder leading to the upper deck, and can be shut off from the hospital-deck preper (i.e. the men's hospital) by a curtain. This has not been used, nor have the curtains on the men's deck been used at any time. The ventilation of the sick officers' cabins is effected by ports, venetian blinds communicating with their saloon, and the perforated zinc plates in the sides of the ship already referred to. The saloon is ventilated by three stern ports, 3 feet 10 inches in height by 3 feet 5 inches in breadth, and by a cowled tube opening 8 inches above the floor, immediately abaft the companion ladder. It was designed that upcast ventilation should be promoted by perforated zinc plates opening into the well of the screw, but as these plates appeared to form inlets for disagreeable smells from below, where the screw-well communicated with the bilges, they were closed at an early period by shutters with which they were provided. There are four water-closets for officers, constructed after Stone's patent with Baker's disinfectant. It should be noted here that the accommodation designed for sick officers in the 'Victor Emanuel' was quite disproportionate as compared with that provided for men. On several occasions provision had to be made for ten sick officers, and in an emergency as many as 15 were accommodated by screening off compartments of the hospital-deck. The available cabins in the other troop-ships and transports in the harbour were also turned to account. As a rule the more severe cases were retained in the hospital ship, and only the less serious ones were sent elsewhere.

Table of Measurements for Cubic Space.

Number	Description	Dimensions				Of each		Total		Grand total	
		Length	Breadth	Height		Cubic contents	Superficial area	Cubic contents	Superficial area	Cubic contents	Superficial area
		ft. in.	ft. in.	ft. in.	ft. in	ft.	ft.	ft.	ft.	ft.	ft.
	Main deck	180 6	42 0	7 0	—	—	—	—	—	53,067	7,581
	Fore „	24 0	32 10	7 0	—	—	—	—	—	5,516	768
2	Ventilating ridges	80 0	1 4	1 2	1 10 of ridge	160	106	—	—	320	—
										58,903	8,349
	Deduct:—										
2	Water-closets	9 3	4 10	7 0	—	312	44	624	88		
2	„ „	9 6	3 10	7 0	—	255	36	510	72		
2	„ „	10 0	3 10	7 0	—	268	39	536	78		
2	Lavatories	15 8	1 9	7 0	—	16	27	32	54		
10	Ventilating shafts	1 8	1 6	7 0	—	14	1½	140	15		
2	Ventilating shafts	1 2	1 2	7 0	—	7	1	14	2		
2	Ventilating shafts	1 0	1 0	7 0	—	5	1	10	2		
2	Bits	2 3	2 3	3 9	—	14	4	28	8		
2	„	2 3	2 3	3 4	—	12	4	24	8		
1	Ice-chest	3 10	2 0	2 0	—	—	—	15	7		
1	Filter	4 0	2 0	2 0	—	—	—	16	8		
2	„	4 6	4 0	2 0	—	36	18	72	36		
1	Mast	5 2	3 7	7 0	—	—	—	52	8		
1	„	3 4	3 4	7 0	—	—	—	58	8		
1	„	1 9	1 9	7 0	—	—	—	16	2		
1	Capstan	4 6	4 6	4 6	—	—	—	67	15		
1	„	4 6	4 6	4 9	—	—	—	72	15		
2	Fixed beams	3 0	1 6	0 6	—	2	4	4	8		
2	Stanchions	1 0	1 0	7 0	—	7	1	14	2		
2	„	0 10	0 10	7 0	—	4	½	8	1		
	Sundries, pipes, &c.	2 0	2 0	7 0	—	—	—	28	4		
6	Baths	6 3	1 10	2 0	—	—	11	—	66		
50	Beams	42 0	0 11	0 11	—	35	—	1,750	—		
142	Beds and bedding	6 0	2 0	0 8	—	8	12	1,136	1,704		
2	Ladders way	8 4	6 0	7 0	—	350	50	710	100		
1	„ „	8 4	10 0	7 0	—	—	—	583	83		
1	Surgery	18 3	10 6	7 0	—	—	—	1,341	191		
1	Shaft-engine room	20 0	13 0	7 0	—	—	—	1,820	260		
1	Shaft-engine room	23 6	11 4	7 0	—	—	—	1,864	266	11,534	3,109
										47,369	5,240
3	Gangways	26 8	5 6	5 6	—	—	—	—	—		

'I am indebted to Surgeon W. H. Steele, M.D., Army Medical Staff, and to Lieutenant W. H. Brown, Army Hospital Corps, for the very careful and accurate measurement of the hospital-deck (see preceding table).

'Supposing the maximum of beds (142) to have been utilised, the following were the dimensions:—

>Average cubic space each bed, 333·58.
>„ spherical „ „ 36·90.
>Total superficial area of ventilation, 446 feet.

'The convalescent deck, which communicates with the hospital and upper decks by trunked hatchways, is 100 feet 6 inches in length, by an average of 45 feet in width and 7 feet 6 inches in height, extending from the stern as far as the foremost part of the main mast, where a bulk-head (with two doors opening through) shuts it off from that part of the vessel occupied by the ship's company. It has two stern ports, 3 feet 2 inches in height and 2 feet 1 inch in width. Downcast ventilation is promoted by two large cowled tubes, and by two smaller tubes of the same kind proceeding to the orlop deck, but communicating with this deck by means of a small opening with a sliding shutter; and upcast ventilation is intended to be carried out by means of numerous orifices in the roof, opening into the iron boxes in the floor of the hospital-deck, which, as before stated, communicate through air-tight wooden boxes with the hollow masts. A similar arrangement exists in the floor of this deck for the purification of the orlop deck underneath. However admirable in theory this plan may be its practical efficacy is open to doubt.

'We notice here, as elsewhere, perforated zinc plates in the sides of the ship, communicating with the bilges below, and with the external air above through small louvred openings. The objection stated elsewhere to these plates applies with more force the lower we descend. An examination showed these plates to be inlets on the orlop deck, where they had

for this reason been pasted over by the occupants of s
cabins.

'At the stern part of the convalescent deck are situat
quarters of the non-commissioned officers and men
Army Hospital Corps, the former to port and the lat
starboard. Between the two are presses for the nava
military libraries. The latter, in addition to the regu
allowance of books, received so many contributions fror
vate sources in England and Ireland before leaving, tha
sides providing for our own wants, we were enabled to s
both light and serious literature to the invalids on boar
various transports leaving Cape Coast Castle for St. V
Cape de Verde Islands, and for England.

'Further forward on the port side were several small
partments, furnished with tables, and screened off by cu
during the day, which did duty during the day as office
the senior medical officer and lieutenant of orderlies.
night the curtains had to be unshipped and hammocks
over these tables, as during the latter part of our st:
Cape Coast Castle, and on the homeward voyage, every a
able spot was required for sleeping accommodation.

'Instead of 65 of the Army Hospital Corps, as was
nally intended, only 37 embarked at Portsmouth, a nur
that barely sufficed for the duties devolving upon the
when the hospital began to fill.

'A tabular form is appended showing the number of
grade which it is considered should be provided for the
ferent duties of a hospital-ship constituted like the "V
Emanuel."

'Number of Hospital Servants, &c., required for the Efficient Working of the Hospital Ship "Victor Emanuel."'

How employed	Staff-serjeant	Serjeants	Corporals	2nd corporals	Privates	Total
Serjeant-major (or acting rank)	1	—	—	—	—	1
Compounders	—	2	—	—	—	2
Steward	—	1	—	—	—	1
Assistant wardmasters	—	—	2	—	—	2
Clerk, principal medical officer	—	1	—	—	—	1
Clerk, captain of orderlies [1]	—	1	1	—	—	2
Pack stores	—	1	—	—	—	1
,, storeman	—	—	—	—	1	1
Steward's ditto	—	—	—	—	2	2
Barber	—	—	—	—	1	1
Carpenter and medical storeman	—	—	—	—	1	1
Tailor	—	—	—	—	1	1
To work laundry	—	—	1	—	6	7
Orderlies, hospital-deck	—	—	—	—	14	14
,, convalescent	—	—	—	—	3	3
,, sick officers	—	—	—	—	4	4
To replace casualties	—	1	2	2	6	11
Total	1	7	6	2	39	55

Section F.—*Passenger Steamers.*

These vessels are divided and classified in the following manner by the Board of Trade:—

I. Seagoing
{
1. Plying beyond home limits ('foreign-going ships').
2. Plying within home limits ('home-trade ships').
}

II. Excursion
{
3. Coasting within home limits (usually by daylight).
}

III. Rivers
{
4. Plying in partially smooth waters (rivers).
5. Plying in smooth waters (rivers and lakes).
}

[1] 'One exclusively for diets and stoppages.'

The owners, agents, or masters must take out correspon<!-- cut -->ing certificates, and special instructions are issued for t<!-- cut --> guidance of surveying officers, whose duty it is to ma<!-- cut --> declaration in every case of inspection that all the provisi<!-- cut --> of the Mercantile Marine Acts in relation to vessels so certif<!-- cut --> are fully carried out.[1]

(a) *Passenger Accommodation.*

The upper weather-deck and the upper surface of t<!-- cut --> poop, forecastle, and spar-deck, being exposed to the weath<!-- cut --> are never to be included in the measurements for passeng<!-- cut --> in foreign-going steamers; nor are the poop, round house, <!-- cut -->deck-house to be measured for passengers, unless they fo<!-- cut --> part of the permanent structure of the vessel; but they shou<!-- cut --> in all cases be railed round the top, to prevent children fr<!-- cut --> falling overboard.

Care should be taken that the means provided for ve<!-- cut -->tilation are sufficient to allow of a good supply of air in t<!-- cut --> event of the hatches being closed in bad weather. Pla<!-- cut --> ventilated by hatches only, or in which provision is not ma<!-- cut --> for a sufficient supply of air and light under all circumstanc<!-- cut --> should not be measured for passengers.

1. *Foreign-going Steamers* are to be measured as f<!-- cut -->lows:—

Saloon, or first-class: The number of properly construct<!-- cut --> fixed berths or sofas that are fitted determine the number <!-- cut -->passengers to be allowed, if sufficient light and ventilation is pr<!-- cut -->vided and a reasonable amount of floor-space. Second-clas<!-- cut --> The number is found in the same way as the first-class. T<!-- cut --> number of third-class passengers may be determined in li<!-- cut --> manner if berths are fitted; if not, the net area of the de<!-- cut --> (that is, after deducting all hatches and encumbrances) mult<!-- cut -->plied by the height between decks, and the product divid<!-- cut -->

---

[1] See *Instructions to Surveyors of Ships appointed by the Board of Tra*<!-- cut --> from which the selections here given have been taken.

by 72, gives the number to be allowed. Six feet between decks is little enough height.

The breadth of the deck is taken inside the water-way, or at the greatest tumble-home if the sides do tumble home.

When cargo or stones are carried in the space measured for passengers, one passenger is to be deducted for every 12 superficial feet of deck-space so occupied.

2. *Home-trade Ships.*—The deck-space set apart for deck or third-class passengers is always to be measured from abaft the windlass (as at present) to a mark which, in paddle-steamers, shall be placed over the shaft, and in other vessels shall be an arbitrary line marked vertically on the house or bulwarks amidships, or as near thereto as convenient. From this mark aft the deck-space is to be measured as far as the deck or third-class passenger accommodation extends, whether to a break or raised quarter-deck, to a poop, or the entire after-length of the deck to the wheel, as the case may be. The breadth for measurement shall be to a point which affords good and convenient foot-room.

Spaces on deck for first- or second-class passengers are to be measured in a similar way.

As each deck passenger is entitled to nine superficial feet of clear space, the whole area of the available part of the deck in square feet divided by 9 will give the number allowed to be carried in summer.

In the case of excursion (3) and river steamers (4 and 5) the superficial area available is divided by 3, 6, and 3 respectively, to obtain the legitimate number of passengers, only that the clear space of the after-saloon must be divided by 9 in all cases, and the two quotients added together.

(b) *Crew Space.*

The Act of 1867 (section 9) provides that every place in any ship occupied by seamen or apprentices and appropriated to their use 'shall contain a certain cubical space (72 cubic feet) and a certain superficial surface (12 feet) for each seaman.'

This place must be securely constructed, properly li[ghted,] ventilated, properly protected from weather and [as] far as possible shut off and protected from effluvi[a that] may be caused by bilge-water and cargo.

The Act does not specify that the space occupi[ed by] crew should be of any particular height, but pro[vides,] 'every such place shall be such as to make the place [fit] for the proper accommodation of the men who are to o[ccupy it.]

In relation to the question of passenger accom[modation,] the two following rules should be specially stated:

1. *Rule for determining the Superficial Area of a g[iven] space.*—First measure the whole middle length of [the space,] then divide it into several, say four, equal transverse [parts;] two extreme and three intermediate measurements [from side] to side. Next multiply the two extreme widths [by 1, the] second and fourth by 4, and the third by 2. N[ext mul-]tiply the sum of these products by one-third of the [common] interval between the widths. From this a deduction [is to be] made for hatches, ventilators, or encumbrances of [any kind.] For example, if the middle length is 30 feet, the [interval] between the breadths will be 7·5 feet, and one-thir[d of the] latter 2·5 feet. Further, let the successive widths b[e as fol-]lows, *in feet and decimals:*—

1. $2·2 \times 1 = 2·2$
2. $10·5 \times 4 = 42·0$
3. $18·5 \times 2 = 37·0$ } 204·7 the sum of products
4. $24·0 \times 4 = 96·0$ $\times 2·5$ (7·5⅓ common int[erval])
5. $27·5 \times 1 = 27·5$

10235
4094
———
511·75 gross area of floor.
−73·10 deductions.
———
438·65 clear area of floor.

12 square feet being allowed to each individual,
$438 \div 12 = 36$, the legal number of passengers.

DETERMINATION OF CUBIC SPACE. 231

2. *Rule for determining the Cubic Capacity of a given Deck-space.*—Having discovered the superficial area by the first rule, we have simply to multiply this by the height between decks.

For example, the clear area of the floor being 438·65, and the height between decks 6·5 square feet, 438 × 6·5 = 2847 the cubic capacity; 72 cubic feet being allowed to each individual,

$$2847 \div 72 = 39 \text{ persons.}$$

36, obtained by the former computation, being less than 39, would be accepted by preference.

The surveyor is enjoined to see that the place appropriated to crews is of sufficient height for men of ordinary stature to stand and move about in in an upright position—that is to say, at least 5 feet 6 inches between the floor and the under side of the beams—and also of such height that if the sleeping bunks are built in two tiers the bottom of the lower tier will be about 12 inches from the floor, and the bottom of the upper tier a sufficient distance from the bottom of the lower tier, as well as from the deck overhead.

For efficient ventilation it is suggested that an iron pipe with a revolving cowl (which in lower forecastles must be as high as the bulwarks) should be fitted at each end or side of the crew-space, so that while impure air escapes at one pure and fresh air will enter at the other, and thus establish a constant circulation. Where such means of ventilation is adopted, one of the ventilators should pass through the deck to at least the lower side of the beams. These pipes may be fitted to unship, and caps may be fitted over the holes when the forecastle is being worked. *Mushroom ventilators* may be fitted for ventilating deck-houses, but must not be fitted to forecastles unless they are at least 30 inches high for topgallant forecastles; but if fitted to lower forecastles they should be at least as high as the bulwarks. Mushrooms should be discouraged in every case except deck-houses.

Under existing circumstances, however, no particular p[lan]
can be insisted upon.

Scuttles, companions, and doors are not to be conside[red]
as efficient means of ventilating crew-spaces. There m[ust]
always be two ventilators in forecastles and deck-houses, a[nd]
in lower forecastles they should always come at least to [the]
upper side of the rail. When a topgallant forecastle is divid[ed]
by two fore and aft bulkheads, with an open space betwe[en]
them, and where cowl ventilators are objected to and can[not]
be conveniently fitted, two mushroom ventilators of sufficie[nt]
height may be fitted, placed a few feet abaft the breast-bea[m,]
each ventilator being a short distance on each side of t[he]
centre line of the ship. Openings of sufficient size must [be]
made in the top and bottom of the bulkheads, covered wi[th]
perforated zinc or other material, and fitted with slides or sm[all]
hinged doors at the top, opening inwards, and so arranged t[hat]
they can be opened or shut at any time, and fitted with su[it-]
able fastenings. If the entrances to the crew-spaces are [not]
in the open passage, jalousies or other ventilating openin[gs]
with slides to close them, must be fitted in the doors.

Drainage holes are usually made through the cant or coa[m-]
ing of upper forecastles or deck-houses, and it is part of [the]
surveyor's duty to see that they are of sufficient number a[nd]
size to admit of a ready escape of water, and that there a[re]
plugs with lanyards or chains attached fitted to each ho[le,]
and that in lower forecastles the scuppers are of such size a[nd]
are so situated that any water may be readily drained off.

When such drainage passes through a privy or other co[m-]
partment, it will be necessary to have a pipe for the drainage [to]
pass through such privy or compartment, with the ends ma[de]
perfectly tight through the cant or coaming of the forecastl[e.]

In many cases it will be found that lower forecastles ha[ve]
simply a hole bored through the floor in each after corner, a[nd]
that filth is allowed to drain through these holes, to adhere [to]
and accumulate upon the timbers, planking, and ceiling, a[nd]
to become stagnant amongst the chain-cables, coals, or ston[es]

which may be stored below. This should not be allowed. There should be proper scuppers or pipes leading from the floor of the forecastle to the limbers, so that the drainage may be readily pumped out by the ship's pumps.[1]

Such drainage pipes are also directed to be trapped efficiently, and every available precaution is to be taken to shut off all effluvia that may arise from the cargo or bilge-water and pervade the berth-place of the seamen.

(c) *Sanitary Provisions in relation to Water-closets, &c.*

Irrespective of the closets for cabin and saloon passengers, closets are to be provided for the *exclusive use of deck passengers* in the ratio of three for every two hundred deck passengers allowed by passenger certificate, and a fair proportion are to be allotted for the sole use of women and children, and so marked outside. Clear passages to these closets must always be maintained. In no case is a less number than two to be provided. These closets should be clean, well lighted, and well drained, and must be of sufficient height and size and effectually protected from weather and sea. In carrying this regulation into effect there need never be more than six water-closets set apart for the exclusive use of the deck or third-class passengers, whatever be the number of those passengers, provided there is one suitable and accessible urinal for the use of male passengers of the deck or third class.

The cubic contents of water-closets and urinals on deck in home-trade steamers are not to be included in the tonnage of the ships, provided each is permanently and conspicuously marked outside as 'water-closet' or 'urinal for deck passengers only.' It will be the duty of the surveyor to see that the privy accommodation is as required by the Act in the cases to which this provision of the Act applies, viz. those in which a

---

[1] So says the law, but the terrible results of such a provision, in case of yellow fever or any infectious malady visiting the ship, must be at once apparent to those who have had the least experience of the subtilty and pertinacity of specific causes, whatever their intrinsic nature may be.

deduction from tonnage is sought. In small vessels wi[th]
bulwarks it may be difficult to arrange an enclosed
such as may be easily fitted in larger vessels; but still a
seat, with a shoot or pan passing over or through th[e]
side, may be fitted, and this may be protected from the w[eather]
by a fixed or folding wooden or iron hood, with suitabl[e]
or doors to enclose the space when occupied. The su[rveyor]
should see that the privies are so built, fitted, and s[ecured]
that no unpleasant smell from them will enter the
occupied by the crew; that the seat and pan are s[o]
fixed; and that the scupper or shoot is so made, fitted,
and secured, and is in such condition, that it will effi[ciently]
answer the purpose for which it is intended.

If the spaces are certified for twenty men, there sho[uld be]
two privies, or one double one, and so on in proportion
number certified for.

(d) *Survey of Distilling Apparatus.*

In emigrant ships the distilling apparatus must be
to pieces every voyage, except in the case of steamers h[olding]
passenger certificates, which must be taken to pieces
once every six months, or oftener, if the surveyor
necessary. The water must be perfectly cool, pure,
drink immediately it is drawn off from the filter, w[hich]
be of suitable size and charged with animal charcoal.

The charcoal must be taken out, cleansed, and re[newed]
every voyage or six months as under the above conditi[ons]
reference to the other parts of the distilling apparatus.

SECTION G.—*The Influence of the Kind or Type of Ship [on] the Health of the Crew.*

There can be no doubt whatever that the health of a
will very largely depend upon the rating and character
ship to which they happen to belong.

The yearly ratio per 1,000 of sick invalided, D. to ho[spital,]
and D.D. in the four classes of vessels employed in the
terranean in 1834, 1835, and 1836 is shown in the foll[owing]

table.¹ The figures on the whole are in favour of ships of the frigate type:—

	Class of vessels	Ratio of sick	Invalided	D. to hosp.	D.D.
1	Ships of the line	1032·0	22·1	39·9	9·9
2	Frigates	892·7	17·5	30·0	8·0
3	Corvettes	1157·8	20·1	48·4	7·4
4	Steamers	1122·8	13·0	94·6	5·6

Dr. Leroy de Méricourt says,² 'In the months of November and December, 1859, 18 ships (13 screw and 5 sailing) left, carrying a small army destined to avenge the insult to the French and English flags at the mouth of the Peiho river. This flotilla anchored in the roads of Chefoo in July the following year.

'Whilst traversing the immense distance which separates France from the Celestial Empire, out of a total of 20,000 sailors and soldiers 109 died. The five sailing ships, with a total of 3,765, lost 45; they only dropped anchor once during the voyage.

'The steamers, out of a total of 8,117, had only 64 deaths to record; but then they called in at from three to seven ports.

'The difference of a third in the rate of mortality in favour of the steamers is undoubtedly owing to the increased speed with which the voyage was accomplished, and in great part to more frequently putting into port.' This authority further adds as an inference, 'Were the same transports by any accident reduced to their sails alone, they would no doubt have presented the same rate of sickness and mortality as the sailing frigates.' The last remark is applicable to our own Indian troopships so far as the time occupied in their voyages is concerned; for, should any untoward circumstance necessitate a delay of three weeks or a month over the usual period of transit to India, it would be attended with very serious con-

¹ See Dr. Saunders's *Hygienic Hints*, p. 34.
² *Modern Naval Hygiene*, translated by Dr. Buckley, S.S.R.N.

sequences. Thus evils which are usually cut short or rap
counteracted at the close of a moderate voyage would t
have full time to develop themselves, with a correspond
increase in the sickness and mortality.

SECTION H.—*Lead Poisoning in the French Navy and in con*
tion with the Treatment of the Double Bottoms of Iron Ship

Some of the more important hygienic regulations in
French navy are of comparatively recent date. Thus b
and basins for the use of stokers forward of the engine-r
were only established by order in 1855, and the reg
issue of lime-juice as an antiscorbutic only instituted in A
1856. A commission composed of three chief apotheca
was ordered to assemble at Toulon, and report on the 1
method of preparing and preserving lime-juice, and a p
was awarded for the process of adding 2 ounces of alcoho
a quart of lime-juice in its natural state.

Lead poisoning seems to have existed in some form
other in the French navy for a considerable time without
tinctive recognition, until the real nature and cause of
symptoms were thoroughly investigated by M. Lefèvre,
on his representation the Minister of Marine issued the foll
ing regulations, October 1858:—

'1. All pipes used in ships of war to convey fresh w;
are to be made of iron, except when the curves are so sharp
to positively require the employment of lead.

'2. The custom of coating the inside of water-tanks, as d
in certain dockyards, is strictly forbidden.

'3. The police regulations of February 1853, regarding
tinning of cooking utensils, will be strictly enforced in the na

'4. The suction-pipes in the main-deck tanks are to
manufactured of wood and readily removable.' These pi
were originally made of lead and of inconveniently large s
which latter defect was remedied by a special order. Ot
circulars, having a similar bearing, were issued from time
time, referring to cooking utensils, the tubes of condense

and the use of a charcoal filter devised by Professor Ortolan, which was intended to retain any particles of brass or lead that might be present.

Instead of red lead, which is so much used in our engineer's department, a substance named mastic or serbat, said to contain about 50 per cent. of sulphate of lead incorporated with gutta-percha, is used with great advantage in the French service. The general adoption of this and one or two other preparations of the kind is interfered with by patent rights, but it would be highly desirable that some substitute should be found to supplant red lead, so constantly used for preserving iron from superficial corrosion.[1] The consideration of this subject has led us insensibly to that of the double bottoms of iron ships, and the evils attending the periodical scraping and painting of their interior.

From the structure of the double bottoms of iron ships it will be easily understood that a constant chipping or scraping off old paint and putting on new in such a confined space must be trying to the health of the men so employed. The entrance to the double bottoms is through narrow manholes, of which there are several in different parts of the ship's inner lining. On entering a manhole, the men have to pass through similar openings from one cell or compartment to another, and while at work scraping or painting they maintain a position either on the back or front of the body, as there is not sufficient room to sit or kneel.

Independently of the presence of lead vapour, the air in these cells is often exceedingly impure, so as to render its inhalation injurious to the health.

While men are employed on this duty they are usually supplied with lime-juice as a pleasant acid drink and prophylactic, and air-pumps are kept constantly in use pumping fresh air down to them. There can be no doubt, however,

---

[1] It appears that a paint the basis of which is oxide of iron is now being used for painting the double bottoms of ships, but it has not yet been sufficiently tested or tried to form a just idea of its merits.

that a system of extraction, if properly arranged or provided for, would be far better than the plenum principle at present so much in vogue in the service; for, although a considerable amount of fresh air is forcibly introduced, stagnation under great pressure must happen in many places, while the foul air is simply diluted without effective removal.

The men should be medically examined from time to time, and on exhibiting any signs of poisoning, however slight, should be taken off the duty.

Special clothing should also be provided for this work, and a supply of fresh water given to the men, to wash themselves before putting on their ordinary dress. (*Anderson.*)

SECTION I.—*The importance of dryness and cleanliness of the ship to the health of the crew* is now so generally admitted that it would almost appear to be unnecessary to adduce further argument in support of it. Still, as single facts are worth heaps of theories, two or three good instances selected from many may be chosen for special reference. Thus, allusion may be made to the case of H.M.S. 'Centurion,'[1] which within a space of nine months lost 292 out of a crew of 506 from cold damp and scurvy, or a culpable neglect of hygienic principles. On the other hand, the sickness in Collingwood's flag-ship during double that time at sea scarcely ever exceeded one per cent., due attention having been paid to the cleanliness, dryness, and proper ventilation of ship, as well as the health and comfort of the crew.

The 'Vernon' and the 'Eagle,' two vessels of the same class, were both commissioned at the same time, and manned to the eastward, the one at Chatham and the other at Sheerness.

While off the river Plate the decks of the former were cleaned by the wet method, and those of the latter by dry stoning; the sick-list of the first exceeded that of the second

[1] Anson's flag-ship.

so much as to attract the observation of the officers of both ships. After the admiral shifted his flag to the 'Vernon,' however, the practice of wetting her lower deck was discontinued, and from that time the standard of health in the ship's company began to rise, until it gradually approximated that of the 'Eagle.'

In 1833 the 'Brisk' spent six months in the river Gambia, and six more in the Bights of Biafra and Benin, as the natives on the Barra shore were rather hostile, but, owing to the bygienic economy adopted, the health of the crew was exceptionally good the whole time.

Captain Murray, of the 'Valorous,' states that when, on his arrival in England in 1823, after two years' service amid the icebergs of Labrador, the ship was ordered to sail immediately for the West Indies, he proceeded to his station with a crew of 150 men, visited almost every island in the West Indies and many of the ports in the Gulf of Mexico, and, notwithstanding the sudden transition from extreme climates, returned to England without the loss of a single man. He also adds that every precaution was used, by lighting stoves between decks and scrubbing with hot sand, to ensure the most thorough dryness. When in command of the 'Recruit' gun-brig, which lay about nine miles from Vera Cruz, the same means preserved the health of the crew when other ships of war anchored around him lost from 20 to 50 men each; and although constant communication was maintained between the 'Recruit' and the other vessels, and all were exposed to the same external disease, no case of sickness occurred on board the 'Recruit.' This case has been quoted by Dr. Hunter, U.S.N., in his late excellent work on the hygiene of the naval and mercantile marine.

The experience of every thinking man afloat is quite to the effect that preventive medicine has hitherto been wofully neglected, but that great things are even now being effected through its instrumentality, and much more will be wrought by it in the future.

SECTION K.—*The Ill Effects of Sleeping on Shore in]*
Districts.

Dr. Saunders, R.N., remarks that 'in all malario and countries the inhabitants of ground floors are affected in a greater proportion than those of the upper and he instances a late sickly season at Barbadoes which 'the proportion of those taken ill with fev lower apartments of the barracks exceeded that of t by one-third throughout the whole course of the epid

To this might be added that the mortality amongst officers at the naval hospital, Port Royal, Jamaica, wl at one time very considerable, has been reduced to a since their quarters were raised upon arches, thus r them from the more direct influence of the ground ai fact, however, must not be confounded with the case ings upon high ground as compared with those h relatively lower position, when both are, so to speak, into continuity by a common system of drainage. U former circumstances fever is much more likely to veloped, as we commonly see at Malta, for example. other hand, comparing one site with another having n connection with it, the higher ground will in general salubrious. Now, it has been abundantly proved tl larious emanations are more vigorous and potent a than by day, and also that they are largely absorbed cepted by an intervening sheet of water. It is alway therefore, in sickly districts to sleep in a boat at some from the shore than on the banks of a river, and still if possible, to return to the ship before nightfall. duces the following interesting case :—

The 'Phœnix' ship of war was returning (1766) fr coast of Guinea with her officers and men in perfect until after having touched at St. Thomas'. Here ne the officers went on shore, and sixteen out of the num mained several nights on the island. Every one of tho slept on shore contracted fever, and thirteen out of the sixteen died.

The rest of the crew, consisting of 280 men, went in parties of twenty or thirty on shore in the daytime, and rambled about the island, hunting, shooting, and so on, but they returned to the ship at night, and not one of those who so returned suffered the slightest indisposition. Exactly similar results occurred the following year with the same ship, at the same place, when she lost eight men out of sixteen who had imprudently remained all the night on shore during the sickly season, while the rest of the ship's company, who, after spending the greater part of the day on shore, always returned to their vessel before nightfall, continued in perfect health.

In May and June 1792 one of the principal causes of disease prevalent in the fleet at Jamaica was the watering duty, which was carried on at Rock Fort. It was the practice of many ships to leave the water casks on shore all night with men to watch them, and many were seized with fever of a bad type, which was fatal in some instances; but the ships that followed a different practice were a little longer watering, but saved the lives of their men. Even the negroes are susceptible of this fever when engaged on the same duty.

In this connection the case of the 'North Star' may be mentioned as showing the prophylactic power of quinine in relation to malarious disease. Twenty men and one officer belonging to this ship were employed on boat-service at Sierra Leone. They all took wine and bark with the exception of the officer, and he was the only individual who was seized with fever, the rest of the party having enjoyed an immunity. Futhermore, in the year 1844 two boats were sent from the 'Hydra' to examine the Sherbro river; the whole of the men were supplied with bark and wine, and not one of them was taken ill, while the whole of the gig's crew, with the exception of the captain, who were similarly exposed for two days only without being supplied with the prophylactic, contracted fever of a dangerous character.

To complete this general idea of the more important hygienic precautions connected with ships, the necessity of running into a colder latitude immediately on the first appearance yellow fever on board may be noticed with one or two cases point. This has now become so much a matter of fact a duty that nothing but the most imperative service requirements should be permitted to oppose it.

When the 'Vestal' was at Port Royal, Jamaica yellow fever appeared amongst the crew, and did not cease although she was shifted from the inside to the quays on the other side of the harbour, nor until she had gone far beyond the precincts of the island and entered the 27th degree of north latitude on her way to Bermuda. The crew of the same vessel, although not the same men (she having been paid off and recommissioned) were again attacked by fever whilst cruising among the windward islands of the West Indies in the latter part of 1839. Instead of running at once to the northward, she proceeded to Carlisle Bay, where she remained a fortnight. During that time the disease evidently increased in malignancy and carried off a considerable number of men. She was then directed to proceed to the northward, and again the disease disappeared in a few days after they had crossed the tropic. The ship's company of the 'Vesuvius' were promptly relieved of an invasion of yellow fever by her being ordered immediately from Sacrificios, where it was contracted, to Halifax Nova Scotia.

DIVISION III.

REMEDIAL OR CORRECTIVE HYGIENE.

CHAPTER I.

'THIS subject,' as already stated, 'embraces attention to all internal sources of disease that may exist on board ship, or such as may have been introduced from without demanding correction or removal.'

Under the first clause would naturally come: 1st, the correction of bilge effluvia; 2ndly, the wholesome conservancy of water-closets, heads, and bow-galleries, and in connection with these the use of antiseptics and deodorants; while under the second clause we have to consider—1st, the segregation of the sick on the first appearance of infectious or contagious disease; and 2ndly, the use of disinfectants and other means under such circumstances.

SECTION A.—*The Treatment of Bilges and Bilge Effluvia.*

When a ship is newly commissioned, the bilges usually present a deceptive appearance of cleanliness, and it is common to say that you might eat your breakfast off the keelson. A few hours at sea, however, will dispel this illusion, and if the accumulation of water, which is inevitable, should extend beyond the influence of the pump-suckers, stagnation, decomposition, and offensive odours will follow one another in quick succession.

In modern ships the flooring of the square or central body is so flat through a considerable extent that, even though the pump-tube may reach the bottom of the well, considerable lodgments of stagnant water remain in the most suitable condition not only for rapid decomposition, but for the free evolution of the offensive results of this change.

If the lines of the ship admit of the complete flow of water from all points into the pump-well, and the latter is kept free from the accumulation of cotton-waste and all other refuse that may choke the grating of the pump, even a chronic leak in such a ship may be looked upon as salutary. Hence the old adage that a 'leaky ship is a sweet one.' This was certainly the case with H.M.S. 'Herald' (Captain, now Admiral Sir H. M. Denham, F.R.S.) during a nine years' commission in the South Seas. A difference of opinion, however, must exist on all debatable subjects, and Dr. Joseph Wilson, of the United States navy, in his excellent work on 'Naval Hygiene,' remarks that he has 'had the misfortune to be on board a vessel in which it was attempted to imitate the leaky ship in this particular, by introducing sea-water every day and pumping it out again. The evil was horribly aggravated, and, so far as I have been able to learn, was not effectually subdued afterwards during a cruise of four years.' The cases cited, however, were very different, and a permanent lodgment had, no doubt, by some means taken place in that noticed by Dr. Wilson.

Should accumulations of water take place in the fore or after cant bodies, the application of a special pump should be made, and the timbers dried up as soon as possible.

Chips and shavings of wood, remaining after dressing the timbers inboard, should be carefully removed whenever they can be reached; but unhappily they are often retained in crevices from which even the most assiduous use of the bilge chain or rope cannot effect their removal. They thus not only undergo decomposition themselves, but materially assist in setting up the same changes in the bilge-water in which they are immersed. The decay of vegetable matter, which would, in stagnant fresh water, evolve light carburetted hydrogen, is, in this case, attended with the production of sulphuretted hydrogen at the expense of the sulphates contained in the sea-water. Now, as this latter will take up about three times its own bulk of sulphuretted hydrogen, the gas further evolved must be delivered into the air-space above it. When sea-water has been long pent up in wooden casks as ballast, serious illness and even fatal results have been recorded as arising from the escape of foul air on removal of the bung. Whether such effects may be attributable to the inhalation of sulphuretted hydrogen alone, but in a highly concentrated state, or to some other but unknown concomitant principles, has not been determined. It is certain, however, that, although that gas is known to be very fatal to horses and dogs, human beings are much more tolerant of it within certain limits.

In the process of washing out the bilges it is evidently a waste of any disinfectant to mix it first with the bilge-water and then immediately pump it into the sea. It would be much better to carry the pumping as far as it is practicable, flush again with sea-water, and finally, after having pumped this out, add the disinfectant.

SECTION B.—*Conservancy, Water-closets, Heads and Bow-Galleries, Deodorants and Antiseptics.*

In the construction of water-closets for ships' use the simpler the whole arrangement is the better. Much woodwork or boxing-up is objectionable. The fall is always good, and the water supply, with a little attention, may be plentiful enough. In most instances, however, deodorants and antiseptics cannot be altogether dispensed with. A small portion of the permanganate of potash may be dissolved in the water of the cistern, and thus, at a trifling cost, an excellent deodorant is always at hand. When required, carbolic acid as an antiseptic may be used immediately after the per[...] with great advantage.[1] If, on the contrary, the car[...] should be used first, it will not only fail as a deodorant its[...] but it will materially interfere with the action of the [...] manganate in this respect.

It is scarcely necessary to describe what is known as *head* of a ship in the more usual sense of the word. In old wooden ships it occupied a very considerable space; [...] since the complete, or almost complete, abolition of the k[...] of the head, and the remarkable configuration of the stem [...] modern ships, the fore part of the topgallant forecastle [...] been turned to account for the accommodation of the cr[...] The use of long collapsible canvas shutes is for several cog[...] reasons objectionable, even where this system is still per[...] tuated. The permanganate of potash and carbolic acid m[...] also be used, in the manner already described, to keep t[...] locality sweet. In modern ships, as a rule, the *head* has b[...] superseded by a much better arrangement known as *b[...] galleries*, by which the disagreeable effect of the old syste[...] especially with a head-wind, is entirely obviated.

The accompanying drawings (Plate XXVIII., fig. [...] A, B, and C) respectively show a front elevation uncovered, [...] athwart-ship section, and the covering-house of this sche[...] in its primitive form, as carried out in H.M.S. 'Egmo[...] In other cases a round shot, with a chain attached als[...] acts as a valve, so as to hold water pumped in while [...] apposition, and permit of being raised for the periodi[...] removal of the contents.

Having thus far noticed some of the principal intrin[...] sources of discomfort and illness on board ship, we may n[...] profitably enter more fully into the subject of correcti[...] agents, named antiseptics, deodorants, and disinfectants.

---

[1] Dr James Lilburne, R.N., has invented an ingenious arrangement effecting this purpose by simply pulling up the handle in the ordin[...] way.

BOW-GALLERY OF H.M.S. 'EGMONT.' 247

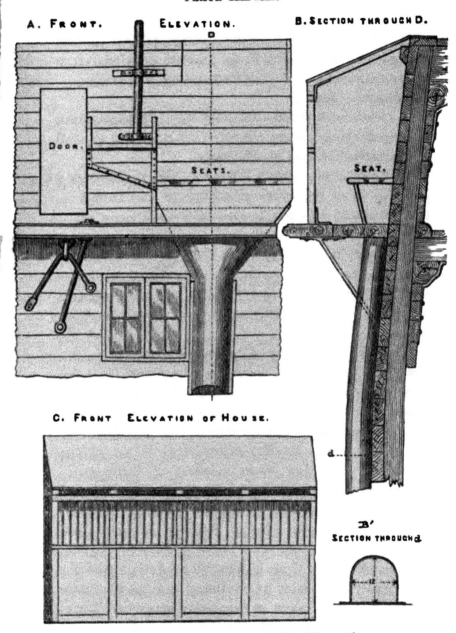

Fig. 40.—Bow-Gallery of H.M.S. 'Egmont.'

Though a better example might be taken from a more modern ship, this will answer the purpose sufficiently without going into minor details.

has been already said that much difference of opi
exists, even amongst medical men, as to the precise
of these terms.

1. *Antiseptics are* chemical agents which prevent
position of organic structures, whether animal or v
by forming a chemical combination with one or
constituents (*Royle*).

2. *Deodorants* oxidise the products of decomposit
recting offensive odours already produced, and tend
vert putrefaction into simple decay.

3. *Disinfectants* absorb certain specific products of
position, or of the effete principles of organic life,
thus supposed to exert a corrective influence on th
matters of infection.

It must be borne in mind that any one of thes
applied to corrective agents can only bear reference
most distinguishing property, for no substance can b
be purely or restrictedly antiseptic, deodorant, o
fectant.

Alcohol is certainly a powerful antiseptic, on
account it is used for anatomical preparations; but
from being a deodorant, it is the ordinary vehicle
fumes, which it preserves in all their integrity. M
but little can be said of its disinfecting qualities.
ganate of potash, on the other hand, is an instan
deodoriser, especially where sulphide of hydrogen
cerned, and by its oxidising property may also be assu
be disinfectant, but its antiseptic power is small i
parison with that of alcohol, chloride of zinc, or c
acid.

The chloride of zinc, or Burnett's solution, was fo
years the disinfectant in ordinary use in the nav
accidents with it were of frequent occurrence, chief
ing from the absence of any definite odour and its
form.

The annual allowance was as follows :—

ANTISEPTICS, DEODORANTS, AND DISINFECTANTS. 249

For first-rate	.	.	. 224 lbs.	
,, second ,,	.	.	. 224 ,,	In all climates the quantity may be extended with the approval of the captain on the application of the medical officer.
,, third ,,	.	.	. 168 ,,	
,, fourth ,,	.	.	. 168 ,,	
,, fifth ,,	.	.	. 112 ,,	
,, sixth ,,	.	.	. 84 ,,	
,, sloops .	.	.	. 56 ,,	
,, cutters	.	.	. 28 ,,	

By Circular No. 37S, August 31, 1867, chloride of zinc was superseded by carbolic acid in the crystalline form, and it was calculated that a supply of 1 lb. per man would, under ordinary circumstances, be sufficient for a year; but the quantity might be doubled in tropical climates and where fevers are prevalent.

Directions as to the Use of Carbolic Acid.

'The crystallised carbolic acid is soluble in water, and 1 lb. to every 5 gallons of water is sufficient for deodorising purposes.

'The bottles, when opened, should be placed in the water for about an hour (according to its temperature), 4, 8, or 12 of the bottles, which contain a pound, being used for a tank of either 20, 40, or 60 gallons. The bottles should be cleared of all adhering crystals, and the solution should be well stored previous to use.

'A solution of this strength is applicable for deodorising purposes, and may be freely sprinkled about decks, or urinals, or any place in the ship where malaria exists; and being neither alkaline, acid, nor corrosive, no injury need be apprehended to wood, iron, metal, or clothes. In a concentrated form the acid acts as a caustic; but its action on the skin may readily be arrested by rubbing with sweet oil.

'From experiments made, by order of the French Government, by MM. Forestier and Marin, all decay of wood arising from moisture or insects is entirely arrested by the application of carbolic acid. The solution may, therefore, be applied to the bilges when fetid bilge-water exists, or be poured into air-openings or any place emitting and unpleasant odours.

'To prevent any effluvium arising from the decomposition of organic matter in the bilge-water, add 1 gallon of solution to every 50 gallons of bilge-water, and whenever effluvia arise therefrom add fresh carbolic acid as may be necessary. The water so treated may be used with safety in the boilers so far as carbolic acid is concerned, as it will not exert an injurious action on any metal, leather, or indiarubber valves.

'Chamber utensils in the sick-bay may be deodorised by about half a pint of the solution.

'When small-pox, typhoid fevers, &c., occur, the spread of contagion may be prevented by a proper use of this disinfectant. In such cases the acid should be used in the crystalline form, viz. 1 lb. of the crystals to 5 or more lbs. of wet sand, placed in shallow vessels in various parts of the sick wards.

'In case of any epidemic breaking out on board, the same mixture is to be used as a sanitary precaution throughout the ship.

'These "Directions" will serve to indicate the uses to which this chemical ingredient (of recent introduction) may be applied; and, from its properties, there is every reason to anticipate that, judiciously applied, it will prove of great value in promoting the sanitary condition of the ships, especially in warm climates; but it is of importance that medical officers should study its action, and make themselves acquainted with the circumstances and cases where its use may be beneficially resorted to.'

It may be stated here that other disinfectants, chloride of lime and permanganate of potash, affect not only the gaseous products of putrefaction, but all organic matters with which they may come in contact; whilst carbolic acid, on the contrary, merely destroys the causes of putrefaction without acting on the organic substances. Thus the former agents mentioned deal with effects, so to speak, whereas carbolic acid exerts itself upon the causes of those natural changes; and it is to this circumstance its remarkable antiseptic power is attributable. With the view of comparing the properties of carbolic acid with those of several other agents in corresponding proportions, a series of experiments were made with a putrid infusion of linseed meal swarming with bacteria, and the results were briefly as follows :—

1. *Chloride of lime* destroyed the putrefactive odour, and the bacteria were precipitated in flocculent masses with their gelatinous matrix.

2. *Carbolic acid* subdued the putrefactive odour, while the bacteria themselves remained quite free in the field, though exhibiting but little movement, and in many instances became punctate or rounded.

3. The *permanganate of potash* acted in the same way as the carbolic acid, but the activity of the bacteria suffered less change up to this stage.

4. *Cupralum* also destroyed the odour and precipitated the bacteria in fleaky masses, leaving, however, some few inactive ones in the field.

5. In the case of *chloralum*, both liquid and in the form of powder, the microscopical characters were similar to those stated in the cupralum experiment, but the odour was affected only to a small extent.

6. Finally, the *universal disinfecting powder* in the proportion used did not seem to correct the odour, nor check the activity of the bacteria to any very appreciable extent.[1]

Odour	Bacteria destroyed or wholly precipitated	Bacteria partially precipitated; some free and active	Bacteria free and active
Destroyed . .	Chloride of lime	—	—
" . .	—	Cupralum	—
Suppressed .	—	—	Carbolic acid
" .	—	—	Condy's fluid
Feebly affected	—	Chloralum (liquid)	—
" "	—	Chloralum (solid)	—
" "	—	—	—
" "	—	Universal disinf.	—

[1] In subsequent experiments, however, better results were obtained.

The foregoing statements may be more concisely expre[ssed] in the preceding table.

If the total destruction of bacteria and their reproduc[tive] energy be regarded as the most reliable evidence of disinf[ect]ing power in accordance with our present attainments in [this] difficult inquiry, the agents above tabularised are given in [the] order of their importance. On the other hand, while, un[der] ordinary circumstances, the impressions of the olfactory se[nse] awaken the apprehension of danger, some of the virulent m[or]bific matters or influences are so subtle as to be quite im[per]ceptible to that faculty. On reviewing the table we find t[hat] the correction of the offensive odour and the suppressio[n or] destruction of the *bacteria* do not hold that close correla[tion] that might be supposed *à priori*. But here is in truth t[he] nice line of demarcation between deodorisation and disin[fec]tion; and until it can be shown that mere deodorants, [so] called, do not at the same time correct morbific agents ot[her] than corporeal bacteria, we should do well to be guided by [the] premonitions of the sense of smell.

The nitrate of lead, or Ledoyen's fluid, has been l[ong] known as a disinfectant, or rather deodorant, for ships' bil[ges,] its effect upon sulphuretted hydrogen being always reli[able] when fairly tried, but Dr. Goolden very recently called [the] attention of the Admiralty to this important agent from [his] own experience of its practical utility. Fleet-Surgeon Eust[ace] made some successful experiments with it, which led him [to] suggest its substitution for the permanganate of potash. [He] recommended a strong solution, i.e. 10 oz. to the gallon, [a] pint of which was to be added to 40 gallons of sea-w[ater] = 1·25 oz. to the pint = 546·8 grs., which being added [to] 40 gallons = 13·6 grains per gallon, instead of 10 grains, recommended by Dr. Goolden, whose formula is :—

Nitrate of lead	30 grs.
Chloride of sodium	120 ,,
Water	3 gals.

This strength was found to be inadequate for the correcting a moderately strong solution of sulphuretted hydrogen, but, on adding three or four times that amount of the agent, it proved to be most effective, throwing down the sulphide of lead as a dense black precipitate.

Three gallons of Dr. Goolden's strength were experimented with at Netley in various ways, and it was found necessary to double it to get a more satisfactory result. The sulphuretted hydrogen was then corrected, and a saline smell substituted for the cadaveric odour.

The chemical change resulting from the admixture of nitrate of lead with chloride of sodium, and of the resulting chloride of lead with sulphuretted hydrogen, may be thus tabularised :—

$$\text{Nitrate of lead} \begin{cases} \overbrace{\text{Nitric acid} \quad \text{Lead}}^{\text{Nitrate of lead}} \\ \underbrace{\text{Sodium} \quad \text{Chlorine}}_{\text{Sodium chloride}} \end{cases} \text{Chloride of lead}$$

$$\text{Hydrochloric acid} \begin{cases} \overbrace{\text{Chlorine} \quad \text{Lead}}^{\text{Chloride of lead}} \\ \underbrace{\text{Hydrogen} \quad \text{Sulphur}}_{\text{Sulphuretted hydrogen}} \end{cases} \text{Sulphide of lead}$$

Hofmann has shown that chloride of zinc acts especially upon the sulphide of ammonium instead of the sulphuretted hydrogen.

It is highly probable, however, that the use of this agent would be even more injurious to iron ships than the permanganate of potash.

The *terebene preparations* deserve some notice in this connection; the principal articles are the following :—

1. *Terebene Powder, Var. A.*—A green-coloured powder, with the odour of pine-wood, partially soluble in water, a whitish sediment forming in a transparent rich green fluid, and the whole becoming opaque by mechanical mixture when shaken.

2. *Terebene Powder, Var. B.*—A yellow powder rese
damp mustard, with a pine-wood odour, partially sol
water, a whitish sediment forming in a transparent
yellow fluid, and the whole becoming opaque and of
yellow hue on being shaken.

Under the microscope var. B presents what would
to be terebene in minute globules surrounded by the
lar matter of the powder with which it is mixed;
the case of var. A these globules were not apparent,
pulverulent matter is more minutely divided.

3. *Terebene Liquid.*—A dense rich brown
fluid, having the odour of turpentine, and quite inso
water.

4. *Sanitas.*—A limpid transparent fluid of a light
tint, like that of lime-juice, having the odour of new
wood and being freely miscible with water.

Abstract of Experiments.

10 per cent. solutions of the above agents were respe
added in different proportions to 10 cc. of beef i
swarming with bacteria. 12 preparations thus obtaine
separately examined under the microscope, and the o
merit in subduing the bacteria was as under :—

1. Terebene powder, var. A.
2. „   „   ., B.
3. „   liquid.
4. Sanitas.

Aften ten days the bacteria had recovered much of
activity in the sanitas vessel, and a large amount of
was present in the field.

In the terebene vessel the bacteria were largely tak
by the oily substance at the bottom, but they were

active, and in some instances excursive in the clearer parts or intervals.

In terebene powder, var. B, the bacteria exhibited very little activity, and none were excursive.

In terebene powder, var. A, on the other hand, motion was only just recognisable, the bacteria being matted together or precipitated.

In a second series of experiments 10 per cent. solutions were added to 20 cc. of strong-smelling sewage matter, in bottles with hollow stoppers armed with moistened lead-papers and numbered in the above order.

In 1 and 2 (terebene powders A and B) no perceptible effect was produced, while in 3 and 4 (terebene liquid and sanitas) they were darkly coloured.

In another bottle with 20 cc. of sewage matter alone but little change had taken place in the lead-paper.

A similar set of experiments was then made, using, however, papers moistened with Nessler's fluid instead of acetate of lead, and in all but little change had taken place, except in the bottle with sewage matter alone, in which the Nessler paper was highly coloured.[1]

Tested by the sense of smell in both experiments, the rather agreeable odour of pine so greatly masked the offensiveness of the fæculent matter as to render it difficult to determine the relative effectiveness of the four agents; but several opinions were in favour of the order being just as above given in relation to their effect on bacteria.

Although the terebene liquid has taken a superior place to sanitas, the varnish-like plasticity and insolubility would effectually preclude its use in many cases in which sanitas would be quite harmless, on account of its complete solubility in water and the ease with which it can be washed away

---

[1] These facts would seem to show that at least some part of the sulphuretted hydrogen was in combination with ammonia, and liberated, just as has been observed in the case of carbolic acid, by the affinity of the terebene preparations for ammonia.

after having been applied to bedding, clothing
although Terebene powder var. A has taken
rapidly destructive effect upon iron wire, with
of copper, would preclude its use on a large
ships.

Section C.—*Infected Ships.*

To quote from the Report of the Havana C
Yellow Fever, ' the annals of medicine
many vessels which, once infected, have
Cape Horn, on to the frozen regions of
infection apparently destroyed—to reapp
renewed activity, on the return of such ve
afterwards, to regions of elevated tempera
ally arises the question, Under what conditions
regarded as ' infected ' ?

It is admitted on all hands that the simple
cases of yellow fever on board cannot with rigid
the ship this character, ' unless further cases sha
developed on board within the time, say six day
attacked had opportunity to become infected by
thing, or person outside the ship.'

A palpable instance of an infected ship is
' Niagara,' of which Dr. Chaillé, Chairman of
Commission, writes under date of July 24,
" Niagara," of a line of steamships from New Yor
left this harbour about July 9, and arrived a
Quarantine with one or more cases of yellow
steamer left New York on the 19th, and arrived in
of Havana on the morning of the 24th, having
cases of yellow fever, one of which was attacked
of the 19th, and the other on the 24th, before the v
the harbour. These facts indicate that the " Niag
infected.' From Dr. D. M. Burgess the followin
obtained relative to the ' Niagara ': ' The steamer
is a first-class iron passenger steamer, and made

in June 1876. Notwithstanding due cleanliness, &c., she went into New York with yellow fever on board on her fourth trip, about September 1876, and has had cases on board every season since that time.' These facts were obtained from the captain, and are attributed by him and Dr. Burgess to faulty construction and continued infection, which both gentlemen deem remediable. The result of this faulty structure is, that some two inches of bilge water cannot be pumped out. Two cases developed upon her last trip from New York, prior to her entering the harbour of Havana.

The following example, as a type of many that may be submitted for the opinion of the naval hygeist, may be worth inserting here :—

The iron ship ' Jorawur ' was unladed by Lascars at the port of Guadaloupe, where she remained, apparently unnecessarily, for about two months, and in consequence suffered an invasion of yellow fever, commencing on July 12, 1880, and terminating on September 7 following. There were fifteen or sixteen cases altogether, and four deaths, two in harbour and two at sea.

Assuming that September 7 was the date of the last case (though this has not been definitely stated) it is clear that this and at least some of the preceding ones had been contracted on board, either by taking it (1) from individuals previously affected, or (2) from the ship itself having thus become contaminated. From the study of the particulars, however, as to the latter possibility, it would appear that the invasion, which had undoubtedly been primarily derived from the shore, had simply run its course, without necessarily implying any contamination of the ship. Nevertheless, the question has arisen whether the vessel above named, after thorough cleansing and fumigation, and the lapse of many months, could be regarded as a safe transport for passengers from Calcutta to the West Indies.

Weighing well all the available information connected with the outbreak, a favourable report was made under two heads,

258   REMEDIAL OR CORRECTIVE HYG

viz.: (1) the facts of experience given abov
the question one of serious importance, and
relation to this special case; fairly indicating
no sufficient proof to show that the ship its
infected, and (b) the consequent improbability
of the disease without fresh exposure to infec

The following favourable conditions were

1. The ship being constructed of iron, not
fact that the 'Niagara' was also an iron ship.

2. The cases having been altogether confin
house.

3. Their complete insulation, and the imm
of excreta, which were always thrown ove
delay.

4. Besides all necessary attention to clea
siduous use of disinfecting agents.

5. The further disinfection and sulphur fun
ship conducted by the health officers of Trini
sequently gave her pratique.

6. The complete immunity of the officers,
were attacked, and the arrest of the disease
crew, none of whom were attacked after the o
communication with its specific cause were tal
would most probably be otherwise if any inte
evil had been developed and persistent in tl
practical proof is perhaps the most cogent of
be perceived from the facts already quoted, th
impossible to give a medical guarantee of exen
the support of such practical proof. In the cae
awur,' however, it was ruled to be more prud
another vessel for the purpose intended.

CHAPTER II.

SECTION A.—*Segregation of the Sick on the First Appearance of Infectious Disease.*

In case of infectious or contagious disease breaking out on board ship, the speedy removal of the first case to hospital or to the shore is the primary object to be attained. Should no hospital or suitable place exist ashore for the reception of the sick, an insulated spot should be chosen, or one on the mainland, as distant as possible from human resort, and a strict quarantine should be instituted. A tent is the most convenient erection that can be made in an emergency of this kind, and with a little attention to external conditions it may be made to suit almost any climate. On the other hand, if the ship is at sea, our resources are so far cut off, and we must effect the isolation of the case from the ship's company as completely as may be practicable. The most convenient part of the ship for this purpose is perhaps under the topgallant forecastle, or the foremost part of the main deck, which should be screened off with canvas, all access being strictly prohibited by placing a sentry near the spot, with the necessary instructions to be transmitted to his relief.

In a passenger steamer belonging to one of the public companies, a case of small-pox has been safely brought home in one of the boats hanging over the ship's side covered with an awning. The passengers knew nothing about it, and no ill effects whatever supervened. When a ship is in motion her bow cleaves the air as well as the water, and any noxious principles that may pass into the air outside the hammock

netting, especially to leeward, hanges off without c
board.

A good strong solution of carbolic acid should
in the bed-pan or other vessel before it is used by th
and some more should be added immediately a
thorough mixture with the evacuations should b
before they are thrown overboard, and care shoul
that portions of the discharges do not remain
patient's body, bedding, or clothing. Pieces of f
saturated with carbolic acid should be freely suspend
the hammock or cot of the sick person, and between
the canvas screen, while the same disinfectant
largely sprinkled about in the immediate vicinity
always been found that cases of yellow fever are m
factorily treated on deck in the open air, or only
awning spread, than either between decks or in the
a hospital; and as the virulence and the consequ
effect of this disease are much increased, in tem
ranging above 72° Fah., the medical officer should
this matter to the captain, that he might take immedi
to run into a colder latitude.

This measure will always be justified by the a
at home unless some very imperative duty shall p
In all cases of specific disease occurring on board s
advisable that the dejections should be thrown direc
board rather than down through the sick-bay water
no matter what the apparent guarantee of disinfection
In the Royal Victoria Hospital at Netley typhoid st
separately dealt with, and never permitted to er
common drainage system, and not a single case of
has ever taken its origin in the institution itself. E
the converse of this are of too common occurrence
special notice here.

SECTION B.—*Disinfection of the Bedding, Clothing, and effects of the Sick.*

The articles and appointments of the sick requiring disinfection may be conveniently divided into two classes:—

1. *Linen and Washing Apparel.*
2. *Woollens, Bedding, and Clothing that cannot be Washed.*

The first class may be treated by immersion in a mixture of the clear solutions of chloride of lime or soda with water, in the proportion of one or two ounces to the gallon. Another simple method is to plunge them in boiling water, and afterwards boil them in the washing water.

It is usual to submit the articles included in the second class to the action of dry heat (210° to 250° F.) where this is possible, with suitable apparatus at hand; but where this cannot be done, as on shipboard, we must have recourse to the natural disinfecting process of prolonged exposure to air, sun, and rain.

Both classes of articles may, however, be subjected to the action of disinfectant gases, either specially applied, or when used in a more general way, to fumigate the ship itself.

It must be remembered as a rule that the length of exposure either to the action of heated air or of disinfectant gases, must bear an inverse relationship to the degree of temperature in the one case, and the degree of concentration in the other.

Thus, for example, an exposure of four hours' duration at a comparatively low temperature would be equivalent in its effect to one hour's exposure at a much higher temperature. We are not yet in a position to say what the precise relationship may be; this is no doubt a purely experimental question, and may be settled at some future time.

262 MANUAL OF CORRECTIVE HYGIENE

SECTION C.—*The Fumigation of Ships with Disin*

The more important disinfectant gases availab
fumigation of ships are:—
1. Sulphurous acid.
2. Nitrous acid.
3. Chlorine.

1. *Sulphurous Acid.*—Sulphur fumigation
very early times for disinfection. This is clearly
the often quoted passage from Pope's 'Homer':—

> 'Bring sulphur straight, and fire,' the monarch cries
> She heard, and at the word obedient flies.
> With fire and sulphur, cure of noxious fumes,
> He purged the walls and blood-polluted rooms.

The plan here resorted to is perhaps the simplest means of evolving sulphurous acid. 1 ounce of sul yield ·732 of a cubic foot of the gas, so that nearly must be used to produce 10 cubic feet. Now when sider Mr. Letheby's proportion of ½ oz. of sulphur 10, or 50 oz. for every 1,000 cubic feet of space, require 1 cwt. of sulphur to fumigate a space of cubic feet, or one deck only of a very ordinary shi proportion, 3·66 per cent., is very much greater than monly supposed to be necessary; but actual exp seems to bear it out, and show that it cannot be reduc than one-third for real efficiency. We are much indebt Baxter for determining by his own experiments, and out so clearly, that carbolic acid and the ordinary disin used after the manner commonly suggested in book very doubtful efficacy, only inspiring a fancied secur the same may be said of fumigation. To burn one ounces of sulphur in a pipkin, with the hope of disin a space of more than 600 or 800 cubic feet, is a mistake, and only creating a nuisance for little or no benefit whatever.

Thus Dr. Lind speaks of lighting 'a number of charcoal fires in different places,' upon each of which 'a handful or two of brimstone' is to be thrown. 'The steam which arises (sulphurous acid) should be closely confined by shutting the ports and hatchways from morning till evening; no person in the meantime being allowed to go below, nor for some time after opening the ports and hatchways, to the end that the steam may be dispersed.'

Very recently a lamp for burning the bisulphide of carbon has been introduced by Messrs. Price and Co., but for the reasons above given this contrivance would be only suitable for fumigation on a small scale, as in the case of officers' cabins or other circumscribed spaces on board ship. Moreover, the storage of sulphur in bulk is attended with much less danger than that of the highly inflammable fluid in question.

The celebrated Sir Roger Curtis has handed down to us a most valuable description of the system adopted by himself in the case of his own ship in which a malignant fever had broken out. The account is so full of instructive matter that it may be studied with much profit by all Naval officers. Though sulphur fumigation was the chief means employed, the precautionary general hygienic measures taken are equally applicable to the use of other gaseous disinfectants.

He commences by observing that 'as seamen have great reluctance in complaining when they find themselves but slightly indisposed, and as it is very material that infected persons should be as speedily as possible removed from the body of the ship's company' . . . . 'great attention was observed by all the officers in immediately reporting every man who appeared to have the smallest indisposition, whether it was discovered by day or by night.'

'The whole of the space under the forecastle on the larboard side, including the round house, was appropriated to the sick, and the obtrusion of any other persons absolute prevented. To this place each individual was removed moment it was discovered that the disease had seized hi .... 'He was thence, as speedily as could be, carried hospital, care being had that everything belonging to h was conveyed thither with him. Moisture acting mo powerfully than any other cause in the production of disea as well as in the propagation of it, our first care was t endeavour to remove all humidity and foulness of t bilges.'

'The well was baled out, scraped and swabbed till entire dry, and then a large fire was kept burning in it for seven hours every day, so that the smallest dampness was n suffered to remain. The hold had the upper tier of casks moved from it, and these were sent on shore. Three fir were then kindled in it, and kept burning for many hou every day, confining the smoke as much as possible, and o casionally shifting the fires from place to place. In the fu made use of, as many empty tar barrels were consumed could be collected for the purpose; at other times wood, a occasionally coals intermixed with shakings of tarred rop every precaution being taken to prevent accident. Wh the fires were extinguished the gratings of the hold were moved and the wind-sails let down. Fires were also used the orlop, cockpit, steward's room, and bread-room on ea side of the between decks, and in the manger; the doors all the store-rooms were occasionally thrown open, and t ventilators (probably the 'ship's lungs') worked unrem tingly day and night.'

'The decks were seldom washed, and never but when t weather was such that the people could remain upon de until it was perfectly dry by the fires and the natural curre of air.' ... 'When the deck was not washed, it was kept pe fectly clean by other means; and slops about the decl together with every sort of dampness, were speedily removed

'The sides, beams, carlings, the deck overhead, and eve

part of the between decks, were whitewashed twice or thrice during the prevalence of the disorder.'

'The fumigations in the hold were thus conducted:— Four half-tubs with stands in them were disposed therein; in each of the tubs was placed an iron pot, in which were thrown about 2 lbs. of brimstone, tied up in a piece of canvas. The gratings were laid, and so closely covered with tarpaulins, old hammocks, swabs, &c., that none of the smoke could escape. When everything was prepared, a red-hot loggerhead, or iron lid, was put into each of the pots to set fire to the brimstone, and the men performing this service having instantly left the hold by means of a grating of the main hatchway kept open for the purpose, the hatches were entirely closed.'

'It was the custom to fumigate the hold, orlop, and between decks at the same time; but, as we could not be furnished with a sufficient quantity of brimstone to make use of it in all the different parts of the ship at the same period, it was usual, therefore, to use the brimstone in the hold, orlop, and between decks in rotation; and where this substance was not applied, what are called *devils*, made of powder wetted with vinegar, were substituted. It ought here to be observed that in those parts of the between decks least accessible to the air, and where, consequently, there is a greater degree of contagion, the flashing of powder from pistols is attended with a very good effect, for the shock of the explosion assists very powerfully in dispersing the infectious matter attached to the timbers of the ship.'

'During the fumigation, the men's hammocks were all hung up in their places, with their blankets spread over them, and all the spare apparel was so disposed on the guns, &c., as to receive the full effect of the fumigation. The clothes which the men wore upon deck during the time of one fumigation were changed upon the next and placed below, that all their things might receive an equal fumigation.'

'The gratings on the main deck were laid and covered

with such care that no smoke could escape, and they
were carefully barred in. The brimstone in tubs, they
and other safe precautions were dispersed about the deck
then lighted; the persons who did this having escape
deck and closed the hatches after them, the operation
completed. The smallest crevices of the ship were perv
by the smoke and effluvia of the brimstone, &c., by w
every part of her was affected in a powerful and astonis
manner.'

'Three hours were generally suffered to elapse before
gratings were removed and the ports opened, and a free
culation of air for a considerable time afterwards bec
necessary before a person could remain below without in
venience.'

'The whole of the hull of the ship, together with everyt
contained therein, both animate and inanimate, was stro
impregnated with the fumes of sulphur (brimstone) to su
degree even that it was perceptible when to leeward of
ship at a considerable distance from her.'

'In damp weather these fumigations were practised e
day, and never less than three times a week. The fires
continued daily.'

'The sick berth was attended to with some solicitud
impede or eradicate the infection, as has been described
respect to the other parts of the ship, nor were the per
and apparel of the men disregarded. Every man in the
was washed from head to foot with warm water and s
and more than even our usual pains were taken that
should be cleanly in all respects. If any old and us
clothes were found, they were thrown overboard. S
serviceable apparel as was discovered the least filthy
washed and fumigated, and the men were forbidden to
woollen trousers. On fine days the whole of their bed
was hung upon lines between the masts and on the rigg
and exposed thus to a free ventilation for many h
Their clothes of every kind were treated in the same ma

2. *Nitrous Acid* :—

Sir Gilbert Blane tells us that in 1796, when the medical branch of the naval service was transferred from the Board of Admiralty to the 'Commissioners of Sick and Wounded Seamen,' new instructions for medical officers were drawn up, and amongst other matters of importance Dr. Carmichael Smyth's system of fumigation by the action of sulphuric acid upon nitrate of potash was introduced. The nitrous fumes resulting were found to produce but little inconvenience to the sick, while they very obviously removed the offensive smell of musty clothes and the effluvia of fœtid ulcers.

A more usual method of obtaining nitrous acid fumes is by pouring three parts of concentrated nitric acid over one part of copper filings or wire in a deep jar. Thus one ounce of copper wire and three ounces of nitric acid will produce about one cubic foot of the gas, and in some recent experiments conducted at Netley this proportion was found to be quite sufficient to precipitate and render nearly motionless very active bacteria in 100 c.c. of decaying infusion of beef, included in a circumscribed space of 53 cubic feet. The fluid was rendered quite sweet to the sense of smell, and further development of bacteria had been obviously arrested, and it bore a remarkable comparison with another 100 c.c. of the beef infusion which had been kept aside for this purpose.

Nitrous acid gas is formed by the union of the nitric oxide originally evolved with the oxygen of the air, and this will continue to be given and taken as long as there is any organic matter present upon which this oxidising action can be exerted. At the rate of 2 per cent., the strength used in the above-mentioned experiment, 6 ounces of nitric acid would be required for every 100 cubic feet, or 16 ounces for 266 cubic feet of space, or finally 1 cwt. of strong nitric acid for the disinfection of 25,367 cubic feet. However valuable, therefore, this agent might be on a small scale, it would be a very dangerous commodity in the large quantities that would be necessary for the fumigation of a ship of war.

3. *Chlorine Gas.*—For the preparation of chlorin[e a]
quarter of a pound of black oxide of manganese fine[ly pow]
dered may be treated with half a pint of muria[tic acid]
previously mixed with a quarter of a pint of water, or a [half]
of a pint of muriatic or dilute sulphuric acid may be [poured]
over a quarter of a pound of chloride of lime contain[ed in a]
jar. Either of these methods would, of course, be onl[y fit]
for a limited supply of the gas, but if numerous ve[ssels so]
prepared were distributed at convenient distances apa[rt, and]
to be put in operation with as little delay as possible, i[t would]
effect an equable and general evolution of the chlorine[, which]
should be closely confined by every available means.

Speaking of the disinfection of ships Mr. Simon s[ays:]
'The process should be conducted as distantly as [possible]
from the shore and from other vessels. All the compa[rtments]
of the ship should first be fumigated with some disi[nfectant]
gas, best with chlorine or nitrous acid, and then [all the]
accessible woodwork (in and out) should be wash[ed with]
a solution of chloride of soda or lime. The bilges [require]
particular attention, and before they are first pump[ed]

in precaution against which danger it is desirable that the persons should have complete baths of soap and water, and that their clothes should partake of the general fumigation of the ship. The person who conducts the fumigation of the ship (especially where there is question of yellow fever) ought not at first to enter the hold, but merely to hang down the hatches, or otherwise place within the hold, the vessel which contains his chemical mixture.'

When the help of negroes is available, as on the West Coast of Africa, or in the West Indies, the duty of distributing the disinfecting agents may be safely committed to them, without risking the lives of those who are, from some cause or other, more susceptible of the yellow fever poison.

In the case of H.M.S. 'Icarus' after a severe visitation of yellow fever in the West Indies, a party of negroes who were engaged for some considerable time in cleaning out the hold and disinfecting the ship enjoyed a complete immunity from the disease, while the boat's crew, who pulled these men to and from the ship, mainly boys from the 'Imaum,' were individually seized with yellow fever, which proved fatal in several cases. It seems, moreover, to be a matter of experience that unless the cleansing process is most perfectly carried out, it would be far better to defer all abortive efforts of the kind until a colder latitude has been reached. It is much easier to stir up infectious filth in the hold and bilges than to remove it as thoroughly as the nature of the case would demand. Indeed it has even been observed that the foulness of ships which have nominally undergone this cleansing has been rendered more apparent than before.

DIVISION IV.

OR APPENDIX.

CHAPTER I.

To the subjects treated in the foregoing
pended (1) a review of the character, habits, and dut
man-of-war's man, with whom the naval medical o[f]
have more especially to do in the exercise of his
afloat; (2) leading particulars in relation to the d[uties and]
responsibilities of medical officers, matters of ro[utine on]
board ship, and (3) medical instructions and enactme[nts more]
or less bearing on the subject of hygiene.

SECTION A.—*The Physique of the Sailor.*

The duties of the man-of-war's man are of such [a nature]
as to call for a light, active, and muscular frame. H[is physi-]
cal condition should approximate as nearly as possibl[e that]
of the athlete, and the nature of his training should
bring him into that condition. His hands should b[e large]
and powerful, yet so thoroughly taught that they [are]
capable of executing the very finest work. His arm[s should]
have their muscular development without being red[undant,]
and the same may be said of his legs. The eye sh[ould be]
clear, and the sight good. The nervous system shou[ld be so]
well balanced that no situation of peril should easily a[ffect it.]
In order to maintain the human body in such a state [of per-]
fection every consideration should be given to the ma[n's]

which the material of the frame is supplied. On board ship, of course, men of very various physical conditions are to be found. The heaviest and most powerful men are employed about the foremast and jibboom, the duties in the fore part of the ship being the heaviest, and calling for the greatest amount of bodily strength. Those next in size and weight are attached to the mainmast, while the lighter men and boys are told off to the mizenmast and after part of the ship, where the duties are less severe and the gear lighter. Then as regards different work men are cast with reference to their agility and general physical condition into topsail, topgallant, and royal yardmen, the lightest and most nimble being sent to the highest yards.

Men of indifferent physical condition are divided off into after guards, waisters, and idlers, men whose duties are conducted on the deck.

The duties of both sides of the ship being quite distinct, and with the view of preventing the confusion that would naturally arise from persons crossing the decks and interfering with one another during exercise, the ship's company is divided into two watches, distinguished by a red transverse stripe on the right or left shoulder of the frock. Moreover, in regard to the sleeping billets of these watches, or the berthing of the hammocks, a most important hygienic principle (originating in experience alone) is adopted in well-regulated ships. Thus, on the main deck, for example, commencing at the fore part of the ship, the hammocks in each transverse row belong alternately to the port and starboard watches, so that when either watch is on deck there must also be an alternation of full and empty hammocks from side to side of the deck. By this arrangement more breathing space is actually provided for at sea than a superficial observer would imagine, seeing all the hammocks slung so closely together. When this precaution has been neglected, it would be clearly the medical officer's duty to represent it properly, and his interference so far could scarcely be called officious.

Section II.—The Natural Character and [illegible]

As the sailors of all countries [illegible] of the same materials, as a genus vary [illegible] in general, a knowledge of their peculiar [illegible] habits is of importance in a hygienic [illegible]

'The character of a British seaman,' [illegible] 'exhibits so many striking singularities, which is mixes so much with all his habits, that a thorough [illegible] with them becomes necessary to both [illegible] man in their respective stations. These peculiarities [illegible] springing of a sea life, from the little connection it a [illegible] the common manners of society. The love of [illegible] enterprise that so soon discovers itself in his boy [illegible] seems to prompt the first inclination for sea, a long ally keeps it alive, and nothing but a voyage will at la the youthful argonaut, to which the parent consent hope that a life of danger and difficulty will soon [illegible] unexperienced sailor and make him wish to live [illegible] This, however, seldom happens; and the first cruise [illegible] makes him fix for a future sea life to the young adven. The voyages of Drake and Anson round the world a: in their way,' but Dr. Trotter says that Robinson Cr made more proselytes than all other mariners.

'In a country like ours, which owes her security t [illegible] we see a victory at sea celebrated above all ot rouses the amor patriæ to the highest pitch of enthusi: reminds a free people of their independence, becaus has decreed that this is our element. The names of o admirals are therefore revered as so many tutelary d our island.'

'Hawke, Rodney, and Howe, and the heroes of the Nile and Rubicon, shrink into insignificance when co with those of April 12 and of June 1. Hence, from [illegible] cannon, the naval spirit of Great Britain descends as in hereditary succession. That courage which distinguishes our seamen, though it is in some degree inherent in their natural constitutions, yet it is increased by their habits of life, and by associating with men who are familiarised to danger, and who from natural prowess consider themselves at sea as rulers by birthright. By these means, in all actions there is a general impulse among the crew of an English man-of-war either to grapple the enemy or lay him close aboard.'

'It is only men of such a description that could undergo the fatigues and perils of a sea life, and there seems a necessity for their being inured to it from an early age.' . . . 'Excluded by the employment they have chosen from all society but that of people of similar dispositions, the deficiencies of education are not felt, and information on general subjects is not courted. Their pride consists in being thought a thoroughbred seaman; and they look upon all landsmen as being of an inferior order. Having little intercourse with the world they are easily defrauded, and made dupes to the deceitful wherever they go. . . . With minds uncultivated, uninformed, they are equally credulous and superstitious; the appearance of the sky, the flight of a bird, the sight of particular fishes, the sailing on a certain day of the week, with other incidents, will fill their minds with omens and disasters.'

The large-heartedness and generous feelings of the genuine sailor are quite proverbial, and need no further exposition in this place. The sailor of the present day, however, is in many particulars a different man from the beau ideal so graphically described by Dr. Trotter. His education is more carefully attended to, and his moral training and social advantages are of a superior description. Some of the lovers of old institutions have declared that there never has been a sailor of the right sort in the navy since all this mental and moral culture has been introduced; but we have proof enough to show that neither loyalty nor fighting qualities suffer any deterioration by social improvement.

Speaking of the character of the sailor, Dr. Wilson, of the

United States Navy, says: 'If we expose his faults, w[hich] indeed, are apparent enough, let us consider the circumst[ances] of his life which have deprived him in some degree o[f the] habit of self-control, and give him some credit for such vi[rtues] as he actually possesses. His life is a life of contrasts. [His] intemperance is partly the consequence of long periods o[f] forced abstinence. His life of privation seems to relieve [him] so much from the necessity of self-control that he lose[s the] power to resist temptation. After long periods of monoto[nous] and unsavoury food, he suddenly has spread before him a pro[f]use feast. There is so little pleasure in his way tha[t he] denies himself no indulgence. His life brings all the pas[sions] into vivid contrast—hope immediately succeeding to desp[air;] excessive labour to idleness; sadness to joy; in fact, plea[sure] to pain and pain to pleasure in every imaginable form. He is as unstable as the sea. He is the creature of imp[ulse] and habitually of generous impulses.' This graphic acc[ount] closes with an incident illustrative of the last statement, [and] many others will be familiar to everybody.

What a good seaman ought to be is well set forth i[n an] excellent address given by Captain Harris of our own ser[vice] to the men under his command, and from which the follo[wing] extracts are taken:—

'On entering a profession which holds out so many adv[an]tages, your duty will be to give your Queen and cou[ntry] your best services, especially when by doing so you [are] benefiting yourselves at the same time.... Sobriety is of [the] utmost importance to a seaman; a steady eye, a ready h[and] belong only to those who are in possession of their reas[on;] hundreds of lives are sacrificed every year on the water f[rom] drunkenness.

'Respectful conduct to your superiors, both on board [and] on shore, is a proof of education and intelligence. Men [who] look forward to rise in the service will show to their superi[ors] the respect they will one day expect from those bene[ath] them; and each of you should hope to rise, for by good c[on]duct you are sure to do so.

'A good seaman is always well dressed—it is a mark of self-respect. I am sure most of you will feel with me how discreditable it is for a seaman to be seen rolling about the streets without shoes, ragged, and dirty.

'A good seaman has his hammock always well lashed up, his laniards and lashings pointed and clews whipped; his bag is never found full of dirty clothes and rubbish, but he has a natural pride in seeing everything belonging to him clean and tidy; he is always smart in his duty, and strictly obedient to orders. It is from such men that petty officers are selected. Who would select a person to govern others who was a sloven or a drunkard, and unfit to govern himself?

'Again, the comfort of your messes depends upon the individual conduct of every man in the mess; never, therefore, use blasphemous or disgusting language, which is contrary to the 'Articles of War,' and inconsistent with the duties you owe to others. A few may laugh at you; but the greater part of those who possess common sense will despise you. The days have happily gone by when it was thought seaman-like to drink, to swear, and be profligate.

'When you obtain leave be sure always to return to it; it is a breach of faith not to do so. Leave-breakers prevent officers from giving the indulgence they frequently desire to give, because they cannot be sure of getting men back at the time their services are required.

'Leave-breaking is occasioned by the indulgence of those vices which ruin half our seamen; hundreds of noble fellows, who have weathered many a storm, and escaped many a bullet, are wrecked in port, and fall victims to a glass of grog from the hands of a designing person. A man gets drunk, loses his money, sells his clothes, loses respect for himself, and, of course, the respect of his officers. Instead of spending his time on shore in healthful recreation and amusement, he spends it driving nails into his coffin, in wasting his money, and losing his character; and, instead of being better fitted for his duties, he is drugged and stupefied, and unfit for anything. Dissatisfied with himself, he quarrels with others, becomes a discontented man.'

That advice of this kind is of hygienic importance is demonstrated by the fact that, in flagships and others in which

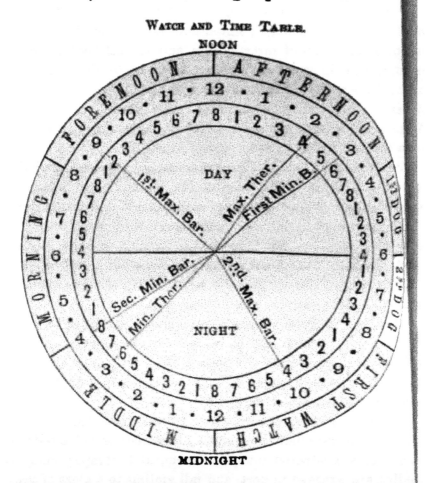

Watch and Time Table.

from an appropriate *esprit de corps*, and the laudable effect of setting an example, high-toned principles are encouraged, the daily sick list is comparatively small.

Section C.—*The Daily Duties of the Sailor.*

In a well-regulated ship there is always enough for everybody to do, with a certain allowance for recreation and rest.

DAILY ROUTINE.

The twenty-four hours of the day and night are divided into five watches—namely, the first, middle, morning, forenoon, and afternoon watches of four hours each, the first commencing at eight o'clock in the evening; and the first and second dog watches of two hours each, namely, from four to six, and from six to eight in the evening.

In the annexed diagram, the hours included in each watch are shown, with the number of bells corresponding with them in the inner circle, and also the maximum and minimum of the thermometer, and the first and second maximum and minimum of the barometer, in radiating lines.

The dog watches were instituted to enable three watchkeepers to interchange their watches, which would be impossible with six equal divisions of the twenty-four hours.

A good idea of the daily duties on board ship may be formed from the routine of one day, say Thursday, in harbour, during the winter months.

4.30 A.M.		Call boatswains, mates.
5.0	,,	Call hands, lash up hammocks.
5.5	,,	Hammock stowers, when present, pipe up.
5.15	,,	Bugle for cooks.
5.30	,,	Breakfast.
6.0	,,	Watch below clean lower and orlop decks.
,,	,,	Forenoon watch clean and stow bags.
,,	,,	Duty boat, clean out.
6.15	,,	Watch fall in, idlers to the pumps.
7.0	,,	Watch below clean and stow bags.
,,	,,	Sub. of the day clean copper on masts.
7.15	,,	Watch below fall in; when present, down ropes, clean wood- and brass-work.
7.30	,,	Upper yardmen fall in, drop duty cutter.
8.0	,,	Evolution; square yards.
8.15	,,	Quarters clean guns.
8.45	,,	Clean arms.
9.0	,,	Inspection, muster, as ordered, or drills.
11.0	,,	Dismiss drills.

11.30 A.M.	Clear up decks.
11.45 „	Bugle for cooks.
Noon.	Dinner.
1.15 P.M.	Quarters.
1.30 „	Retreat; hands make and mend clothes.
3.50 „	Upper yardmen fall in.
4.0 „	Down top-gallant yards, clear up decks, down ropes, up clothes lines.
4.30 „	Quarters, up boats, reeve clothes lines.
5.0 „	Bugle for cooks.
5.15 „	Supper, shift clothing.
7.15 „	Down steerage hammocks.
7.25 „	Call young gentlemen, petty officers.
8.30 „	Out lights, clear up lower and main decks.
8.50 „	Out pipes, clear up upper deck.
9.0 „	Rounds.
10.0 „	Out steerage lights.
11.0 „	Out ward-room lights.

On special occasions half-an-hour's lights may be allo to the gun-room officers, and the smoking hour may also extended with the permission of the captain.—N.B. Wl any special duty is going forward—calling the hands deck during the smoking time—pipes, lights, and cigars m be put out *pro tem.*, as it is unseemly for officers to sm while the men are employed.

The physical exertion put forth by the sailor in his or nary duties is far greater than that required of the soldi and, as before intimated, the potential energy derivable fr food should hold a corresponding proportion (*see* chapter Diet and Exercise). The movements of men on a dead le in the barrack square, even though encumbered with accout ments to some extent, can scarcely be compared with runni up the rigging, furling sails, and sending down masts a yards. Again, some of the sailor's most arduous duties performed in heavy weather, during which the soldier wo

THE MARITIME LIFE. 279

most probably find some shelter. Indeed, the influence of the maritime life, with all its hardships, discomforts, and tests of endurance, is such as to develop an early senectude, and shorten the register of life.

The latter remark, though quite true even to this day, is nevertheless more especially applicable to former times, when the principles of hygiene were neither so well known nor practically carried into effect as they are at present.

The death rate has thus exhibited a considerable diminution during the last few years, and better things still may be expected in the future.

CHAPTER II.

DUTIES AND RESPONSIBILITIES OF MEDICAL OFFICERS,]
OF ROUTINE, ETC.

SECTION A.—*Leave and Interchange of Duties,*

IN small vessels, bearing a single medical officer, staff surgeon, or a surgeon in charge, though he is cally responsible at all times for what may transpire tion to his duty, he cannot be always on board. He i fore, placed under no restriction, except that in the his not being able to attend the sick at the morn evening visit hour, he shall arrange with some other officer to do so for him ; and also that when he absents from the ship, he shall leave notice as to where he found in case of necessity.

Though in all ships the question of leave is regul the fleet or staff surgeon, where two medical offic borne, the senior and the junior take duty on alterna Again, in large ships bearing a fleet or staff surgeon surgeons, the latter take duty on alternate days—i.e the morning visit of one day to that of the next.

The forenoon duties in all ships of war are very ge uniform, but in some instances certain differences exis more or less affect the time at which the sick may be niently seen in the morning. Moreover, according particular views of the fleet or staff surgeon, the sick visited either before or after the ward-room breakfas which latter is usually at eight bells, namely, eight o'clc Thus six or seven or one bell may be chosen. Perh: bells, i.e., seven o'clock, would be the most convenient; ai with a very large sick list there will be time enough to furnish a statement of it to the captain and commander respectively by the fleet surgeon and senior surgeon at divisions, i.e. nine o'clock A.M.

As the medical officers are enjoined [1] to visit the sick at least twice a day, or as often as the respective cases may require, they are seen again at evening quarters, i.e., four or five o'clock P.M.

At the morning visit the fleet or staff surgeon sees and prescribes for the patients already on the sick-list *seriatim*, discharging any who may be fit for duty, and entering new cases. Any matters of minor surgery which he may not think necessary to attend to himself, he hands over to the senior surgeon, who is careful that all instructions given to him in relation to the patients are fully carried out. The discipline and internal management of the sick bay, and the issue of wine and extras for the sick, are also under his supervision.

The junior surgeon, besides attending to the dressing and bandaging, &c., is responsible for the compounding of medicines prescribed by the fleet or staff surgeon. He also sees that the stock-bottles, and other medicines in general use, are replenished, and in no case should dangerous drugs be dispensed by the sick-berth steward, however trustworthy he may be. Neglect in a matter of this kind partakes of the character of recklessness, making culpability doubly culpable, and evil consequences are sure to fall upon the shoulders of those who are legally responsible.

The surgeon on duty remains on board to meet any emergency that may arise, and attend to the administration of the sick bay, more particularly as to the cleanliness and proper ventilation of the place, the tidiness of the bedding and movable articles, and the personal appearance and comfort of the patients themselves. He also inspects the food at meal-times, so that any cause of complaint might be either speedily recti-

---

[1] Instructions for Medical Officers, p. 12, art. 12.

fied or shown to be without sufficient foundation, often is the case.

The officer on duty pays a final visit to the sick P.M., to see if anything is required, and that go preserved. He also sees that all documents cont the medical returns, or accounts of the ship passi his hands, are properly kept. By careful atten simple particular day after day, there can be no neatly filling up every paper and form for the cor which the fleet or staff surgeon of the ship is respo

Patients sent to hospital, firing parties, boa and armed, and accidents or sickness befalling me are attended by the surgeon off duty or by the sen officer if necessary.

SECTION B.—*Medical Documents and List-books i Requisition on Board Ship.*

These are the following:—

1. The *Staff Surgeon's Rough Journal* of practice the symptoms and progress of each case, with the prescribed, and all injunctions as to treatment, entered.

This is perhaps the most important document in the medical officer's charge. It is, in fact, a kind *in parvo* from which, if need be, most of the return in the instructions may be compiled.

2. *The Daily Sick-list*, in which the number on books, name, age, rating, date of entry and discha ber of days' sickness, whither discharged, and disea of every case, are entered in the order of their occur

3. A book sufficiently large, with a comprehensi betical index, to serve as a medical history book o and to facilitate the drawing up of the alphabetical of the fair journal, No. 11. This is made up periodi the entries in the Daily Sick Book, and has now

most useful document for reference, affording ready and precise information respecting individuals, so often required by the captain or commanding officer.

4. A Case Book for recording the cases of men sent to hospital, invalided, or who have died, as also those of any particular interest, both medical and surgical. The cases inserted in the fair journal are selected from this book.

5. A special List Book of moderate size, ruled faintly, and divided into three parts. The first for a list of men sent to hospital, invalided, or dead; the second for a list of trusses issued or of pension certificates granted; and the third for a venereal list. The first list should be in the form of the Daily Sick Book, but with an additional column for the date of discharge from hospital, of invaliding, or death, as the case might be. The third, or the venereal list, should be as in the printed form No. 275, in which the returns are made quarterly.

Surgeons should keep a copy of the Daily Sick Book, both for their own use and to check the staff surgeon's list. They should be also very particular in keeping their own journals creditably, as they are actually responsible for no other official documents but the certificates of conduct from the captain and the fleet or staff surgeon with whom they serve.

SECTION C.—*Manning and Arming Boats.*

This constitutes an evolution of much importance, as in actual warfare it is always called into requisition. In the 'Boat Signal Book,' p. xix., it is provided that the senior officers ship off the boats summoned by signal, and the captain of each ship whose boats contain more than eighty men is to send a fast-pulling boat in addition, having a medical officer on board, to attend in rear of the line; and this is repeated at p. xxv., art. 3, thus: 'A fast-pulling boat with the medical officers will attend in rear of the line.' At p. xxvi., art. 8, it is specified that, 'According to the exercise or service on which men may be ordered to proceed, additional men told off to carry provisions, spare ammunition, and str for the wounded,' but no particulars are given as to the of these stretchers.

From the 'Manual of Gunnery of H.M.'s Fleet' (p nary chapter), we learn that a case for small stores is carried by the boom boats and smaller boats, con amongst other things two tourniquets, and that each of boats will have a medical officer.

The quotations here given embrace, perhaps, written law on the subject, and it would appear that officers who have been actually engaged under the c stances in question have followed their own view instincts in making provision for the exigencies of e ticular case. Carrying amputating instruments in a b anything very cumbersome, may do very well for parad it is doubtful whether the performance of a capital ope in a boat could be undertaken with even the faintest success. Besides, should such an emergency happen, a mon scalpel in the hands of a good anatomist is capa accomplishing greater things than are commonly conce it. One might, therefore, trust to a good pocket-case o service, being also furnished with a haversack containin *sponge, lint, plaster, bandages, anodynes, and restoratives.*

The pads of ordinary tourniquets are so small and fective that most unhappy results are known to have att the indiscriminate use of these instruments in action. whole circulation in a limb, venous as well as arteria in numerous instances been arrested for many hours tog where the temporary application of the point of the fing a judiciously applied compress, would have answered a purpose.

SECTION D.—*General, and Fire Quarters.*

The great object of general quarters, and indeed of

and men with the duties that may at any time devolve upon them, both in preparing for battle and actually engaging the enemy. Therefore the more distinctly those duties are defined, and the more perfectly they are carried out in periodical exercises, the more efficient must be the discipline and fewer the difficulties likely to present themselves in actual warfare.

In case of action or fire the principal medical officer should immediately proceed to the sick bay, muster the sick, and send such as are at all fit for duty in such heavy emergency to their quarters, reporting his having done so to the captain or commanding officer. He should then select the absolutely helpless and have them conveyed to a place of safety appointed by the executive, the surgeons taking charge of them to their boats in case of fire. Under such circumstances the sick should be so distributed that each medical officer shall have an equal number in his boat, to prevent the embarrassment of having the boats incapacitated by being over-crowded with sick.

In case of action men not absolutely helpless should be utilised to provide blankets, sling the steerage hammocks, bring fresh and salt water, sand and swabs, to the cockpit under the supervision of the inferior sick bay men.

For general quarters a drawer should be set apart in the dispensary to contain a certain number of bandages of different kinds, calico, strapping towels, tourniquets, waxed ligatures, &c., and it may remain always in readiness. This drawer, along with a tray containing carbolic acid, tincture of opium, chloral, chloroform, olive oil, &c., and two sick bay beds with clean sheets, should be conveyed to the cockpit. The operation table is then to be set up, and a large tray covered with a white cloth placed conveniently for instruments, &c. Drinking water and pannikins are to be provided by the convalescent sick told off for the purpose. The ward-room steward should be in charge of such stimulants, soda water, &c., as the staff surgeon may demand, placing himself under the orders of the paymaster and chaplain, who should assist in the adminis-

286

tration of drink and support to the wounded. The as[sistance of the]
paymaster and clerks would also render valuable aid [to the]
medical officers, but their special duties under circum[stances]
of this kind should be accurately defined so as to a[void]
misunderstanding.

Section E.—*Ambulance Lifts for Ships of War.*

An efficient and expeditious means of conveying w[ounded]
men from one deck to another, or even from one ship [to an]other, while at sea, has always been a great deside[ratum,]
especially during action, and numerous schemes hav[e been]
suggested from time to time. A simple bowline on the [end,]
arm-chairs properly slung, or flour casks with the sta[ves]
cut as to receive a man in the sitting posture, are among [the]
earliest plans adopted on board ship, where the 'servic[e cot,']
from its inconvenient size, would be inapplicable. As [well]
the hatches of a ship are too small to permit the des[cent of]
the ordinary cot through them without altering the hori[zontal]
position of the frame, any deviation from which towar[ds the]
head, foot, or either side would be attended with pai[n, and]
possibly with much injury to a patient badly wounded.

The defects here noticed have been very satisfactoril[y met]
in the ambulance cot devised by Surgeon Albert C. G[orgas,]
U.S.N., an account of which (though without a drawi[ng) is]
given in the appendix to the work on 'Naval Hygien[e' by]
Surgeon Joseph Wilson, U.S.N. The leading idea in th[is cot]
is the introduction of a double inclined plane, whi[ch is]
fastened upon the frame, and a band of canvas secured [to the]
upper part of the same.

'The thighs and legs of the patient are flexed ove[r the]
double inclined plane, and the canvas band is tied aroun[d his]
chest beneath his arms, his head resting upon a pillow.['] 'In
this ambulance lift the sliding down of the occupant is arr[ested]
by his buttocks and thighs being supported by the [inclined]
surface of the double inclined plane, and his body is
further held by a strap.

Ships' cots are at least 6 feet long by 28 inches wide. The flexion of the legs over the double inclined plane permits the shortening of the cot to 5 feet 8 inches, and as it is an advantage to have the canvas sides embrace the patient closely, it is narrowed so as to be but 21 inches wide.

The proportions of the inclined plane are such as to adapt it to both tall and short men and even boys.

It should be stated here that the cot is principally suspended by a whip attached to the head clews, while a guiding line is connected with those of the foot, by which means the descent is regulated as required. Or it is suggested that both sets of clews may be secured to the ends of a short pole with an eye in the centre, and the whole apparatus lowered by a double whip.

This contrivance has been practically tried during the late war with perfect success. It has also been used in our own service at general quarters, and Dr. Davis, Fleet Surgeon, R.N., reports very favourably of its utility in comparison with other means tested by him.

Fig. 41, Plate XXIX., exhibits another form of ambulance lift for ship or shore, in which the ordinary sailor's hammock is utilised, having the head and foot clews secured to a short pole (between four and five feet long), to which again a span is attached above, with an eye in the middle for the lower hook of a double whip, or fixity to a longer pole when the apparatus is used on shore. The easiest possible movement is thus effected, either in lowering a patient from one deck to another, or carriage from place to place on shore. Nothing more is required when the injuries are confined to the head, trunk, or upper extremities; but by the addition of a small transverse ham-piece placed under the hammock, and connected by a lanyard at each end with the pole above, provision is made for fracture of the leg or of the thigh, with the whole effect of a double inclined plane.

A drawing of this ambulance lift is also given in Surgeon-

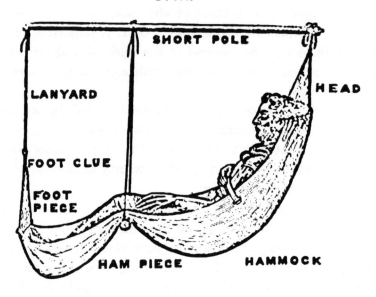

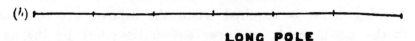

Fig. 41.—Ambulance Lift (Macdonald).

method of transporting wounded from deck to deck, exhibited at Paris in 1878 by Dr. J. Maréchal of Brest. The hammock is strengthened externally by a kind of cradle of wood, and the patient is laced up in it quickly, and conveyed to a shute which is fitted to the hatchway, and capable of being loosened at one end so as to permit the hammock with the patient to slide as it were from the deck above into the hands of carriers on the deck below, where it may be slung in the usual way without loss of time.

In boat service a very good stretcher may be extemporised by lashing the eyelet holes of a hammock to an oar on either side, and rolling it up to make it sufficiently narrow. Two boats' stretchers will then form the head and foot of the frame, and afford additional security to the patient.

Other simple forms of stretchers will be found in the little work already referred to.

APPENDIX

OF

MEDICAL INSTRUCTIONS AND ENACTMENTS.

SELECTIONS FROM THE QUEEN'S REGULATIONS AND ADMIRALTY INSTRUCTIONS BEARING ON THE PROVINCE OF 'NAVAL HYGIENE' (1879).

I. SCALE OF VICTUALLING IN HER MAJESTY'S NAVY.

	When to be issued	Articles		Seamen: Officers, Crew, and others, at a Seaman's Full Allowance	Seamen: Supernumeraries at two-thirds of a Seaman's Allowance	Troops
1	Daily. See note *, p. 292.	Biscuit or	lb.	1¼	5/6	3/4*
2		Soft bread	"	1½	1	1*
3		Spirit	pint	1/8	1/12	..
4		Porter	"	..	..	1
5		Sugar	oz.	2	1⅓	2
6		Chocolate	"	1	2/3	..
7		Tea	"	1/4	1/6	1/2
8	Weekly. See note †, p. 292.	Oatmeal	"	3	2	..†
9		Mustard	"	1/2	1/3	1/2
10		Pepper	"	1/4	1/6	1/4
11		Salt	"	..	..	2
12		Vinegar	pint	1/4	1/6	1/12
13		Pickles (various)	oz.	..	..	6
14	Daily, when procurable. See note ‡, p. 292.	Fresh meat	lb.	1	2/3	3/4‡
15		Vegetables	"	1/2	1/3	1/2
	When fresh provisions cannot be procured:—	—				
16	Every other day, as regards seamen, and twice a week in the other cases	Salt pork	lb.	1	2/3	3/4
17		Split peas	"	1/3	2/9	3/8
18		Compressed mixed Vegetables	oz.	..	..	1
19		Celery seed	½ oz. to every 8 lbs. of Split Peas put into the coppers.			

SCALE OF VICTUALLING IN HER MAJESTY'S NAVY—*continued.*

	When to be issued	Articles		Seamen: Officers, Crew, and others, at a Seaman's Full Allowance	Seamen: Supernumeraries at two-thirds of a Seaman's Allowance	Troops
20	On the alternate days to regular seamen, and twice a week to marine troops	Salt Beef	lb.	1	⅔	¾
21		Flour	oz.	9	6	6
22		Suet	"	¾	½	1
23		Raisins	"	1½	1	2
7		Sugar	"	..	..	2
24		Preserved potato	"	..	..	2
25	On the other alternate days to regular seamen. Troops are to have preserved meat thrice, preserved potato twice, and rice once a week	Preserved meat with either	lb.	¾	½	¾
24		1. Preserved potato or	oz.	4	2⅔	2
26		2. Rice or	"	4	2⅔	4
24		3. Preserved potato and	"	2	1⅓	..
26		Rice or	"	2	1⅓	..
21		4. Flour	"	9	6	..
22		Suet	"	¾	½	..
23		Raisins	"	1½	1	..

SCALE OF SUBSTITUTES.

In case it should be necessary to issue substitutes for any of the articles in this scale of victualling the following substitution is to be adopted, viz.:—

Biscuits	1 pound	are to be considered equal to each other.
Flour	1 pound	
Rice	1 pound	
Wine	½ pint	do. do.
Spirit	¼ gill	
Porter	1 pint	
Coffee	1 ounce	do. do.
Cocoa	1 ounce	
Chocolate	1 ounce	
Tea	¼ ounce	

The following, when issued with meat rations are to be considered equal to each other:—

		Seamen	Troops
1	Split peas	½ pound	⅜ pound
	Peas whole	½ pint	—
	Flour	½ pound	⅜ pound
	Calavances	½ pint	⅜ pint
	Dholl	½ pint	⅜ pint
	Rice	½ pound	⅜ pound
2	Vegetables		½ pound
	Compressed mixed vegetables		1 ounce
	Preserved potato		2 ounces
3	Oatmeal		¼ pint or 5 ounces
	Split peas		⅜ pound

NOTES.

* Soft bread is to be issued to troops four days in the week, and biscuit the remaining three days.

† When troops are on fresh meat victualling, a sufficient quantity of oatmeal may be issued for thickening their soup.

‡ When fresh meat is issued to troops, bread or biscuit, in addition to supplies, according to above scale, is also to be issued at the rate of 4 oz. of bread or 3 oz. of biscuit for each man.

NOTE.—When women and children are carried they are to be victualled in accordance with scale for victualling in her Majesty's troop ships.

SCALES OF VICTUALLING, WATER, AND FORAGE FOR HER MAJESTY'S TROOP SHIPS.

Troops.

SCALE OF RATIONS PER MAN.

Days of the Week	Daily															Weekly				
	Salt Beef	Flour	Suet	Raisins	Salt Pork	Split Peas	Preserved Meat	Compressed mixed Vegetables	Biscuit	Fresh Bread	Rice	Porter	Preserved Potatoes (uncooked)	Sugar (unrefined)	Tea	Vinegar	Mustard	Pickles (of various descriptions)	Pepper (ground)	Salt
	oz	oz	oz	oz	oz	pint	oz	oz	oz	lb	oz	pint	oz	oz	oz	pint	oz	oz	oz	oz
Sunday . .	12	6	1	½	..	..	..	..	12	..	..	1	2	4	½					
Monday .	..	..	..	..	..	..	12	..	..	1	4	1	..	2	½					
Tuesday .	..	..	..	..	12	⅜	..	1	12	..	..	1	..	2	½					
Wednesday .	12	6	1	½	..	..	..	..	..	1	..	1	2	4	½	⅛	½	6	⅛	2
Thursday .	..	..	..	..	..	..	12	..	12	..	..	1	2	2	½					
Friday . .	..	..	..	..	12	⅜	..	1	..	1	..	1	..	2	½					
Saturday .	..	..	..	..	..	..	12	..	..	1	..	1	2	2	½					

NOTE.—Spirit is not to be issued except in special cases on certificate of the medical officer in charge.

SCALE OF RATIONS PER WOMAN.

Days of the Week	Daily															Weekly				
	Salt Beef	Flour	Suet	Raisins	Salt Pork	Split Peas	Preserved Meat	Compressed mixed Vegetables	Biscuit	Fresh Bread	Rice	Porter	Preserved Potatoes (uncooked)	Sugar (unrefined)	Tea	Vinegar	Mustard	Pickles (of various descriptions)	Pepper (ground)	Salt
	oz	oz	oz	oz	oz	pint	oz	oz	oz	lb	oz	pint	oz	oz	oz	pint	oz	oz	oz	oz
Sunday . .	8	6	1	2	..	..	..	..	8	..		½	2	4	½					
Monday .	..	..	..	..	..	..	8	..	..	¾	4	½	..	2	½					
Tuesday .	..	..	..	..	8	⅜	..	1	8	..	..	½	..	2	½					
Wednesday .	3	6	1	2	..	..	..	..	..	¾	..	½	2	4	½	⅛	½	6	⅛	2
Thursday .	..	..	..	..	..	..	8	..	8	..	..	½	2	2	½					
Friday . .	..	..	..	..	8	⅜	..	1	..	¾	..	½	..	2	½					
Saturday .	..	..	..	..	..	..	8	..	..	¾	..	½	2	2	½					

SCALE OF RATIONS PER CHILD OF FIVE TO TEN YEARS OF AGE.

Days of the Week	Salt Pork, or Salt Beef *	Flour	Suet	Raisins	Soup and Bouilli	Rice
	oz.	oz.	oz.	oz.	pint	oz.
Sunday	6	3	½	3	..	2
Monday	..	..	..	..	..	..
Tuesday	..	..	..	..	½	2
Wednesday	6	3	½	2	..	..
Thursday	..	..	..	..	..	..
Friday	..	..	..	..	½	2
Saturday	..	..	..	..	..	..

* Either salt pork or salt beef is to be issued at the direct[ion of the officer] in charge.

† If preserved milk is used, sufficient to make half-a-pint.

SCALE OF RATIONS PER CHILD UNDER FIVE [YEARS OF AGE.]

Days of the Week	Biscuit Powder, or Rusks	Sugar (unrefined)	Fresh Milk.*	Soup and Bouilli, Essence of Beef, or Mutton Broth †
	oz.	oz.	pint	pint
Sunday	4	2	2	Sufficient to make
Monday	4	2	2	
Tuesday	4	2	2	
Wednesday	4	2	2	
Thursday	4	2	2	
Friday	4	2	2	
Saturday	4	2	2	

NOTE.—Each infant under one year of age [is to be supplied] with milk, corn-flour, sago, or arrowroot, and sug[ar, at the] discretion of the medical officer in charge.

* If preserved milk is used, sufficient to make 2 pints.

† These articles are to be provided in equal quantities, and are soup and bouilli 5½ ounces, cooked with ¼ pint of water; essence [in] pint canister, cooked with ¼ pint of water; and mutton broth 4 o[unces; a] quantity of boiling water, will make the half-pint required.

SCALE OF SUBSTITUTES. 295

NOTES.

a. Boys of 10 years and under 14 years of age, to receive the woman's ration, but without porter. Boys of 14 years of age, or upwards, to receive the man's ration, but without porter. Girls of 10 years of age, or upwards, to receive the woman's ration, but without porter.

b. Boys and girls, of 17 years of age or upwards, are to be considered in all respects as adults.

c. Temperance men not receiving porter (or spirit, as a substitute), are each to be allowed, daily, one ounce of sugar, and a quarter of an ounce of tea, in addition to the quantities of those articles specified in the scale of rations; those men who do not receive these additional quantities will be credited in office with a penny a day.

d. Temperance women not receiving porter, and other women to whom it may not be practicable to supply porter, are to be granted a similar additional allowance of sugar and tea.

e. Neither porter nor spirit is to be issued to prisoners or 'punishment men,' except under military advice, and with the sanction of the military commanding officer.

f. Preserved meat is to consist of beef and mutton, which are to be provided in equal quantities, and to be issued alternately.

g. Fresh meat and fresh vegetables are to be issued, whenever practicable, 1 lb. fresh meat being considered equal to 1 lb. salt meat; but 8 oz. of fresh vegetables are to be the ration for men, women, or children. When fresh vegetables are not procurable, preserved potatoes (uncooked) 2 oz., or compressed mixed vegetables 1 oz., are to be issued in lieu.

h. Fresh vegetables are to be issued, whenever procurable, with salt or preserved meat, in lieu of the flour, suet, raisins, peas, compressed vegetables, preserved potatoes or rice, specified in the scales.

i. Fresh meat and fresh vegetables are also to be obtained, for 2 days' consumption after leaving port, should the weather admit of their keeping sweet.

j. In cases in which it may be impossible to provide fresh bread, biscuit is to be issued as the ration in the proportions shown in the respective scales for men, women, and children.

k. When fresh meat is issued, bread or biscuit, in addition to supplies according to the above scale, is also to be issued at the rate of 4 oz. of bread or 3 oz. of biscuit for each man and woman.

l. Oatmeal may be issued for thickening soup, when fresh meat is issued, to such extent as may be considered necessary, and the extra issues are to be separately certified to.

m. Any articles in the foregoing scales of rations may be stopped or changed, but only in individual cases, upon the special requisition of the medical officer.

n. The scales of rations are to be regarded as generally applicable to invalids, as well as to persons in health; invalids are, however, to be provided with fresh bread, every day.

o. In ships conveying invalids, there is also to be provided a liberal proportion of live stock (oxen, sheep, and poultry, but not pigs), with provender and water for their subsistence. In lieu also of the regulated supply of salt meats, an equivalent in preserved meat, as well as an extra quantity of prepared soup, is to be shipped for the invalids. They are to be replenished, as far as may be practicable, at any ports at which the ship may touch. Issues are to be made at the discretion of the medical officer in charge.

SCALE OF SUBSTITUTES.

The above scales of rations being sufficiently varied for health, are to be adhered to, except as regards the substitution of fresh for salted or preserved provisions, whenever practicable, in the proportions shown below. In order, however, to meet cases in which it may be actually necessary to depart from the scale, a list of equivalents is appended :—

Fresh bread . 1 lb. ⎫
Flour . . ¾ lb. ⎬ To be considered equal to ¾ lb. biscuit.
Rice . . ¾ lb. ⎭
Fresh meat . 1 lb. ,, ,, ,, 1 lb. salt meat.
Spirit . . ½ gill ,, ,, ,, 1 pint porter.

Coffee (roasted and ground)	1 oz.	To be consi…		
Chocolate	1 oz.		½ oz.	
Fresh vegetables ½ lb. To be considered equal to . .		2 oz. preserved cooked) or 1 …		

Flour . .	.	½ lb.
Split peas .	.	⅛ pint
Calavances	.	⅛ pint
Dholl .	.	⅛ pint
Rice . .	.	⅛ lb.
Oatmeal . .	⅛ pint	,, ,,

MEDICAL COMFORTS.

Such articles as may be necessary for the use of t… be supplied, as required, from the general mess stock provisions. Lime juice, with sugar, is to be issued … tion of the medical officer in charge; a sufficient … obtained to provide for the issue of 1 oz. of lime ju… per diem for each person from the 9th day at sea inclu… end of the voyage. A sufficient supply is also to b… carbolic acid and Condy's Fluid, as well as of articl… comforts in Table N, see p. 297, that may not be i… mess stores.

WATER.

Water is to be issued on the most liberal scale pos… minimum daily allowance of water (distilled or filter… for each individual embarked, including the crew of th… when out of the tropics, and 1 gallon when within … which quantities are to suffice them for all purposes.

SCALE OF WATER, FORAGE, ETC., FOR HORSES OR …

8 gallons of water .		Each anima… eight tim… follows :—
½ peck or 5 lbs. of oats .		
1½ ,, 5 ,, bran .	for each animal daily	Four times with
10 lbs. hay . . .		
1 ounce of nitre . .		And, in th… four times hay.
1 gill of vinegar . .		

A supply of carrots is to be provided in addition.

The full quantities of the daily ration should not l… in the opinion of the military commanding officer t… actually required.

All the articles are to be served out by Imperial w…

SCALE OF MEDICAL COMFORTS.

For the Complement.

Class of Ship	For all Seagoing Ships			For Ships proceeding to foreign Stations
	Essence of Beef	Extractum carnis	Egg Powder	Wine
	¼ pints	ozs.	lbs.	dozens
1st Class	40	20	8	7
2nd Class	30	15	6	6
3rd Class	25	12½	5	5
4th Class	20	10	4	4
Sloops and Gun Vessels	15	7½	4	3
Smaller Vessels	10	5	3	3

- a. Preserved meat . . . 1 lb., or
- b. Common soup . . . 2 pints, or
- c. Concentrated soup . . ½ pint
- d. Preserved carrots . . ¼ lb.
- e. Cocoatina . . . 1 oz.
- f. Preserved potatoes or rice . ¼ lb.
- g. Mutton broth . . . ½ pint

for each person of the complement.

For Ships proceeding to the undermentioned Stations the following Articles are, in addition to the above, to be demanded:—

Class of Ship	East Indies, China, and Australia			Cape of Good Hope and West Coast of Africa, North America and West Indies, and Mediterranean			Pacific and South-East Coast of America			Cape of Good Hope and West Coast of Africa, East Indies, and China	
	Calves' foot Jelly	Preserved Milk	Preserved Fowl	Calves' foot Jelly	Preserved Milk	Preserved Fowl	Calves' foot Jelly	Preserved Milk	Preserved Fowl	Egg Powder	Cocoatina for each person in the Complement
	lbs.	pts.	lbs.	lbs.	pts.	lbs.	lbs.	pts.	lbs.	lbs.	
1st Class	60	230	240	30	115	120	15	57	60	8	
2nd Class	48	200	200	24	100	100	12	50	50	6	
3rd Class	36	160	160	18	80	80	9	40	40	5	1 oz.
4th Class	24	130	120	12	65	60	6	32	30	4	
Sloops and Gun Vessels	12	100	80	6	50	40	3	25	20	4	
Smaller Vessels	6	50	40	3	25	20	2	12	10	3	

II. REGULATION KIT FOR THE SHIP'S COMPANY.

CLOTHING OF THE SHIP'S COMPANY.

Articles in accordance with the prescribed Pattern for the respective Ratings		Chief Petty Officers, Seaman Class	Master-at-Arms, Naval School-masters, Ships' Stewards, &c.	Engine Room and Skilled Artificers	Ships' Corporals, Writers 2nd Class, Sick-Berth Steward, &c.	Bandsmen	Servants	Other Petty Officers, Seamen, Boys, &c.	Remarks
Articles of Uniform Regulations referred to	.	XLVI.	XLVII. to XLIX.	L. to LIII.	LIV. to LV.	LVII. to LVIII.	LVI.	LIX.	
Frock coat	No.	:	1	:	:	:	:	:	
Long jacket, cloth	,,	1	1	1	:	:	:	:	
,, serge	,,	1	:	1	:	:	:	1	
Round jacket, cloth	,,	:	:	:	1	:	1	:	Not for boys.
,, serge	,,	:	:	:	1	:	:	:	
Trowsers, blue cloth	Pairs.	2	2	2	2	:	2	2	
,, white duck	No.	2 or more for all ratings, according to climate.							
Waistcoat, blue cloth	,,	2	2	1	1	:	1	:	
,, white ,,	,,	:	:	:	1	:	:	2 or more, according to climate	
Blue serge frock	,,	:	:	:	:	:	:	2	
,, serge jumper	,,	:	:	:	:	:	:	1	
Drill frocks	,,	:	:	:	Optional with all ratings.	:	:	2	
Duck jumpers	,,	:	:	:	:	:	:	2	
Pea jacket	,,	2	2	2	2	2	2	2	
Black silk neckerchief	,,	:	:	:	:	:	:	1	
Hat, black	,,	:	:	:	:	:	:	1	
,, white	,,	:	:	:	:	:	:	2	
,, ribbons	,,	:	:	:	:	:	:	2	
Cap, blue cloth *	,,	2	2	2	2	:	2	:	
,, ,, with peak	,,	:	:	:	:	:	:	:	Devices as directed

* Men in Troop Ships when actually employed in trooping, or when coaling, may wear caps; on all other occasions they are to wear the established uniform of the service.

REGULATION KIT FOR THE SHIP'S COMPANY—*Continued.*

Articles in accordance with the prescribed Pattern for the respective Ratings		Chief Petty Officers, Seaman Class	Master-at-Arms, Naval School-masters, Ships' Stewards, &c.	Engine Room and Skilled Artificers	Ships' Corporals, Writers 2nd Class, Sick-Berth Steward, &c.	Bandsmen	Servants	Other Petty Officers, Seamen, Boys, &c.	Remarks
Articles of Uniform Regulations referred to		XLVI.	XLVII. to XLIX.	L. to LIII.	LIV. to LV.	LVII. to LVIII.	LVI.	LIX.	
				Optional with all ratings.					
Comforter	No.	4	4	4	4	4	4	4	
Flannels	„	3	3	3	3		3		
Shirts, white	„	4	4	4	4	4	4	3	
„ blue check	„							1	
White working suit	„	1			1			1	
Serge night suit	„	1	1	1	1		1	1	
Socks or stockings	Pairs.	2	2	2	2	2	2	2	According to climate.
Towels	No.	2	2	2	2	2	2	2	
Type	„	1	1	1	1	1	1	1	
Knife with two lanyards	„							1	
Knife	„	1	1	1	1	1	1	1	
Shoes	Pairs.	1	1	1	1	1	1	1	
Half Boots	„	1	1	1	1	1	1	1	
Bed Covers	No.	2	2	2	2	2	2	2	
Bed	„	1	1	1	1	1	1	1	
Blanket	„	1	1	1	1	1	1	1	
Band—Tunic, blue	„					2			
„ serge	„								
„ white	„								
Cap	„								

III. CLOTHING, CLEANLINESS, AND PRESERVATION OF HEALTH.

496. He (the captain) is to divide all the ship's company, exclusive of the marines, into divisions, and appoint a lieutenant to command each division, who is to have under his orders as many sub-lieutenants and midshipmen as the number on board will admit. He is to take especial care that the divisional officers conform in every particular to the directions contained in Chapter XIV., p. 184.

497. He will cause the men's clothing and bedding to be inspected by the divisional officers, before each issue of clothing materials, or oftener if necessary—taking care that the inspections are so conducted as not to be unnecessarily irksome to the men. The general issue of clothing is to take place every month, and the officers of divisions are to prepare lists, specifying the quantities required by each man, entering the men's names thereon, consecutively, as they stand on the ship's books. The lists are to be delivered in time for the accountant officer to satisfy himself that the value of the articles required by each man will not, even in the case of a new entry, bring the individual in debt to the Crown more than the amount of two months' pay; and subsequent issues are to be so regulated as to leave a balance in the man's favour.

2. The issue of clothing to boys is to be so regulated that they may generally be kept clear of debt.

3. The captain will not sanction large issues of clothing to a man, whereby his wages are dissipated and many irregularities arise; but he will assure himself, before approving the list, that the articles demanded are really necessary for the man's use and comfort—remembering that he will be held liable to reimburse the Crown should anyone under his command, on quitting the service, be in debt beyond the extent authorised by the foregoing instructions and those relating to pay. See Art. 1684, and also 1686, as to casual issues.

498. He is to permit all the officers and men, including the Royal Marines, to wear beards and moustaches.

2. In all cases when the permission is taken advantage of, the use of the razor must be entirely discontinued. Moustaches, except in the case of marines (Article 1118), are not to be worn without the beard, nor the beard without moustaches.

3. The hair of the beard, moustaches, and whiskers, i
kept well cut and trimmed, and not too long for cleanlines
captain is to give such directions as seem to him desirab
these heads, and is to establish, as far as may be practicab
formity as to length of the hair, beards, moustaches, and w
of the men; observing that those men who do not avail the
of the permission to wear beards and moustaches will wea
hair and whiskers as heretofore.

4. Officers of divisions will take special care that the pro
of Clauses 2 and 3 are strictly attended to by such of their
may avail themselves of the permission to wear beards and
taches, and failure in these respects will render the offende
to summary punishment.

499. The captain will use his best endeavours to ensure
liness, dryness, and good ventilation throughout the ship'
pany and throughout every part of the ship; that she is
pumped dry, the pump-well frequently swabbed, and a f
down to dry it, proper precautions being taken to guard
accidents. He is to take care that there is a free passage fo
aft for the water; that those places where, from the trim
ship, there may be a lodgment, are baled out and dried; that
possible means are taken to ensure a free and thorough circu
of air, and that room be left for a man to get down upon the
to clear the limbers. He will frequently examine the state
holds, and the lower parts of the ship, in company with the n
officer, and when not perfectly clean and free from obn
smells, he will cause a thorough examination to be made to
and remove whatever may be likely to engender disease.

2. He is to cause an officer to inspect the holds, and all p
the ship below, every morning, and to report to him whethe
are in a clean and well-ventilated state or otherwise.

3. He will take care that the holds are whitewashed eve
months, or oftener if necessary.

4. If the weather should prevent the ports from being o
for a considerable time, fires are to be lighted in the stove
windsails are to be freely used, so that the lower decks may b
as dry and as well ventilated as possible.

5. He is to see that the men are properly clothed, in the
lished uniform, according to the nature of the climate in
they may be serving; that they are generally cleanly in thei
sons and dress, and that they are never suffered to rem

wet clothes, or sleep in wet bedding, when it can possibly be avoided.

6. The bedding is to be aired once a week when the weather will permit, each article being exposed separately to the air by being tied up in the rigging or upon girt lines. Twice in every year the blankets are to be washed with soap, in warm water; and once a year the bed-tickings are to be washed, and the hair beaten and teazed.

7. No poison or poisonous acid is to be used to clean mess traps.

500. The captain will take care that the regulation kit (Appendix VIII., page 687) for petty officers, seamen, and boys, is strictly adhered to; he will not permit the slightest deviation from the established patterns or drawings, so that, on transfer, men and boys may be spared the expense of alterations.

2. The number of articles may, however, be exceeded when of the authorised pattern, if they can be conveniently stowed.

501. He will take care that the officers and men are permitted to avail themselves of the special fittings provided in the ship for personal washing; that when practicable fresh water be issued for the purpose; that the bath-room when so fitted is kept supplied with both hot and cold water; that it is open for the use of those who desire it every evening after quarters; and that proper times are appointed for washing the person, so that it may be a part of the daily routine.

502. He will, before the ship leaves England, or any port where there is a naval hospital, take steps to ascertain whether any of the men are suffering from disease requiring hospital treatment; the officers of the divisions, accompanied by a medical officer, are to go carefully round the divisions, and are to call upon the men to inform the medical officer of any complaints, however trifling, they may be labouring under; and should there be reason to fear from the appearance of any man that he may be suffering from concealed disease, he is to be medically inspected.

2. No man discharged from the sick list after venereal disease is to be allowed to go on leave till eight days have elapsed from the date of his discharge.

3. Should the captain find, on inquiry in any port abroad which his ship may occasionally visit, that venereal disease is notoriously prevalent, he may exercise his discretion in withholding leave during his stay at the place, should due regard for the health of

APPENDIX.

3. The hair of the beard, moustaches, kept well cut and trimmed, and not too lon; captain is to give such directions as seem t these heads, and is to establish, as far as formity as to length of the hair, beards, of the men; observing that those men who of the permission to wear beards and hair and whiskers as heretofore.

4. Officers of divisions will take special of Clauses 2 and 3 are strictly attended to may avail themselves of the permission to w taches, and failure in these respects will rend to summary punishment.

499. The captain will use his best end liness, dryness, and good ventilation throu pany and throughout every part of the ship; pumped dry, the pump-well frequently swab down to dry it, proper precautions being take accidents. He is to take care that there is a fre aft for the water; that those places where, fro ship, there may be a lodgment, are baled out and possible means are taken to ensure a free and th of air, and that room be left for a man to get dow to clear the limbers. He will frequently examin holds, and the lower parts of the ship, in company officer, and when not perfectly clean and free smells, he will cause a thorough examination to be and remove whatever may be likely to engender dis

2. He is to cause an officer to inspect the holds, the ship below, every morning, and to report to him are in a clean and well-ventilated state or otherwise.

3. He will take care that the holds are whitewas months, or oftener if necessary.

4. If the weather should prevent the ports from for a considerable time, fires are to be lighted in th windsails are to be freely used, so that the lower deck as dry and as well ventilated as possible.

5. He is to see that the men are properly clothed, lished uniform, according to the nature of the clim they may be serving; that they are generally cleanly rons and dress, and that they are never suffered

the officers and men, and the duty on which he is en
such a precaution necessary. In every case of ref
this ground he is to report the fact to his commande
ing his reasons for having done so.

IV. MEDICAL INSTRUCTIONS.
§ I. Hospital and Sick Quarters.

1004. When practicable, a medical officer is al
pany a patient to hospital.

1005. No officer, except in a case of urgency,
hospital without the previous approval of the senior
who before giving it will satisfy himself with the
doing. Should, however, the medical officer in cha
pital consider any particular patient so sent not to be
he is still to be received, but the medical officer
opinion, with the grounds for forming it, to the seni

1006. No officer is, for his own convenience, t
vant to attend upon him while sick in a naval hospit
is a staff of nurses or other attendants provided ;
cases, when it may be necessary to permit a servant
his master to hospital, the victualling of the ser
arranged from afloat.

1007. All persons serving in ships afflicted with
disease are, if practicable, to be sent to the nearest h
as possible.

1008. Officers are to be allowed to take with th
such clothes or effects as they may desire ; but men a
whole of their clothes and effects ; marines, in additi
and accoutrements when on the home station.

1009. As far as practicable, every patient sho
him from his ship all necessary clothing ; but if he a
to take up a supply at the hospital, the value will
directed by Arts. 1477 and 1478, when provided w
otherwise, as directed by Art. 1504.

1010. Captains will receive from the hospital autl
culars of patients from their ships who may die, or b
invalided, run, or be otherwise disposed of, so that
tions may be made on the ship's books.

1011. When patients are cured, they are to be re
ship to which they belong, if she be in port ; but, if

to be received as supernumeraries, and retained either for passage or for disposal, in such ship as, in the absence of general local orders on the subject, the senior officer present may specially direct.

2. Should any patients on being so discharged from hospital be deemed unserviceable, or if there should be urgent reasons why they should not be received and reference to a senior officer be impracticable, they may be sent back, but with the returned patients the principal medical officer of the hospital should receive from the captain and the medical officer of the ship a statement of the grounds for refusing to receive them, and full particulars are also to be at once furnished to the superior authority under whom the captain may be acting.

1012. When men are invalided from a hospital, the principal medical officer of the establishment will certify to the fact by his signature on the parchment certificate.

1013. In case the necessity should arise for landing sick at a place where there is no hospital, the senior officer is to make the best arrangements in his power. If the services of a private practitioner are necessary, he is to enter into a contract with him for the attendance and medicines for each patient; and the victualling also, if deemed expedient, on such terms as may, with due regard to the comfort and care of the patients, be best for the public service.

2. The practitioner so appointed is to be required to render any returns or reports that may at the time be deemed necessary. He should be informed that he will receive the usual documents with the patients, and when they are returned to their own or to any other ship, he is to send back the documents, and obtain from the captain a certificate that the patients have been received. If any patient dies or deserts, he is to note the date on his ticket, and send it with a statement showing how his effects have been disposed of to the Admiralty, for the Accountant-General, and a duplicate thereof to the commander-in-chief, for the information of the captain.

3. Before approving of the payment of these accounts, the senior officer will assure himself that they have been carefully examined by competent officers.

1014. When patients are sent to sick quarters on shore other than those of established surgeons and agents, a statement showing why the case could not be safely treated on board is in each instance to be forwarded to the Admiralty, for the Direc[tor?] approved of by the captain. When there is no medica[l] ship, the captain will obtain the information from the to whom the patient is sent for transmission in like m[anner].

1015. The subsistence of patients of either the [mili]tary service in the hospitals of the other, at home or [abroad] be paid for at the following rates:—

For officers	2s. 6d. per die[m]
For men	7d. ,,
For boys	6d. ,,

2. In the case of naval patients the accountant office[r] these payments on the approval of the captain.

1016. Patients from hospital as well as from the si[ck] if necessary, to be treated as convalescents so long as t[he] officer of the ship may think it necessary.

1017. Distressed British subjects arriving home in be sent to naval hospitals until they can be received into workhouses as casual poor, or conveyed to their proper parishes.

1018. When a person dies in a ship at a place where naval hospital, the body is to be sent to the hospital for i[nterment] but if the friends of the deceased desire to undertake th[is at] their own expense, the body is to be delivered up to the[m].

2. When a body is sent to hospital for interment, t[he] officer of the ship is to forward a certificate, approv[ed by the] captain, of the deceased's age, date of death, and the which he died.

1019. Officers and men of ships, including any on le[ave] at a place where there is no naval hospital or burial gro[und] unless their friends wish to undertake the burial, be inte[rred at] public expense; but in no case will the Admiralty sanc[tion pay]ment of more than 14l., from the public funds, for the fu[neral of an] officer; or 6l. for that of any other person. Proper vo[uchers for] such payments as the captain may direct to be made u[nder this] head, are to be transmitted by the accountant officer wit[h his] account.

2. Coast Guard officers are also instructed to make [neces]sary arrangements when such persons die near to their st[ations]

§ II. THE INSPECTOR-GENERAL OR DEPUTY INSPECTOR-GENERAL OF A FLEET.

1020. He is, on appointment for service afloat, to perform such medical duties as may be required of him by the commander-in-chief or senior officer of the fleet, squadron, or station, or by the captain of the ship in which he may be serving, or other his superior officer, and he will comply with all orders he may receive from the Admiralty, or from the Director-General.

1021. He is, when in a hospital ship, to have medical charge of all the patients, and he is to visit them regularly morning and evening, or oftener if necessary. All arrangements relating to the part of the hospital ship appropriated for the sick and wounded are to be entirely under his control; and when necessary he will propose to the captain any measure likely in his opinion to conduce to the comfort of the sick or to the acceleration of their cure.

1022. He is, under the direction or with the sanction of the senior officer on the spot, to visit from time to time the ships present, to inquire into their sanitary state and the treatment of their sick. He will examine the medical officers' journals, and correct any errors of practice he may detect; and with this object he may call on the medical officers of ships for written statements as to the prevalence of any disease, or as to the treatment or progress of any particular case or cases. He will also make himself thoroughly acquainted with the conduct and abilities of the several surgeons.

1023. He is occasionally to examine the instruments, medicines, and necessaries in the ships, and when from any cause he finds remedial measures necessary, he will suggest them to the senior officer.

1024. He is to report in the prescribed forms to the commander-in-chief or to the senior officer weekly, or oftener, if required—

a. The state of the sick in the hospital,
b. The general condition of the sick of the fleet,

sending duplicates to the Director-General.

1025. He will suggest to the commander-in-chief or senior officer any measures which he may deem calculated to improve the health of, or check the progress of disease in, particular ships, and to preserve the health of the fleet generally.

1026. He will report annually in the prescribed form to the Director-General upon the health of the fleet; he will enter fully

into the sanitary state of the respective crews as re[
effectiveness, and also into the medical topography of [
He will report fully upon any epidemic that may have [
or any disease that may have been unusually prevalent.
that he may be fully informed on these subjects, t
officers will furnish him quarterly with duplicates of
logical returns.

1027. When on a foreign station he is, if required
the senior officer, to visit the naval hospitals or sick quar
not in charge of a medical officer senior to himself, and
the medical treatment, diet, and comfort of the patien
the general economy of the establishment, as well as up
penditure and condition of the stores, and the general e
the officers and others employed therein.

1028. He will, when directed to attend a survey on
men, assist the surveying officers with his opinion.

1029. He will forward his correspondence in the
manner:—

a. Returns and accounts . . .	Direct to th ant-Gener case may
b. Reports relative to the medical and surgical treatment and care of the sick and wounded . . .	Direct to th General.
c. Suggestions as to the fittings and internal arrangements of the hospital ship, and correspondence relative to individual officers and men borne on her books, on subjects other than (b) . . .	To, or thr captain of
d. Reports and returns relative to the fleet generally, or to ships other than the hospital ship . .	Direct to th der-in-chi officer pro

§ III. THE MEDICAL OFFICER.

1030. He is to obey not only all orders he may re[
his captain or other his superior officer, but also any
relating to—
    a. The administering of medicines,
    b. The treatment of the sick, or
    c. To his accounts and returns,

which he may receive from the Director-General, the A

General, or from the inspector or deputy-inspector in commission attached to the fleet or squadron to which his ship belongs; he will furnish them, or any of them, through his captain, with any information that may be required of him respecting—

  d. The patients under his care, and
  e. The measures adopted for their cure;
  f. his accounts and returns;

but any suggestions, explanations, or observations he may have to offer, connected with his particular duties and not of a purely medical or surgical character, which directly or indirectly concern the duties and responsibilities of others than medical officers, and which obviously lie beyond the province of the medical department to remedy or to deal with adequately, are to be made in duplicate to his captain, who will forward the original to the Commander-in-Chief, and the duplicate to the Director-General, noting in each case his approval, or such observations as he may wish to offer on the medical officer's representations.

1031. The medical officer is to provide himself with, and keep in proper repair at his own expense, a complete set of surgical instruments, as set out in the established form; on first fitting out he will obtain a certificate from the naval hospital as to their number and condition, and send it to the Director-General.

2. He is to examine frequently the surgical instruments with which the surgeons are hereby required to provide themselves, to see that they are in good repair and according to scale, giving annually certificates of their number and condition.

1032. On first fitting out he will apply to the nearest hospital or depôt for the established supplies of medicines and medicine chests, utensils, necessaries, bedding, and appliances specified in Established Scales A and B.

2. The contents of one of the medicine chests when more than one are supplied, and of the grocery and necessary chests, are to be stowed away in the Dispensary, and the empty chests immediately returned into store addressed to the officer in charge of the depôt from which they were issued. The other complete medicine chests will be placed in a safe place, so that the medical officer may have ready access to them, and from these chests the medicines required from time to time in the dispensary are to be drawn, the empty bottles and jars being returned into the spaces from whence the full ones are taken.

3. Where only one medicine chest with one or t
chests are supplied, they are to remain on board,
where there is no dispensary, the medicines and nec
be kept in their respective chests. Diagrams showi
of the medicines are supplied with the articles on fit

4. The medicine chests will not be struck down
or spirit room upon any pretence whatever, nor
situation where they may sustain injury. Accomr
provided for the due care of all medicines and med
medical officer will be held responsible for their pres

5. He is annually, or oftener if necessary, to mak
in the established forms, showing the quantities r
the quantities required to complete the establishe
according to the scales. These demands, when ap
captain, are to be taken, with the medicine chests,
or depôt, in order that the requisite supplies may
and, to prevent inconvenience or delay, demands
sented there, if possible, before three o'clock in the t
no stores are to be returned after that hour. Dema
be repeated for medicines, utensils, or necessaries
nor for groceries within six months, unless the ship
detached service, or extraordinary circumstances shal
or are likely to cause, an unusual expenditure, th
which is to be explained on the demand, and to be r
Director-General by letter at the same time. Trus
are to be completed as often as necessary. As to
Art. 1766.

6. The medical officers of stationary ships at home
there are no hospitals or medical depôts, are not,
their demands, to send the empty chests and bottle
plies will be sent in contractors' bottles, which are t
and retained until an opportunity offers of sending
issuing depôt free of expense.

1033. In a small vessel not bearing a medical
officer in command is to have charge of the medicine
stores, which, with the medical and surgical handboo
the quantities allowed, instructions for using the m
directions for applying tourniquets, will be suppli
nearest naval hospital on demand when fitting out ;
care to replenish the medicines or the stores as occa
quire ; and he will bear in mind that although the n

supplied by avoirdupois weight, they are to be dispensed by the weights and measures of the British Pharmacopœia, according to which the doses specified in the medical handbook are regulated.

2. A quarterly return, in the established form, of the sick and wounded, is to be forwarded from all ships not bearing a medical officer, to the Commander-in-Chief, for the Admiralty.

1034. On a ship being commissioned, the medical officer is to make an immediate detailed application in duplicate through his captain, to the Director-General, for such other articles not particularised in Scales A and B in the Book of Forms, including stationery and printed forms not included in the established list, as he may consider to be necessary for the use of the sick bay.

2. On receiving the Director-General's sanction to the demand, he is to purchase, on the lowest possible terms, such of the articles as cannot be obtained from the naval hospital or depôt. The expense of such articles is to be defrayed by the accountant officer in the same manner as those provided under Art. 1036. With regard to any stores which may subsequently be obtained for the sick bay, no purchases of articles obtainable out of the store are to be made at ports where there are medical depôts for the service afloat; and if purchases of regulation medicines or stores allowed by the established scales are at any time made, a statement showing the reasons for making them, and why a proper stock of articles was not obtained when the ship was last at a medical depôt, is to be sent at the time when the articles are bought to the Director-General.

3. Demands for sick bay stores for Indian troop ships are to be sent to the director of transports.

1035. The medical officer will superintend the sick mess, which is to be formed in each ship for the comfort of the sick and wounded. He will cause the accountant officer to be informed when any man in the sick list is to join the sick mess, so that the man may be checked of his provisions.

The medical officer is to demand from the accountant officer, with the approval of the captain, such articles of diet, medical comforts, &c. (including wine and spirit), as he may consider necessary for the use of the sick, including invalids; but, while fully providing for the due comfort and subsistence of those for whom the ordinary ration is unsuitable, he is to guard against profuse expenditure or unnecessary indulgence, and he will adhere

312   APPENDIX.

as closely as may be to the following daily scheme of d
sick :—

	FULL DIET	HALF DIET
Soft bread (when procurable) . .	1 lb.	12 oz.
Beef	1 ,,	8 ,,
Vegetables (when procurable) . .	1 ,,	8 ,,
Broth	1 pint	1 pint
Barley for ditto	12 drachms	12 drachms
Or rice, in lieu of barley . .	10 ,,	10 ,,
Pot herbs (when procurable) . .	24 ,,	24 ,,
Salt	8 ,,	8 ,,
Vinegar	16 ,,	16 ,,
Tea	3 ,,	3 ,,
Sugar	14 ,,	14 ,,
Milk (when procurable) . .	½ of a pint	½ of a pint
Wine	At the discretion of the medical	
Cocoa (as a substitute for tea) . .	1 oz.	1 oz.

N.B.—Medical comforts, and such articles of the men's daily allowance
deem advisable, are to form part of the diet for the sick.

3. For these supplies he is to grant receipts quarter
obtain from the accountant officer counterparts or issue 1
his signature thereto. It is, however, to be understood
medical officer is not to give receipts to the accountant
any articles forming a part of the authorised scale of r
men, unless the quantities supplied may have exceeded
portions allowed for the number victualled in the sick m
being taken that in regard to tea, sugar, and other article
in Scale B, the excess, if any, is limited by the proportio
by that scale, except on extraordinary occasions, which
stated by the medical officer in his reports.

1036. The medical officer will, in accordance with A
demand of the accountant officer on first commissioning o
such sum of money as he may think necessary to provide
fresh diet, washing, and other small occasional expenses
of the sick. At the end of each quarter, or sooner if the
is nearly exhausted, he will render to the captain a detai
ment of the payments made, to be accompanied when p1
by receipts or sub-vouchers; he will then receive, on the
approval, from the accountant officer a sum equal to the
actually accounted for, so as to have in his hands the
originally advanced. On being superseded, or on the ship b
off, or in case of his death, the balance of this public mone
returned to the accountant officer, with the accounts and
for the intervening period since the accounts were last ren

1037. An account of the medicine and medical stores is to be rendered for a period of twelve months from the date of the officer taking charge (except in the case of the Indian troop ships, which are specially provided for), and for each ensuing twelve months from the date of completing the last account; or for any shorter period on giving up charge or on the ship being paid off.

1038. Medicines and medical stores supplied from a regular establishment will be accompanied by invoices in the prescribed form, which are to be preserved by the medical officer for future reference, and by which he is to examine the several quantities, and, if correct, they are to be entered in the proper columns of his account.

2. The articles received from the accountant officer, as shown in the issue notes (see Art. 1662), are also to be entered in the account, as well as all articles obtained from any other source or purchased for the sick berth, except diet for the sick; the issue or supply notes are to be preserved by the medical officer for future reference.

3. The articles received are to be administered as occasion requires for the relief of the sick and wounded, and no part of them is to be wasted or applied to any other purpose than that for which they are intended; and if any unusual expenditure of medicines or stores should occur, an explanation of the circumstances causing such expenditure is to be forwarded with the account. Should any articles of medicine, utensils, bedding, necessaries, or appliances become unfit for use, they are not to be taken credit for, nor returned into store, until a survey has been held upon them (Chap. XLVI., page 574). Credit will not be allowed for any bedding or utensil expended, unless under unavoidable circumstances, which must be satisfactorily explained; and an explanation on the established form of the cause of all losses and breakages must be transmitted with the account.

1039. Receipts for trusses issued and for supplies to other medical officers, &c., and for articles returned into store, are to be obtained and to accompany the account.

1040. The account is always to be closed by a survey, as directed in Art. 1826, except when the ship is paid off, when the whole of the remaining stores are to be returned into the nearest medical establishment, and the receipts for the quantities returned into store transmitted as vouchers to the final account; but in the Indian troop ships the survey on the remains is to be held at the end of the trooping season in each year, as well as charge.

2. The account is to be transmitted by the capt accompanied by a schedule prepared by the medic proper form, to be obtained from the accountant o the documents forwarded with it.

1041. When the medical officer shall be superse he is to deliver the whole of the stores in his cl cessor, or in his absence to some authorised perso directed in Chapter XLVI., page 574.

1042. All naval sick quarters on shore which of a resident medical officer, are to be treated as t account as sick bays on shore of the ships from been sent for treatment, or on the books of whi borne if left behind in the quarters in charge of th of another ship.

2. All articles, other than of diet, purchased such sick quarters, and who are treated there by the of their ships, are likewise to be accounted for officers on their annual accounts of medicines an receipt is to be obtained by them from the officer w the sick quarter buildings for any stores which the the sick quarters on the final departure of their v port.

3. These sick quarters being, however, provided sary bedding, furniture, hospital stores, and utens of the officer in charge of the buildings upon the D to whom he is responsible for duly maintaining th stores, medical officers of her Majesty's ships are no chases of any articles of the foregoing description officers and men under treatment in these quarters.

1043. He is to represent to the captain, whenev sider any men from recent illness or impaired healt shore, boat, or detached service which is about to be

1044. He will, whenever he considers it advisal to every person about to form part of a working in unhealthy localities, whether tropical or not, fou phate of quinine in water before landing; and again if any men remain on shore all night, the officer charge should be furnished with a sufficient quantity for each man night and morning. When the medi siders wine or spirit more advisable than water, he will inform the captain, who will direct the accountant officer to make the requisite issues.

2. The formula for making the sulphate of quinia for issue in the manner above directed is given in Appendix V. to the Medical and Surgical Handbook, copies of which will be supplied to ships for boat service.

He will not charge himself with these extra issues of wine or spirit, but he will observe and report very fully on their effects, and note the total quantity so issued at the end of his journal.

1045. He will, if he should consider any newly-raised men, who have been found fit for the service, are likely, from any cause, to propagate any infectious disease, although no such disease may have been developed, inform the captain, who will order them to be well washed, and their clothes thoroughly fumigated, and the men themselves cleansed and kept apart from the ship's company for a reasonable time. Should the disease have developed itself at the place from whence the suspected men came, the captain will, in addition to these precautions, report immediately the particulars to his commander-in-chief.

1046. The medical officer will, whenever necessary, and especially when infectious diseases have broken out or are threatening, suggest to the captain to cause hanging stoves to be placed in parts of the ship where they are required for ventilation or for dryness. He will also make such suggestions as may occur to him as necessary with reference to clothing when going from a warm to a colder climate, or *vice versâ*.

1047. He will, if he learns on arrival at a place that any disease is prevalent which is likely to prove detrimental to the health of the ship's company in his medical charge, inform the captain, so that proper measures may be adopted to prevent its occurring or breaking out, in the ship or among any of the ship's company. Should it break out or occur, or should he have reason to suspect its presence in a latent form, he will, with the captain's sanction, adopt every possible measure to prevent its spread or development. Patients with infectious diseases should be at once removed from the ship, or, if that is not practicable, separated as much as possible from the ship's company, their persons washed, and their clothing changed; the bedding and clothes they have recently worn should be thrown overboard or immersed in boiling water.

1048. Should sloughing ulcer break out, the patients affected

and thoroughly washed, and ...
Each should have a separate ...
directly the ulcer puts on a heal...

1049. When an infectious dis...
apprise the captain, for the infor...
or senior officer present. Should ...
senior officer, the captain will be gui...
diately communicating the particu...
medical officer will also inform the I...
General of the Fleet, if any, and state ...
of the disease, and the health of the ship...
he will give full information on these ...
returns.

1050. The medical officer will, whene...
duties he shall discover that any person ...
concealed, aggravated, or feigned any dis...
the service, report the particulars of the ...
that, if deemed advisable, the offender may ...
case shall deserve.

1051. He will, whenever supplies of water are
the shore, or from rivers, for drinking or cooking
tute as careful an analysis of it as possible with the
supplied, and he will at once inform the captain
exists as to its purity, in order that it may either b
gether, or only used for washing purposes.

2. All such analyses are to be duly recorded i
Journal.

1052. He and the surgeons are to visit the sick
day, and oftener when necessary; he will take care t
or attendants fully understand that day or night he i
called in case any doubtful or unfavourable change t
patient.

1053. The sick berth itself, and the sick berth a
dants, and nurses, are to be entirely under his di
berth is to be kept dry, clean, and sufficiently warm.
and other articles supplied for the use of the sick a
clean, and ready for immediate use. He will judge
should remain in the berth, and will, when necessary

captain for any further requisites that may be needed for the sick, or any additional men as day or night nurses.

1054. His attention is not to be confined to men on the sick list; but he will watch attentively every circumstance likely to affect the health of the ship generally. Should he suspect the presence of disease or indisposition in any man, he is at once to examine and deal with him accordingly.

1055. When directed by the captain, he and the surgeons will inspect the men, to ascertain if they have any concealed diseases requiring treatment. When venereal cases are discharged cured, he will in each case make a particular report, as no man so discharged is, as a precautionary measure, allowed to go on shore till eight days have elapsed from the date of his discharge from the sick list.

1056. He will forward quarterly in the established form a return of venereal disease on board, which is to include only cases that are suspected of being capable of reproducing the disease, and which are inserted under that head in the Nosological Returns.

2. The average number of men on board is to be found by adding up the number victualled each day of the quarter, and dividing the total by the number of days in the quarter. The accountant officer will sign the return with reference to the correctness of this average.

1057. He is to take care that every preparation is made for the accommodation and treatment of the wounded. When clearing for action, he, with the surgeons and others appointed to attend him, will repair to their station, where a platform with every convenience is to be provided.

2. He is, under the authority of the captain, to instruct or cause to be instructed a certain number of persons quartered in different parts of the ship in the use of the tourniquet, and to provide a sufficient number of temporary tourniquets for the different quarters and tops, so that the wounded, while waiting to be medically attended, may not lose more blood than can be avoided.

1058. He is to report at once to the Director-General, and to the superior medical officer in charge of the fleet, if any, the particulars of every death that occurs on board, as well as of any deaths that may occur among persons on leave.

1059. In cases of sudden death, without previous indisposition, he is, with the sanction of the captain, to examine the body to ascertain the cause: should there be any appearances of a suspicious character, he will at once inform the captain that, practicable, an inquest may be held.

1060. He will record in his sick book daily tualled in the sick mess.

1061. He is to represent to the captain whom any officers and men are, from impaired health or objects for survey; he will be very careful not to be deceived by men feigning diseases for the purpo charged or sent home.

1062. When invalids are sent to a ship for a concise statement of each case, in the established the medical treatment to the period of their being accompany them; it is to be handed over to the m the hospital or ship into which they are discharged home. When officers are invalided from foreig medical officer is to deliver to each a detailed statem of the commencement and progress of his compla send it by the first opportunity to the Secretary of noting on the cover, ' Director-General, Medical De

1063. A nominal list of all the invalids embar tablished form, is to be transmitted to the Director should any of the invalids have died during the medical officer is to transmit the original cases receiv accompanied by a detail of the symptoms and mod while under his care.

1064. When men can be conveniently cured on b not to be sent to a hospital, hospital ship, or sick qu labouring under an infectious or contagious diseas wounds or complaints render their retention on board others or injurious to themselves, or if the numbe wounded be so great as to prevent their receiving prope they are to be sent to hospital as soon as possible. therefore, it becomes necessary to send patients to a medical officer is to inform the captain, who will, w give the requisite orders for preparing their pay and a noting upon the latter whether the patient has been board for that day or not, and inserting in both an each man's effects. The patient's effects are to be caref and marked with the name of the ship and the owner. officer will also give as early information as possible cipal medical officer of the number of patients to be hospital, and the probable time at which they will be disembarked, in order that due preparation may be made for their reception. A medical officer will, when practicable, be sent with the patients to see that they are properly received at the hospital or sick quarters, and that they are conveyed thither with as little inconvenience as possible ; and should two boats be required, he is to be sent in the one with the worst cases, in order to afford ready relief on the passage. A detailed statement of each case, sealed up, is to be delivered with the patients at the hospital, showing the manner in which they were first seized, the nature and progress of their disorders, the means used for their cure, and whether there is reason for suspecting any of their complaints to be feigned.

1065. Patients affected with itch are to be received into naval hospitals at home and abroad, provided they are not sent in such numbers as to encroach on the room and accommodation required for the treatment of more serious cases.

1066. The medical officer from whose ship men have been sent to a hospital is to visit them as frequently as the captain may require ; obtaining in every case the previous consent of the principal medical officer of the hospital, who will give such information as may enable the medical officer of the ship to inform the captain when any of them are likely to return to their ship.

1067. The medical officer is to keep a daily sick-book, which is to contain the names of all the sick on board, and which he is to submit to the captain every morning : at the same time suggesting any measures he may consider necessary for the comfort and benefit of his patients.

2. Whenever the name of any person is inserted in the sick-book for a wound or injury, the part of the body injured is to be stated, and, if possible, how the wound or injury was occasioned.

1068. He is also to deliver to the captain weekly, or at such other periods as he may direct, a return of the sick on board in the established form.

1069. He is to forward quarterly to the Director-General a nosological return in the established form of the state of the sick, properly filled up and signed by himself, subjoining to it, under the head of remarks, a clear and succinct account of the several diseases, the state of the weather, of any peculiarities of climate, and the average height of the thermometer ; and he is also to detail every other circumstance that may have had an influence in promoting health or generating sickness in the ship's company.

These returns are to be completed and read
one week after the termination of the pe
made up ; before being transmitted to th
are to be submitted to the captain for his in
in forwarding them is to be fully explained
General. In each return a list is to be giv
certificates have been granted, or trusses is
or, if none have been granted, it is to be
of a continuance of any prevailing sickness
of an endemic or epidemic character, or w
infection, contagion, or other causes of
special report in connection therewith is to
often as opportunities may offer. If there
or Deputy-Inspector-General attached to t
which his ship belongs, a copy of every no
transmitted to him ; and upon the arriva
from abroad, or from a lengthened cruise,
diately transmitted to the Director-General
sede or in any way interfere with the retu
at the regular stated periods.

1070. He is to keep a rough and a fair
in the form established, transmitting the l
General made up to December 31 of each ye
charge within three months of the expiratio
transmit his journal completed to Decembe
year, taking care that the nosological tab
journal are drawn up as follows :—Table
cases of sickness occurring previously to De
year ; Table No. 4 is to include all cases occ
sequent year. In the event of his being s
the Table No. 4 is to contain all cases occurr
and the date of his giving up charge. In T
the number of cases of each class of disease, a
periods of age during the first year ; and in
made of cases during the subsequent year,

the head of General Remarks, a history of the complaints prevalent in the ship during the period of the journal, as well as any information of a professional character, or in connection with the collateral sciences, that he may think of value. If any malignant or infectious diseases make their appearance, he is to endeavour to trace them to their source, to account for their introduction, and to explain the means used for destroying the infection and preventing their reappearance.

2. In Table No. 1 he is to insert the movements of the ship during the period of the journal.

3. In Table No. 2 he is to insert the names of persons who have received wounds or hurts which may partly or wholly disqualify them for the public service, or subsequently, in any way, interfere with their earning a livelihood, specifying those to whom hurt certificates have been given.

4. When the journal is completed, he is to copy his sick-book into the form provided at the end of the journal, arranging it alphabetically, and strictly in accordance with the specimen given in the book of forms.

5. Further, he is to keep his fair journal in such a state of forwardness, that at any time it may be transmitted to the Director-General ; and it is at the latest to be transmitted within six weeks after the period for which it is due. The importance of this injunction cannot be overrated, as pensions and gratuities are often dependent upon the care with which the cases of both officers and men have been recorded in the medical journals of the ships in which they have served.

1072. A medical history sheet in the established form is to be provided for each man or boy on first entry by the medical officer, by whom these documents are to be kept and carefully filled up.

2. Whenever a man or boy is sent to hospital or transferred to another ship or to head-quarters, the medical history sheet is to accompany his certificate, so that it may follow him wherever he goes. When he is finally discharged the service, it is to be sent to the Medical Director-General, and if he re-enters it is to be forwarded to the medical officer of the ship on the captain's application.

3. Should the man or boy be borne as part complement, the medical officer will record 'nil' in case he should never have been on the sick list.

4. In ships without a medical officer, the captain will see that

all necessary entries are made by the medical officers w
called on to give occasional attendance.

5. When men and boys are being medically ...
medical officers will note on the medical sheet all ...
the person or other peculiarities, congenital or ...
would be useful for future identification, or, if already ...
to verify, and, if necessary, amend the previous ...

1073. When directed by the captain to examine m...
he is not only to examine their persons very carefully, t
whether they are fit for the service, but he is also to in
particularly into their previous history, so as to be abl
whether there is any risk of their bringing infection int
He is also to ascertain whether they are pensioned, an
represent the same to the captain. If they come from a r
or receiving ship, and are found to be unfit for the servic
report, in writing, to the captain his reasons for deemin
be so, in order that he may adopt the measures direc
instructions.

1074. When a medical officer is examining any such
admission into the Naval Service, or into the Royal Mar
first to observe whether he has any marks of wounds, or
the bones of the head, whether his eyesight or hearing is
whether he is deformed, lame, or has an impediment
or weakness of intellect ; and should any of these or oth
or physical defects exist to such an extent as might, in t]
of the examining officer, disqualify him for the efficient
of his duty, be is to report him unfit, but in ships spe
nished with the prescribed forms, the examination is t
pleted and the details duly entered.

2. Should the person present no outward appearance
ness, he is to be directed to strip ; and the medical officer
satisfy himself, by a careful inspection of the entire cuta
face, that it is not only in itself free from disease, but th
no evidence or sign of the existence of any internal con
constitutional derangement.

3. He is to ascertain that there is a proper and just
between the different members of the body, that there is
weakness or deformity, that the limbs are of equal lengt
and well developed, that there are no visible marks of
fracture, depression, or disease of the bones of the head
herent cicatrices, that the hearing is perfect in both ears,

is no defect or deformity of the bones of the nose, and that the teeth are good, strong, and sufficient in number.

4. The chest should be carefully examined in reference to its form and capacity, and the condition of the heart and lungs ascertained by percussion and auscultation.

5. The eyes should be clear, intelligent, and expressive of health, the eyesight good.

6. The abdomen is next to be examined for the purpose of detecting any enlargement or disease of the contained viscera, or predisposition to hernia from whatever cause.

7. The examining officer shall next direct the person to extend and slowly raise his arms until the hands meet above his head ; he is then to perform the various movements of the shoulder, elbow, and wrist joints ; to flux and extend, supinate, and pronate the forearm ; to flux and extend the fingers and thumbs ; and, by holding on by a rope, show that he can bear the weight of the body clear of the ground without any difficulty, with each hand, for at least five seconds.

8. In the examination of the lower extremities, the person is to be made to walk backwards and forwards, to hop first on one foot and then on the other, to flex and extend the limbs and feet to show that the movements of the various joints can be freely and rapidly performed.

1075. Persons of whatever class, or age, who are found to be labouring under any of the undermentioned physical defects or infirmities are to be considered unfit for her Majesty's service :—

- a. A weak constitution arising from imperfect development, or weakness of the physical powers of the body, or from chronic disease, constitutional depravity, wounds, or injuries.
- b. Chronic eruptions on the skin or scalp ; syphilis, primary or constitutional ; gonorrhœa ; extensive marks of cupping, leeching, or blistering, or of issues. Marks of punishment are to be reported to the captain.
- c. Malformation of the head, with a dry, harsh, divergent state of the hair of the scalp, fracture or depression of the bones of the skull, disordered intellect, imbecility, epilepsy, paralysis, or impediment of speech.
- d. Blindness or defective vision in one or both eyes, fistula lachrymalis, and ptosis.
- e. Impaired hearing, or discharge from one or both ears, disease

or thickening of the lining membrane of
ear.

f. Disease of the bones of the nose or of its
polypus.

g. Disease of the throat, palate, or tonsils; u
offensive breath from constitutional caus
gums, scrofulous disease of the glands of
neck, external cicatrices, whether from scrof
suicidal wounds.

h. Functional or organic disease of the heart or
deformity or contraction of the chest, flat
sub-clavicular regions, phthisis, hæmoptysi
dyspnœa, aphonia, chronic cough, or other
tubercular exudation into the pulmonary tiss

i. Swelling or distension of the abdomen, undue ob
or enlargement of the liver, spleen, or kid
ture, weakness, or distension of the abdo
stricture of the urethra, incontinence of urin
fistula.

j. The non-descent of one or of both testicles, va
drocele, and sarcocele.

k. Fistula, or fissure of the anus, hæmorrhoids,
or prolapsus of the rectum.

l. Paralysis, weakness, impaired motion, or contr
upper or lower extremities, from whatever
rism, a varicose state of the veins, especiall
Chalky deposits, bunions, distortion, malform
feet, or malposition of the fingers or toes ; no

m. Distortion of the spine, of the bones of the che
from injury or constitutional defect.

2. Whenever test-types are supplied, the power of v
eye separately, as well as together, is to be ascertained
finally rejecting a person who failed to read the types,
tested with objects familiar to him, and at distances corr
the size of the objects, as the inability occasionally arise
causes than defective sight. If they fail to distinguish
they should be tried with brighter and decided colou
purpose red, blue, green, and yellow ribbon flags m
When the sight is found defective, the particulars are to
in the register of physical examination when required
how far short of the normal distances given in the test-

the letters or figures be seen, and when one is more defective than the other, the limit of good vision of each eye is to be noted.

3. As it is clearly possible that some of the preceding defects or disabilities may exist in a minor degree, the examining officers must necessarily, in such cases, be guided by their own judgment as to whether they are of such importance as entirely to disqualify a man or boy for the service; observing, however, that no person is to be reported fit unless he is likely to continue efficient and serviceable in any climate, and under all the vicissitudes of the service, for a period of not less than ten years.

1076. All men and boys entering the service are to be re-vaccinated.

2. All men who have not been re-vaccinated between their first entry in the service and the age of eighteen shall be re-vaccinated as soon as possible, however good their primary cicatrices may appear, or even should they present unmistakable evidence of having suffered from small-pox previous to that age. The re-vaccination is to be made with lymph either taken fresh from the arm of a child, or from supplies to be obtained from the National Vaccine Institution.

3. On the Home Station the medical officer will obtain supplies of lymph by written application direct to the Secretary of the Local Government Board, London; on Foreign Stations, if supplies cannot be obtained at a Naval Medical Depôt, application is to be made to the Director-General.

4. No person shall be considered re-vaccinated who has had the operation performed with lymph taken from the arm of a re-vaccinated person, but all persons so re-vaccinated shall again be vaccinated with lymph taken from the sources specified above.

5. A notation of the date of re-vaccination is to be made by the medical officer on each man's certificate of service, specifying the result, whether a perfect vaccine vesicle, a modified vaccine vesicle, or no result; and he will, with the captain's sanction, occasionally examine the certificates to see that these important precautionary regulations are in no case overlooked or disregarded.

6. The medical officer will, as soon as convenient after he joins a ship, satisfy himself that each officer has been successfully re-vaccinated, and so also with regard to every officer who may subsequently join, except those borne for disposal or as temporary supernumeraries in home ships, and whose stay in them will be but short.

7. When vaccination or re-vaccination cannot be satisfactorily

performed in a ship, resource is to be had to local vaccinators, who will, under the authority of the captain, be paid by the accountant officer for each successful case, on the certificate of the medical officer, or, when none is borne, of the captain.

xxxx. All persons examined for entry into the naval service or marines by a medical officer are to be entered on a list in the medical journal of the ship, in the nosological returns for hospitals and marine infirmaries, and in the weekly returns made by surgeons and agents.

xxxx. When any person on full pay shall receive a wound or hurt in an act of duty, either afloat or on shore, the medical officer will prepare a hurt certificate in the established form, describing minutely the nature of the injury, together with the manner in which it was received, the particular act of duty on which the injured person was employed, and whether he was sober or not at the time; the certificate is to be signed by the captain and by the medical officer, and also if possible by some officer of the military branch, or, if none, by some other person who witnessed the accident. The certificate is to be granted whether the injury disables the individual from continuing in the service or not.

2. These certificates are not to be given for wounds or hurts received on leave (except in an act of duty while on leave), or occasioned by drunkenness or other improper conduct, but shall be confined solely to injuries received in acts of duty.

3. They shall not be granted for rupture unless the individual shall make application immediately after the accident; they should be made out within forty-eight hours of the rupture. In exceptional cases, when this rule cannot be observed, the reasons are to be given on the certificate.

4. Notations of injuries received in acts of duty shall also be made on men's parchment certificates at the same time that the hurt certificates are granted.

5. Men's hurt certificates are to be kept and dealt with in the same manner as their parchment certificates until they are pensioned or otherwise disposed of: officers' hurt certificates are to be delivered to them.

6. When marines are disembarked, the hurt certificate, signed by the commandant and the medical officer, and by some officer or other person who witnessed the accident, is to be granted under the same conditions as when serving afloat.

7. Notices are to be posted up on board all ships and at the

marine divisions, to the effect that no injuries received after August 30, 1870, will be considered when men are finally discharged from the service, unless they can produce proper hurt certificates, and also cautioning men to report immediately any appearance of rupture.

1079. Every medical officer serving on board any of her Majesty's ships is, previously to his sending any letter or any communication whatever relative to his public duty, to the Director-General, to submit it to the captain, who will note thereon his approval, or such observations as he may think necessary.

1080. All unemployed medical officers upon the active list of the navy are to keep the Director-General informed of their permanent addresses, so that they may be speedily communicated with as occasion shall require; and whenever such officers are in or passing through London, on appointment to a ship or after discharge from a ship, they are without fail to communicate personally with the Director-General.

1081. Every fleet or staff surgeon on active service is to forward annually to the Director-General, and for any shorter period on being paid off, superseded or invalided, the original or attested copies of the certificates of his service and conduct, signed by the captain. He is also to transmit regularly all the medical returns, accounts, and other documents required by these instructions, to enable the accounts to be speedily closed.

1082. The medical officer is to grant to the surgeons serving under him at the end of each year, and also when leaving a ship, certificates of their conduct, which are to be approved of by the captain, who, when they are not satisfactory, will call upon the medical officer for a detailed report, which he will forward to the Admiralty through the commander-in-chief with his own remarks.

1083. As medical officers are afforded many opportunities of obtaining a knowledge of the medical topography of the places they visit; of the more prevalent diseases and the approved mode of treatment; of the healing properties, preparations, and uses of medicinal plants or productions, they should report all the information they can collect on these interesting and other cognate subjects that they may believe to be new or but little known; and the senior medical officers should encourage those serving under them to cultivate a taste for scientific observation, which can hardly fail to be of use to the individual himself as well as to the service and to the cause of science.

§ IV. Surgeons.

1084. The surgeons are to make themselves acq the foregoing instructions for the medical officer, a therewith at all times in so far as they may relate to or when they are acting for the medical officer.

1085. They are to provide themselves with the particularised in the established form of certificate, in medical charge they are to keep a surgeon's journa ward it to the Director-General on December 31 in ea

1086. A surgeon is to send to the Director-Genea of every year's service, and on quitting a ship, certifica signed by the captain and medical officer respectively ; from the medical officer in the established form, shc has furnished himself with the instruments required, are in complete order ; if he does not regularly trans tificates, or attested copies thereof, at the periods omission will be regarded as an objection to his prom his being placed on the half-pay list when paid off.

1087. In the absence of the medical officer, or no fleet or staff surgeon is borne, the senior surgeon observe and follow these instructions ; and in the ev validing or death of the medical officer, he will be hel for the medical returns and accounts of the ship until

§ V. General.

1088. Whenever operations are to be performed hospital, timely notice will be given, in order that as sible of the medical officers in port may attend ; and notice that operations are to be performed elsewh officers in charge will attend themselves, and encourag them to do so also, that no opportunity may be lost their surgical experience.

1089. All medicines are to be uniformly received, accounted for by avoirdupois weight of 16 drachms and 16 ounces to the pound, but they will be disp weights and measures of the British Pharmacopoeia.

1090. All medicines or medicinal compounds kept dispensaries are—

    a. If poisonous, to be put into dark blue bottles yellow labels, with the word POISON legibly the name of the medicine :

b. If harmless, into white or pale green glass bottles, or white ware jars with green labels.

2. When supplied to patients, whether for internal or external uses, they are—
   a. If poisonous, to be put in ribbed or fluted bottles of a dark blue colour only, with the yellow POISON label:
   b. If harmless, in bottles of pale green or white glass only, with green labels.

3. No other bottles or labels are on any account to be used.

4. All medicines labelled POISON are to be kept under lock and key and apart from the others in the dispensary.

V. QUARANTINE REGULATIONS.

(*Vide Act* 6 *Geo. IV. cap.* 78, *in sec.* 234 *of the Customs Consolidation Act*, 1876, &c.)

1938. The captain is to direct an officer, when sent to a ship, not to go on board until he shall have ascertained that she did not come from any place which may subject her to quarantine; and if she did come from any such place, to obtain whatever information he is sent for, without quitting the boat. But if any of her Majesty's ships shall, either at sea or in port, have communication with other ships, by which they may be subject to quarantine, the captain is on no account to conceal such communication, but to make it known by at once carrying the proper quarantine flag at one of the mast-heads, and he is to prevent all communication with ships or the shore until she be liberated; while in quarantine he is to observe, in the most strict and particular manner, all regulations for the conduct of ships so situated, as hereinafter explained.

1939. The captain of a ship liable to quarantine shall at all times, when she meets with any other ship at sea, or when within two leagues of the coast of the United Kingdom, or the islands of Guernsey, Jersey, Alderney, Sark, or Man, cause to be hoisted a signal to denote that the ship he commands is liable to the performance of quarantine. The signal in the day time to be, if the ship have a clean bill of health, a large yellow flag of six breadths of bunting at the maintop-mast-head; if she shall not have a clean bill of health, a like yellow flag with a circular mark or ball entirely black in the middle thereof, the diameter of which shall be equal to two breadths of bunting; and in the night time the sign: both cases be a large signal lantern with a light therein (commonly used on board her Majesty's ships of war) at mast-head.

1940. The captain of any of her Majesty's ships of shall meet a vessel liable to perform quarantine coming t port, shall take care to prevent the landing of any articles from on board the same, until the vessel shall be the charge of the superintendent of quarantine, or his or the principal or other officer of her Majesty's Cus thorised to act at any of the out-ports, and the capta Majesty's ships are at all times to furnish such assista officers respectively as may be required of them for enf due performance of quarantine.

1941. All vessels, as well her Majesty's ships of war coming from, or having touched at, any place from w Majesty, her heirs or successors, by and with the advi Privy Council, or any two of the Lords of the Privy Co have declared it probable that the plague or other infecti may be brought, shall be obliged to perform quarantii manner as shall be notified by proclamation, or publisl 'London Gazette.'

1942. All baggage, packets, packages, wearing appa letters, or any other articles whatsoever arriving in vess from infected places, are liable to quarantine in the san as goods, wares, and merchandise. Any person landing ping, or moving in order to land, such baggage or oth from on board a vessel liable to quarantine, shall forfeit 500*l*.; and any person clandestinely conveying, or conc the purpose of conveying, any of the articles above e from a vessel actually performing quarantine, or from shall forfeit the sum of 100*l*.

1943. All her Majesty's ships of war, transports, vessels in the actual service of Government, under the co a commissioned officer of her Majesty's Navy, coming Mediterranean, or West Barbary on the Atlantic Ocea furnished with clean bills of health, shall perform quaran Motherbank and nowhere else, in a separate and distinc pointed and marked out with yellow buoys for that purp centre of which place a floating lazaret is stationed, wit flag constantly flying at the mast-head.

1944. No persons, vessels, or boats whatsoever, other than the vessels or boats belonging to the medical attendant or superintendent of quarantine, or his assistant, or other boats regularly employed under the authority of the Commissioners of Customs in the quarantine service, shall go, under any pretence whatever, within the limits so marked out, except in case of special necessity and emergency, and with permission first had and obtained from the superintendent of quarantine or his assistant.

1945. Her Majesty's ships and vessels liable to quarantine, and furnished with clean bills of health, shall perform a quarantine of fifteen days, commencing on the day that the ship or vessel shall have arrived at the appointed quarantine station; but the Lords of the Privy Council, in consideration of the inconvenience and expense incurred by her Majesty's ships of war arriving from the Mediterranean, in consequence of their detention in quarantine until orders respecting them can be forwarded from London, have given orders that the proper officers shall release all ships of war belonging to her Majesty, or to any nation in amity with her Majesty, which may arrive from the Mediterranean or from West Barbary Coast on the Atlantic Ocean, immediately on their arrival, without waiting for special orders from their lordships; provided the captain shall declare that all persons on board are, and have been, free from any disease of a suspicious nature as to contagion during the voyage. Her Majesty's ships and vessels with foul bills of health shall perform a quarantine of thirty days; and with suspected bills of health (commonly called touched patents or bills), of twenty days.

1946. No article, however little susceptible it may be thought of infection, is to be conveyed from one vessel under quarantine to another, nor is any personal intercourse to be permitted from any such vessel to another, and nothing whatever is to be delivered from on board any vessel under quarantine without an order in writing from the superintendent or his assistant; every such order is to be entered in a book by one of the guardians appointed by the superintendent as quarantine guardians on board each ship performing quarantine.

1947. Every person quitting a vessel liable to quarantine, unless by proper authority, may be apprehended by any constable, and is liable to imprisonment for six months, and to forfeiture of the sum of 300*l*.

1948. Any person or persons liable to quarantine, or having

had any intercourse or communication with a person o
liable to quarantine, who shall refuse to repair to the laza
or other place duly appointed for the performance of quar
shall escape, or attempt to escape, therefrom before qua
duly performed, shall forfeit 200*l*., and the quarantine
use force to compel such person or persons to return to
or other duly appointed place for quarantine.

1949. Communication may be made by persons in q
with others not in quarantine, by letters, under such re
and restrictions as will prevent the spread of infection ;
purpose an officer appointed by the superintendent of q
shall daily, at a fixed hour, go round the different laza
vessels in quarantine to receive letters. Letters may al
ceived under similar restrictions, but no personal comm
or conference is to be had by persons not under quaran
persons under quarantine (except the medical attendant
perintendent of quarantine, or his assistant, or any per
authorised by Order in Council), unless by permission
presence of the superintendent or his assistant, and un
regulations and restrictions as shall be directed by him.

1950. The captains of all her Majesty's ships of w
ports, and other vessels, are subject to all the provision
and regulations concerning quarantine under the Act above
and to all the pains, penalties, forfeitures, and punishm
any breach or disobedience thereof, in the same manne
masters of merchant ships ; each ship is therefore suppl
the special quarantine regulations containing the said Act
Orders in Council issued under the authority thereof.

2. The captains of all vessels, whether liable to quara
not, neglecting to bring to, on being requested by an
Customs, authorised to act in the quarantine service, are
a penalty of 100*l*.

1951. Penalties for any of the foregoing offences aga
quarantine statutes, or for not flying the appointed signal
ceeding 100*l*. for each offence, are in certain cases recovera
marily under Sec. 234 of the Customs' Consolidation A
in default of payment the offender is liable to six mo
prisonment.

1952. Officers in command of fleets, squadrons, or sin
are to be very careful when arriving at a port out of th
Kingdom, whether British or foreign, to comply strictly

local regulations relative to quarantine; in cases of doubt, and when the local regulations may not be known, no communication should be held with the shore, with boats, or with other ships, until a sufficient time has elapsed to allow of the visit of the health officer.

2. If the ship or ships shall have arrived from an infected port, or shall have any infectious or contagious disease on board, or shall have communicated with a ship from an infected port, or with contagion or infection on board, the quarantine flag is to be hoisted and kept flying until pratique is received.

3. Every facility is to be afforded to health officers when performing these duties.

1953. Before a ship sails from a home or any foreign port, the captain will take care to obtain a bill of health.

SELECTIONS FROM THE REGULATIONS FOR THE MEDICAL DEPARTMENT OF THE ARMY (1878).

I. DUTIES OF MEDICAL OFFICERS IN CHARGE OF TROOPS ON BOARD SHIP.

62. When troops are ordered on foreign service, and have been detailed by the commanding officer, they will be at once examined by a medical officer. They will, subsequently, be inspected by the principal medical officer, several days before the date of embarkation, to decide as to their general fitness, so as to give the commanding officer sufficient time to replace those considered ineligible by the principal medical officer.

63. A medical officer will, on the day of embarkation, if possible, or if this be impracticable, on the previous day, make a careful examination of every soldier, woman, and child of every regiment or detachment ordered to embark for foreign service. He will forward to the principal medical officer of the district for transmission to the Director-General of the Army Medical Department a statement of the number of men, women, and children fit to embark, together with a certificate that he has made the examination referred to, and that no case of infectious disease exists amongst them. In all cases where troops, soldiers' wives, or children, are proceeding from one station to another, the sanitary provisions laid down in Part 5, Sec. vii. of these regulations will be followed.

64. The medical comforts required for troops embarked on board her Majesty's ships will be obtained by the paymaster of the ship, and be issued by him on the requisition of the medical officer in charge of the troops. Supplies of medical comforts required from army stores for her Majesty's ships conveying troops or military invalids, will be placed in charge of the paymaster of the ship, who will be accountable to the Admiralty for the quantities remaining unexpended at the conclusion of the voyage.

68. In hired ships a copy of the regulations for her Majesty's transport service will be provided by the Admiralty and kept on board, and access can be had thereto by application to the master of the vessel.

77. They (the medical officers) will also be prepared with information on the following points :—

- a. Date of departure of the vessel from the port where the troops embarked, and the name of the port.
- b. Length of the passage in days.
- c. State health of troops on board.
- d. Whether the ship has been provided with every requisite, with special reference to the amount and quality of provisions in accordance with the scale, and with an adequate supply of water, medicines, instruments, and medical comforts.
- e. Whether the ship has been kept in a good sanitary condition in respect to ventilation, cleanliness, means of ablution, &c.
- f. Whether the accommodation has been good, and whether the superficial area and cubic space per man of sleeping accommodation has been sufficient.
- g. Whether any defects have been discovered during the voyage.
- h. The number of officers, men, women, and children embarked.
- i. The deaths in each class.
- j. The number of births during the voyage.
- k. The prevailing diseases on board and their causes.
- l. The nature of the accommodation for the reception and treatment of the sick, including the superficial area and cubic space for sick bed.

m. When lime juice and sugar have been issued, the quantities of each supplied for each man, for what length of time used, and the total of each consumed during the voyage. A detail of names will not be required.

II. MOVEMENT OF TROOPS BY SEA.

670. Every soldier, woman, and child about to embark will be carefully examined by a medical officer on the day of departure, or if the military arrangements will not admit of this, on the day previous, with a view to prevent any individuals showing symptoms of contagious disease proceeding on board ship. All soldiers' families under orders to proceed to a foreign station should be under medical observation for some weeks before embarkation. Every woman, and every child above three months old, must be vaccinated before proceeding to embark, unless already bearing satisfactory marks of vaccination. Soldiers' wives near their confinement (within two months) will not be embarked on her Majesty's Indian troop ships, or in mail or contract steamers, or other vessels, and the husbands of such women will be detained with them.

671. When a ship is engaged wholly or partially for the conveyance of troops, the inspections prescribed in Section 17, paragraphs 23 to 28 of the 'Queen's Regulations and Orders for the Army, 1873,' will be held, and the senior medical officer on the spot, and, if practicable, the medical officer in charge of the troops, will attend the inspections and report upon the sanitary condition of the ship, and on the arrangements made. When invalids are to be embarked, the senior medical officer will satisfy himself that there is a due proportion of medical officers according to the number and state of the sick.

672. Should the inspecting medical officer discover any defects likely to affect injuriously the health of the troops or the sick during the voyage, he will make his remarks accordingly on the report of inspection, and he will forthwith report the circumstances in writing in such detail as he may consider necessary to the officer commanding at the port, transmitting a copy to the principal medical officer on the station, who will forward the same with his remarks to the Director-General.

673. The medical officer in charge of troops and sick will, during the voyage, keep a constant watch over the ventilation and cleanliness of the ship, the cleanliness of the water-closets, the condition of the bilge, and over all other matters likely to affect in-

juriously the health of the troops or sick [see ' Queen's
and Orders for the Army, 1873,' Section 17, ' Dutie
Ship ']. Should defects arise in any of these matters,
officer in charge will immediately represent the same t
commanding on board, with such recommendations as]
sider necessary for the preservation of health. After
been eight days at sea, or whenever the medical of
necessary, lime juice and sugar will be issued with the
according to the scale of victualling which is to be seen

674. Medical officers embarked with troops on bo
ship, deeming it necessary to make any statement an
upon the sanitary arrangements, or the supplies on
address such report to the officer commanding the t
mitting a duplicate to the principal medical officer at
embarkation. Copies of any adverse remarks embod
usual report of sick must also be furnished to the officer
ing. The sanitary arrangements on board her Majo
ships rests with the naval medical officer under the ca
should the medical officer in charge of the troops consid
sary to make any suggestions on the subject, he wil
report to the officer commanding the troops. Wheneve
any infectious disease has made its appearance amongst
or their families during a voyage, the medical officer in
landing, will make a special report of the circumsta
military and medical authorities at the port of disembar

675. Whenever a disembarkation takes place at a
where there is any law or local ordinance in force for the
of venereal disease, the medical officer detailed to visit a
the vessel will ascertain whether the medical officer in
inspected the troops, with a view to detect and guard a
introduction of these diseases. He will report the res
inspection of the vessel to the principal medical officer
mission to the Director-General, with the return of tl
board, W. O. Form 294 B.

III. HOSPITAL SHIPS FOR AN ARMY CORPS.

423. The relative responsibility of the Admiralty
Office with regard to hospital ships for an Army Corps,
follows.

424. The Admiralty will undertake the lodging, v
and conveyance of the sick, and for that purpose will p

necessary shipping fittings, bedding, food, medical comforts, disinfectants, and mess utensils of every kind.

425. The War Office will undertake to furnish the medical and other attendance necessary for the proper treatment and nursing of the sick, and the washing of all hospital clothing and bedding used by them, and will supply all articles of personal and hospital clothing, medical and surgical appliances, and hospital utensils.

426. Floating hospital accommodation, whether stationary or for transport purposes, will be separate and exclusive of the hospital accommodation for the force on land.

427. The following will be the floating hospital accommodation for an Army Corps:—Each division of an Army Corps will have a depôt hospital ship (with steam power) capable of making up 200 beds or 250 on an emergency.

428. There will be one or more swift powerful steamers, each making up 60 beds, which will be employed as relieving ships for the depôt hospital ships to take the worst cases to England. Despatch vessels, each fitted out with about 30 canvas cots, will carry less severe cases to any available packet station to meet the packets on their way to England.

429. Special arrangements will be made for carrying a small number of invalids in each steam packet.

430. Each depôt hospital ship will have a small steam transport attached as a store ship.

431. Every transport will accommodate temporarily in its sick bay three per cent. of the entire force that it carries.

432. Each depôt hospital ship will be supplied with 400 canvas cots in addition to the cots required for use on board. These will be fitted into transports remaining at the base of operations when additional hospital accommodation is required.

433. The dieting of patients on board depôt hospital ships and their relieving vessels will be conducted in the same way as in station hospitals, and the same War Office forms will be used. Daily requisitions for articles of diet and medical comforts will be made on the paymaster, or, if it be a hired ship, on the master of the vessel.

434. A statement of provisions received, issued, and remaining will be completed on W. O. Form 184, at the end of each month, and forwarded to the head-quarters of the Army Medical Department for transmission to the Surveyor-General of the Ordnance, War Office, London.

435. Each of these hospital ships will be provided with a suffi-

cient staff of the Army Hospital Corps for carrying out th
duties detailed in paragraphs 425, 436.

436. The regulations for medical officers in charge of
board ship [Part L, Section III., Subsection III.] will
despatch vessels, transports, and packets used for the
accommodation of the sick of the Army Corps.

437. When a ship has been taken up by the Admiral
conveyance of troops, either as a transport or a troop fre
an army medical officer (if possible the medical officer
have charge of the troops) will make a careful inspecti
ship's crew, at the time of the first inspection of the ve
will immediately inform the naval inspecting officer of
reporting the same to the principal medical officer.

438. The medical officer in charge of troops on bo
ports and troop freight ships will take medical charge of
crew also when the ship does not carry a surgeon, and
medicines, &c., for their use from the public stock
will have a general sanitary supervision over the ship
make inspections of the quarters occupied both by the t
by the crew.

439. The following is a detail of the medical equipm
will be put on board a transport for the use of troops and

> One medicine chest complete.
> One case of surgeon's instruments.
> One case of tooth instruments.
> One stomach pump.
> One box of fracture apparatus.

440. This equipment will be put on board and hande
the medical officer in charge, who will give a receipt for
to the principal medical officer at the port of embarkation

441. In the event of the medical officer landing with
when transports are employed during military operations,
ment will be left on board the ship under the charge of th
who will give a receipt to the medical officer specifying the
articles, not quantities, contained in each. The master w
nished with a duplicate thereof countersigned by the
officer.

442. The equipment will be handed over again to
medical officer who embarks for duty on board, and who
nish the master with a receipt for the same.

UNITED STATES 'PASSENGER ACT OF APRIL 8, 1880.'

A Bill to regulate the Carriage of Passengers by Sea.

Be it enacted, &c., That it shall not be lawful for the master of a steamship or other vessel, whereon emigrant passengers, or passengers other than cabin passengers, have been taken at any port or place in a foreign country or dominion (ports and places in foreign territory contiguous to the United States excepted), to bring such vessel and passengers to any port or place in the United States, unless the compartments, spaces, and accommodations hereinafter mentioned have been provided, allotted, maintained, and used for and by such passengers during the entire voyage; that is to say, in a steamship, the compartments or spaces, unobstructed by cargo, stores, or goods, shall be of sufficient dimensions to allow, for each and every passenger carried or brought therein, one hundred cubic feet, if the compartment or space is located on the first deck next below the uppermost deck of the vessel, or in a poop or deck-house constructed on the main deck of the vessel; and one hundred and twenty cubic feet for each passenger carried or brought therein, if the compartment or space is located on the second deck below the uppermost deck of the vessel; and it shall not be lawful to carry or bring passengers on any deck other than the two decks above mentioned, and in the aforesaid poop or deck-houses. And in sailing vessels such passengers shall be carried or brought only on the deck (not being an orlop deck) that is next below the uppermost deck of the vessel, or in a poop or deck-house constructed on the main deck; and the compartment or space, unobstructed by cargo, stores, or goods, shall be of sufficient dimensions to allow one hundred and twenty cubic feet for each and every passenger brought therein. And such passengers shall not be carried or brought in any between-decks, nor in any compartment, space, poop or deck-house, the clear height of which is less than seven feet. In computing the number of such passengers carried or brought in any vessel, children under one year of age shall not be included, and two children between one and eight years of age shall be counted as one passenger: and any persons brought in such vessel, who shall have been, during the voyage, taken from any other vessel

wrecked or in distress on the high seas, or have been
sea from any boat, raft, or otherwise, shall not be incl
computation. The master of a vessel coming to a po
the United States in violation of either of the provi
section, shall be deemed guilty of a misdemeanor;
number of passengers, other than cabin passengers
brought in the vessel, or in any compartment, space, p
house thereof, is greater than the number allowed to
brought therein respectively, as hereinbefore prescril
master shall be fined fifty dollars for each and every
excess of the proper number, and may also be imprise
ceeding six months.

§ 2. *And be it further enacted*, That in every such
other vessel, there shall be a sufficient number of be
proper accommodation, as hereinafter provided, of a
sengers. There shall not be on any deck, nor in any c
or space occupied by such passengers, more than two tie
The berths shall be properly constructed, parallel with
the vessel, and be separated from each other by p
berths ordinarily are separated, and each berth shall
two feet in width and six feet in length; and the inter
the floor or lowest part of the lower tier of berths and t
neath them shall not be less than six inches, nor
between each tier of berths, and the interval between
most tier and the deck above it, less than two feet six
each berth shall be occupied by not more than one pas
eight years of age; but double berths of twice the
tioned width may be provided, each double berth to be
no more and by none other than two women, or by
and two children under the age of eight years, or by h
wife, or by a man and two of his own children unde
eight years, or by two men, members of the same famil
male passengers, upwards of fourteen years of age, v
occupy berths with their wives, shall be berthed in th
of the vessel, in a compartment divided off from the spa
appropriated to the other passengers by a substantia
secured bulkhead, without opening or communication w
joining passenger space; and unmarried female passeng
berthed in a compartment separated from the spaces
other passengers by a substantial and well-constructed
the opening or communication from which to any ad

senger space shall be so constructed that it can be closed and secured. Each berth shall be numbered serially, on the outside berth-board, according to the number of passengers that may lawfully occupy the berth ; and the berths occupied by such passengers shall not be removed or taken down until they have been inspected by a customs officer as hereinafter provided. For any violation of either of the provisions of this section, the master of the vessel shall be liable to a fine of five dollars for each passenger carried or brought on the vessel.

§ 3. *And be it further enacted,* That every such steamship or other vessel shall have adequate provision for affording light and air to the passenger decks and to the compartments and spaces occupied by such passengers, and with adequate means and appliances for ventilating the said compartments and spaces. To compartments having sufficient space for fifty or more of such passengers, at least two ventilators, each not less than twelve inches in diameter, shall be provided, one of which ventilators shall be inserted in the forward part of the compartment, and the other in the after part thereof, and shall be so constructed as to ventilate the compartment ; and additional ventilators shall be provided for each compartment in the proportion of two ventilators for each additional fifty of such passengers carried or brought in the compartment. All ventilators shall be carried at least six feet above the uppermost deck of the vessel, and shall be of the most approved form and construction. In any steamship the ventilating apparatus provided, or any method of ventilation adopted thereon, which has been approved by the proper emigration officers at the port or place from which said vessel was cleared, shall be deemed a compliance with the foregoing provisions ; and in all vessels carrying or bringing such passengers, there shall be properly constructed hatchways over the compartments or spaces occupied by such passengers, which hatchways shall be properly covered with houses or booby-hatches, and the coamings or sills of which shall rise at least one foot above the deck ; and the said houses shall have a door on each side, so constructed as to afford the greatest amount of light and air and of protection from wet that the case will admit ; and there shall be proper companion-ways or ladders from each hatchway leading to the compartments or spaces occupied by such passengers ; and the said companion-ways or ladders shall be securely constructed, and be provided with hand-rails or strong rope, and such passengers shall have the free and unimpeded use of the whole of each hatch-

way situated over the compartments or spaces approp
use; and every vessel carrying or bringing such pa
have a properly located and constructed camboose
range, or other cooking apparatus, the dimensions a
which shall be sufficient to provide for properly coo
paring the food of all such passengers. In every vess
bringing such passengers, there shall be at least two
or privies, and an additional water-closet or privy f
hundred male passengers on board, for the exclusiv
male passengers, and an additional water-closet or p
fifty female passengers on board, for the exclusive use
passengers and young children on board. The afo
closets and privies shall be properly enclosed, and lo
side of the vessel, and shall be separated from passe
by substantial and properly constructed partitions o
and the water-closets and privies shall be kept and m
serviceable and cleanly condition throughout the voya

For any violation of either of the provisions of th
for any neglect to conform to the requirements therec
of the vessel shall be liable to a penalty not exceeding
and fifty dollars.

§ 4. *And be it further enacted,* That every such
other vessel shall have on board during the voyage, pr
and secured, a supply of good and wholesome food, pr
water, sufficient to provide for the daily distribution
such passengers while on board the vessel an allowanc
provisions equal, for the first twenty days of the voy
to at least fifty cents, United States money, per head,
good and wholesome character and of sufficient quanti
served on tables with seats around, as now is custo
second cabin of the transatlantic steamships, the con
the fifty cents' value to be made in bulk at the rate of
for every hundred passengers. Mothers with infant
children shall be furnished the necessary quantity of

If any passenger shall, at any time during the voyage, be put upon short allowance of food or water, the master of the vessel shall pay to such passenger three dollars for each and every day the passenger may have been put on short allowance. And for every wilful violation of any of the provisions of this section, the master shall be deemed guilty of a misdemeanor, and shall be fined not more than five hundred dollars, and be imprisoned for a term not exceeding six months. The enforcement of this penalty, however, shall not affect the civil responsibility of the master and owners of the vessel to such passengers as may have suffered from any negligence, breach of contract, or default on the part of such masters and owners.

§ 5. *And be it further enacted,* That in every such steamship or other vessel, there shall be properly built and secured, or divided off from other spaces, two compartments or spaces to be used exclusively as hospitals for such passengers, one for men, and the other for women; the hospitals shall be located in a deck-house constructed on the main deck or on the deck next below the uppermost deck of the vessel, and not elsewhere; the hospital spaces shall in no case be less than in the proportion of eighteen clear superficial feet for every fifty such passengers who are carried or brought on the vessel, and such hospitals shall be supplied with proper beds, bedding, and utensils, and be kept so filled and supplied throughout the voyage. And every steamship or other vessel carrying or bringing emigrant passengers, or passengers other than cabin passengers, exceeding fifty in number, shall carry a duly qualified and competent surgeon or medical practitioner, who shall be rated as such in the ship's articles, and who shall be provided with surgical instruments, medical comforts, and medicines proper and necessary for diseases and accidents incident to sea voyages, and for the proper medical treatment of such passengers during the voyage, and with such articles of food and nourishment as may be proper and necessary for preserving the health of infants and young children; and the services of such surgeon or medical practitioner shall be promptly given, in any case of sickness or disease, to any of the passengers, or to any infant or young child of any such passengers who may need his services. For a violation of either of the provisions of this section, the master of the vessel shall be liable to a penalty not exceeding two hundred and fifty dollars.

§ 6. *And be it further enacted,* That the master of every such

steamship or other vessel is authorised to maintain good ⟨
and such habits of cleanliness amongst such passengers as
to the preservation and promotion of health, and to th
shall cause such regulations as he may adopt for such pur
posted up on board the vessel, in a place or places accessib
passengers, and shall keep the same so posted up d⟨
voyage; the said master shall cause the compartments a
provided for or occupied by such passengers to be ⟨kept⟩
in a clean and healthy condition, and to be, as ⟨often as⟩
necessary, disinfected with chloride of lime, or by ⟨some⟩
efficient disinfectant. Whenever the state of the we⟨ather⟩
permit, such passengers and their bedding shall be mu⟨stered on⟩
deck, and a clear and sufficient space on the uppermost d⟨eck of the⟩
vessel shall be set apart, and so kept, for the use and e⟨xercise of⟩
such passengers during the voyage. For each neglect or ⟨violation⟩
of any of the provisions of this section, the master of ⟨the vessel⟩
shall be liable to a penalty not exceeding two hundred
dollars.

§ 7. *And be it further enacted,* That neither the officers,
nor other persons employed on any such steamship or ot⟨her vessel⟩
shall visit or frequent any part of the vessel provided or ⟨assigned⟩
to the use of such passengers, except by the direction or p⟨ermission⟩
of the master of such vessel first made or given for such ⟨purpose;⟩
and every officer, seaman, or other person employed on boar⟨d such⟩
vessel, who shall violate the provisions of this section, ⟨shall be⟩
deemed guilty of a misdemeanor, and may be fined not e⟨xceeding⟩
one hundred dollars, and be imprisoned not exceeding twe⟨lve months⟩
for each violation; and the master of such vessel who d⟨irects or⟩
permits any officer, seaman, or other person employed on b⟨oard such⟩
vessel, to visit or frequent any part of the vessel provid⟨ed or⟩
assigned to the use of such passengers, or the compart⟨ments or⟩
spaces occupied by such passengers, except for the purpose ⟨of doing⟩
or performing some necessary act or duty as an officer, se⟨aman, or⟩
other person employed on board of the vessel, shall be
guilty of a misdemeanor, and may be fined not more than ⟨one hun-⟩
dred dollars for each time he directs or permits the provision⟨s of this⟩
section to be violated. A copy of this section, written or ⟨printed,⟩
in the language or languages of the passengers on board, ⟨shall by⟩
or under the direction of the master of the vessel, be pos⟨ted in a⟩
conspicuous place on the forecastle and in the several part⟨s of the⟩
vessel provided and assigned for the use of such passengers

each compartment or space occupied by such passengers, and the same shall be kept so posted during the voyage ; and if the said master neglects so to do, he shall be deemed guilty of a misdemeanor, and shall be fined not more than one hundred dollars.

§ 8. *And be it further enacted,* That it shall not be lawful to take, carry, or have on board of any such steamship or other vessel any nitro-glycerine, dynamite, or any other explosive article or compound, nor any vitriol or like acids, nor gunpowder, except for the ship's use, nor any article or number of articles, whether as cargo or ballast, which, by reason of the nature or quantity or mode of storage thereof, shall, either singly or collectively, be likely to endanger the health or lives of the passengers or the safety of the vessel ; and horses, cattle, or other animals taken on board of or brought in any such vessel shall not be carried on any deck below the deck on which the passengers are berthed, nor in any compartment in which passengers are berthed, nor in any adjoining compartment, except in a vessel built of iron, and of which the compartments are divided off by water-tight bulkheads extending to the upper deck. For every violation of any of the provisions of this section the master of the vessel shall be deemed guilty of a misdemeanor, and shall be fined not exceeding one thousand dollars, and be imprisoned for a period not exceeding one year.

§ 9. *And be it further enacted,* That it shall not be lawful for the master of any such steamship or other vessel, not in distress, after the arrival of the vessel within any collection-district of the United States, to allow any person or persons, except a pilot, officer of the customs, or health officer, to come on board of the vessel, or to leave the vessel, until the vessel has been taken in charge by an officer of the customs, nor after charge so taken, without leave of such officer, until all the passengers with their baggage have been duly landed from the vessel ; and on the arrival of any such steamship or other vessel within any collection-district of the United States, the master thereof shall deliver to the officer of customs who first comes on board the vessel and makes demand therefor, a correct list, signed by the master, of all the passengers taken on board the vessel at any foreign port or place, specifying separately the names of the cabin passengers, their age, sex, calling, and the country of which they are citizens, and the number of pieces of baggage belonging to each passenger, and also the name, age, sex, calling, and native country of each emigrant passenger, or passengers other than cabin passengers, and their intended destina-

tion or location, and the number of pieces of baggag[e]
each passenger, and also the location of the compart[ment]
occupied by each of such passengers during the voya[ge]
of such passengers died on the voyage, the list sh[all]
name, age, and cause of death of each deceased pas[s]
duplicate of the aforesaid list of passengers, verified
the master, shall, with the manifest of the cargo, b[e]
the master to the collector of customs on the entry
For a violation of either of the provisions of this
permitting or neglecting to prevent a violation there
of the vessel shall be liable to a fine not exceeding
dollars.

§ 10. *And be it further enacted,* That in case the[re]
occurred on board any such steamship or other ves[sel]
among such passengers during the voyage, the master
of the vessel shall, within forty-eight hours after the.
vessel within a collection-district of the United Sta[tes]
twenty-four hours after the entry of the vessel, pay t[o]
of customs of such district the sum of ten dollars
every such passenger above the age of eight years w[ho]
died on the voyage by natural disease; and the m[aster]
signee of any vessels, who neglects or refuses to pa[y]
lector, within the times hereinbefore prescribed, the s[um]
aforesaid, shall be liable to a penalty of fifty dollars i[n]
the sum required to be paid as aforesaid for each pa[s]
death occurred on the voyage. All sums of money
collector, under the provisions of this section, shall b[e]
into the Treasury of the United States in such mann[er]
such regulations as shall be prescribed by the Sec[retary]
Treasury.

§ 11. *And be it further enacted,* That the collect[or]
of the collection-district within which, or the surveyo[r]
of which, any such steamship or other vessel arrives, s[hall]
inspector or other officer of the customs to make an e[xamination]
the vessel, and to admeasure the compartments or sp[ace]
by the emigrant passengers, or passengers other tha[n]
sengers, during the voyage (and such measurements [shall be]
in the manner provided by law for admeasuring vessels
and to compare the number of such passengers found
the list of such passengers furnished by the master t[o]
officer; and the said inspector or other officer shall

to the aforesaid collector or surveyor, stating the port of departure, the time of sailing, the length of the voyage, the ventilation, the number of such passengers on board the vessel, and their native country respectively ; the cubic quantity of each compartment or space, and the number of berths and passengers in each space ; the kind and quality of the food furnished to such passengers on the voyage, the number of deaths, and the age and sex of those who died during the voyage, and of what disease ; and in case there was any unusual sickness or mortality during the voyage, to report whether the same was caused by any neglect or violation of the provisions of this Act, or by the want of proper care against disease by the master or owner of the vessel ; and the said reports shall be forwarded to the Secretary of the Treasury at such times and in such manner as he shall direct.

§ 12. *And be it further enacted*, The provisions of this Act shall apply to every steamship or other vessel whereon emigrant passengers, or passengers other than cabin passengers, are taken on board at a port or place in the United States for conveyance to any port or place in a foreign country, except foreign territory contiguous to the United States, and shall also apply to any vessel whereon such passengers are taken on board at any port or place of the United States on the Atlantic Ocean or its tributaries for conveyance to a port or place on the Pacific Ocean or its tributaries, or *vice versâ*, and whether the voyage of said vessel is to be continuous from port to port, or such passengers are to be conveyed from port to port in part by the way of any overland route through Mexico or Central America ; and before any such vessel shall be cleared from, or may lawfully depart from, the port or place where such passengers are taken on board, the master of such vessel shall furnish to the officer of customs of the district from which such vessel is about to depart, a correct list of all passengers who have been, or are intended to be, taken on board the vessel ; and the said list shall specify the age, sex, and nationality of each passenger, and whether the said passengers are cabin or other passengers, and the location of the compartment or space in the vessel provided and intended for the use of the passengers other than cabin passengers ; and the said collector of customs may direct an examination of the vessel to be made by an inspector or other officer of the customs, who shall make the examination and report whether the provisions of this Act have been complied with in respect to such vessel, and the said collector is authorised to withhold the clearance of such vessel until

the coming in of such report ; and if the said report
that any of the provisions of this Act have not been com
the collector is authorised and directed to withhold th
of such vessel until the said provisions are complied wi
the master of any such vessel shall wilfully present or
presented to the aforesaid collector of customs any false
lent list or lists of such passengers, or if any such vessel
aforesaid port or place without having been duly clea
collector of customs, the master shall be deemed guilty
meanor, and may be fined not exceeding one thousand
be imprisoned not exceeding one year, and the vesse
liable to seizure and forfeiture.

§ 13. *And be it further enacted*, That the amount of
fines and penalties imposed by any section of this Act
master of any steamship or other vessel carrying or bri
grant passengers, or passengers other than cabin pass
any violation of the provisions of this Act, shall be liens
vessel, and such vessel may be libelled therefor in any
district court of the United States where such vessel sl
or depart.

§ 14. *And be it further enacted*, That this Act shall
operation and take effect on the   day of
hundred and eighty ; and sections forty-two hundred an
to forty-two hundred and seventy-seven inclusive, of th
Statutes of the United States, are, from and after the
repealed ; and this Act may be cited for all purposes as
senger Act, eighteen hundred and eighty.'

MODE OF MEASUREMENT. REVISED STATUTES

§ 4150. The registry of every vessel shall express l
and breadth, together with her depth, and the height
third or spar deck, which shall be ascertained in the
manner : the tonnage deck, in all vessels having three
decks to the hull, shall be the second deck from below ; i
cases the upper deck of the hull is to be the tonnage-d
length from the fore part of the outer planking on the si
stem to the after part of the main stern-port of screw-stea
to the after part of the rudder-port of all other vessels, me
the top of the tonnage-deck, shall be accounted the vesse
The breadth of the broadest part on the outside of the v

be accounted the vessel's breadth of beam. A measure from the under side of the tonnage-deck plank, amidships, to the ceiling of the hold (average thickness), shall be accounted the depth of hold. If the vessel has a third deck, then the height from the top of the tonnage-deck plank to the under side of the upper-deck plank shall be accounted as the height under the spar-deck. All measurements to be taken in feet and fractions of feet, and all fractions of feet shall be expressed in decimals.

§ 4151. No part of any vessel shall be required by the preceding section to be measured or registered for tonnage that is used for cabins or state-rooms, and constructed entirely above the first deck, which is not a deck to the hull.

§ 4153. The register tonnage of every vessel built within the United States, or owned by a citizen or citizens thereof, shall be her entire internal cubical capacity in tons of one hundred cubic feet each, to be ascertained as follows:—

Measure the length of the vessel in a straight line along the upper side of the tonnage-deck, from the inside of the inner plank, average thickness, at the side of the stem to the inside of the plank on the stern-timbers, average thickness, deducting from this length what is due to the rake of the bow in the thickness of the deck, and what is due to the rake of the stern-timber in the thickness of the deck, and also what is due to the rake of the stern-timber in one-third of the round of the beam ; divide the length so taken into the number of equal parts required by the following table, according to the class in such table to which the vessel belongs :—

TABLE OF CLASSES.

Class 1. Vessels of which the tonnage-length, according to the above measurement, is fifty feet and under, into six equal parts.

Class 2. Vessels of which the tonnage-length, according to the above measurement, is above fifty and not exceeding one hundred feet, into eight equal parts.

Class 3. Vessels of which the tonnage-length, according to the above measurement, is above one hundred feet and not exceeding one hundred and fifty feet, into ten equal parts.

Class 4. Vessels of which the tonnage length, according to the above measurement, is above one hundred and fifty feet and not exceeding two hundred feet, into twelve equal parts.

Class 5. Vessels of which the tonnage-length, above measurement, is above two hundred and a hundred and fifty feet, into fourteen equal parts.

Class 6. Vessels of which the tonnage-length, above measurement, is above two hundred and fif teen equal parts.

Then, the hold being sufficiently cleared to quired depths and breadths being properly taken, verse area of such vessel at each point of division follows :—

Measure the depth at each point of division f distance of one-third of the round of the beam or, in case of a break, below a line stretched thereof, to the upper side of the floor-timber, at t limber-strake, after deducting the average thickne which is between the bilge-planks and limber-strak depth at the midship division of the length do not feet, divide each depth into four equal parts ; th inside horizontal breadth at each of the three poi and also at the upper and lower points of the depth, measurement to the average thickness of that par which is between the points of measurement ; number from above, numbering the upper breadth one, and the lowest breadth ; multiply the second and fourt the third by two ; add these products together, and the first breadth and the last, or fifth ; multiply the obtained by one-third of the common interval betwee and the product shall be deemed the transverse ar midship depth exceed sixteen feet, divide each d equal parts, instead of four, and measure, as before horizontal breadths at the five points of division, a upper and lower points of the depth ; number them before ; multiply the second, fourth, and sixth, by third and fifth by two ; add these products togeth sum add the first breadth and the last, or seventh ; quantities thus obtained by one-third of the commo tween the breadths, and the product shall be deemed area.

Having thus ascertained the transverse area at division of the length of the vessel, as required abov ascertain the register tonnage of the vessel in the follow

UNITED STATES PASSENGER ACT.   351

—Number the areas successively one, two, three, and so forth, number one being at the extreme limit of the length at the bow, and the last number at the extreme limit of the length at the stern; then, whether the length be divided, according to the table, into six or sixteen parts, as in classes one and six, or any intermediate number, as in classes two, three, four, and five, multiply the second, and every even-numbered area, by four, and the third, and every odd-numbered area, except the first and last, by two; add these products together, and to the sum add the first and last, if they yield anything: mu'tiply the quantities thus obtained by one-third of the common interval between the areas, and the product will be the cubical contents of the space under the tonnage-deck; divide this product by one hundred, and the quotient, being the tonnage under the tonnage-deck, shall be deemed to be the register tonnage of the vessel, subject to the additions hereinafter mentioned. If there be a break, a poop, or any other permanent closed-in space on the upper decks or the spar-deck, available for cargo or stores, or for the berthing or accommodation of passengers or crew, the tonnage of such space shall be ascertained as follows: —Measure the internal length of such space in feet, and divide it into an even number of equal parts, of which the distance asunder shall be most nearly equal to those into which the length of the tonnage-deck has been divided; measure at the middle of its height the inside breadths; namely, one at each end, and at each of the points of division, numbering them successively one, two, three, and so forth; then to the sum of the end breadths add four times the sum of the even-numbered breadths and twice the sum of the odd-numbered breadths, except the first and the last, and multiply the whole sum by one-third of the common interval between the breadths; the product will give the mean horizontal area of such space; then measure the mean height between the planks of the decks, and multiply it by the mean horizontal area; divide the product by one hundred, and the quotient shall be deemed to be the tonnage of such space, and shall be added to the tonnage under the tonnage-decks, ascertained as aforesaid. If a vessel has a third deck or spar-deck, the tonnage of the space between it and the tonnage-deck shall be ascertained as follows:—Measure in feet the inside length of the space, at the middle of its height, from the plank at the side of the stem to the plank on the timbers at the stern, and divide the length into the same number of equal parts into which the length of the tonnage-deck is divided; measure,

also at the middle of its height, the inside breadth of the
each of the points of division, also the breadth of the sten
breadth at the stern; number them successively one, tv
and so forth, commencing at the stem; multiply the se
all other even-numbered breadths, by four, and the third
the other odd-numbered breadths, except the first and th
two; to the sum of these products add the first and last
multiply the whole sum by one-third of the common int
tween the breadths, and the result will give, in mean s
feet, the mean horizontal area of such space; measure
height between the plank of the two decks, and multiply
mean horizontal area, and the product will be the cubical
of the space; divide this product by one hundred, and the
shall be deemed to be the tonnage of such space, and shall
to the other tonnage of the vessel, ascertained as above
And if the vessel has more than three decks, the tonnag
space between decks, above the tonnage-deck, shall be
ascertained in the manner above described, and shall be
the tonnage of the vessel ascertained as above directed.
taining the tonnage of open vessels the upper edge of tl
strake is to form the boundary-line of measurement, and t
shall be taken from an athwart-ship line, extending from t
edge of such strake at each division of the length. The re
the vessel shall express the number of decks, the tonnag
the tonnage-deck, that of the between-decks, above the
deck; also that of the poop or other inclosed spaces al
deck, each separately. In every registered United Stat
the number denoting the total registered tonnage shall b
carved or otherwise permanently marked on her main be
shall be so continued; and if at any time cease to be so co
such vessel shall no longer be recognised as a registered v
the United States.

MEASUREMENT OF FOREIGN VESSELS. REVISED STATU

§ 4154. . . . If the vessel be double-decked, take the
thereof from the fore part of the main stem to the after par
stern-port, above the upper deck, the breadth thereof
broadest part above the main wales, half of which breadth
accounted the depth of such vessel, and shall then deduct f
length three-fifths of the breadth, multiply the remainder

breadth, and the product by the depth, and shall divide this last product by ninety-five; the quotient whereof shall be deemed the true contents or tonnage of such vessel. If such vessel be single decked, the surveyor, or other person, shall take the length and breadth as above directed in respect to a double-decked vessel, shall deduct from the length three-fifths of the breadth, and, taking the depth from the under side of the deck-plank to the ceiling in the hold, shall multiply and divide in the same manner, and the quotient shall be deemed the tonnage of such vessel.

[N. Y. Cat. No. 1087.]

REPORT OF EXAMINATION

*Of   of   tons burden, Capt.   , from
Arrived at   ,   , 18   . Date of sailing,   .
Length of voyage,   days. Number, diameter, and description
of ventilators,   .   Height of ventilators above Upper
Deck,   .   Number of Decks,   .*

PASSENGERS		Males	Females	Total No. of Passengers
Cabin passengers	Class 1.			
	Eight years of age or over			
	Under eight years of age			
	Total			
Passengers, other than cabin	Class 2.			
	Eight years of age or over			
	Under eight and over one			
	Under one year of age			
	Total			

SPACE FOR PASSENGERS, OTHER THAN CABIN PASSENGERS.

	Height between Decks	Superficial Capacity, in Feet	No. of Passengers, other than Cabin Passengers, allowed by Law	No. of Statute Passengers brought, other than Cabin Passengers
Main Deck				
Lower Deck				
Deck-houses				
Total				

Food (kinds and daily allowance)_____

How cooked (whether well or badly, etc.)_____

Number, capacity, and arrangement of hospitals_____

Number of tiers of berths .
Distance between berths and deck beneath . . .
Dimensions of single berths .
Dimensions of double berths
Number of physicians on board . . . .
Locality and separation of latrines_____

Number of houses over hatchway . . .
Number of cabooses . .
Number of latrines for males
Number of latrines for females . . . .

NATIVE COUNTRY OF PASSENGERS, OTHER THAN CABIN.

DEATHS AND BIRTHS AMONG PASSENGERS, OTHER THAN CABIN.

	Deaths	Males	Females	Births	Number
Passengers	Above eight years, from natural disease . .			Males .	
	Above eight years, from other causes . . .				
	Under eight years of age .			Females .	
	Total			Total .	

Causes of mortality during voyage_____

Receipts under § 4268, Revised Statutes of the United States_____ .

REMARKS.

_____, 187____ _____, *Examiner.*

To_____

FORM A.

No.____.   Port of _____.

THE UNITED STATES OF AMERICA.—NATIONAL BOARD OF HEALTH.

Bill of Health.

I,_____ (consul, consular agent, or other officer empowered by law to sign), at the port of _____, do hereby state that the vessel hereinafter named clears from this port under the following circumstances :—

Name of vessel : _____.   Tonnage :_____ .

Apartments for passengers, No._____.   Destination : _____.

Name of medical officer (if any) : _____ .

Total number of passengers : 1st cabin,_____; 2nd cabin, _____; steerage,_____ .

Nature (vessel-of-war, ship, schooner, etc.) :_____ . Guns :_____ .

Where last from : _____.   Name of captain :_____ .

Total number of crew :_____.   Cargo : _____ .

Sanitary history of the vessel :—

1. Sanitary condition of vessel (before and after reception of cargo, with note of any decayed wood). Note disinfection of vessel :

2. Sanitary condition of cargo :

3. Sanitary condition of crew :

4. Sanitary condition of passengers :

5. Sanitary condition of clothing, food, water, air-space, and ventilation (to be in quantity as required by Revised Statutes) :

6. Sanitary condition of port and adjoining country—

   a. Prevailing diseases (if any) :

   b. Number of cases of and deaths from yellow fever, Asiatic cholera, plague, small-pox, or typhus fever during the week preceding :

b. Number of cases of—		b. Number of deaths from—	
Yellow fever	———	Yellow fever	—
Asiatic cholera	———	Asiatic cholera	—
Plague	———	Plague	—
Small-pox	———	Small-pox	—
Typhus fever	———	Typhus fever	—
Relapsing fever	———	Relapsing fever	—

7. Any circumstances affecting the public health existing in port of departure to be here stated :

CLEAN.

I certify that I have personally inspected the said vessel, that the above statements are correct ; that good health is enj[oyed] in this port and the adjacent country, without any suspici[on of] yellow fever, Asiatic cholera, or plague ; that neither small-po[x or] typhus fever exists as an epidemic ; that the sanitary conditi[on of] the vessel, cargo, crew, and passengers is good ; that the rules [and] regulations prescribed by the National Board of Health have [been] complied with, and that the [name of vessel] leaves this port in *pratique*, bound for_____, United States of America.

[Signature of medical officer.]

Or,   FOUL.

I certify that I have personally inspected the said vessel, that the above statements are correct, and that she leaves this bound for_____, United States of America, *in quarant*[ine].

[Signature of medical officer.

I certify that the foregoing statements are made by_____ _____, M.D., who has personally inspected said vessel ; I am satisfied that the said statements are correct ; and] further certify that the said vessel leaves this port bound _____, in the United States, in _____ *pratique* [or in [qua]rantine].

In witness whereof, I have hereunto set my hand and the [seal] of office, at the port of_____, this____ day of_____ 18___, ___ o'clock.

[Seal.]   _____ _____

[*Consul-General, Consul, Commercial Agent, Sanitary Officer, et*[c.]

INDEX.

ABI

A BILL to regulate the carriage of passengers by sea, 339
Abstract of Admiral Sir Michael Seymour's orders (Hong Kong, 1857), 211
Admiralty instructions and Queen's regulations, selections from, 291
Afterhoods, 19
Air, apparatus required for analysis of, 131
— chemical and microscopical examination of, 130
— method of estimating the CO_2 in, 132
Alcohol an antiseptic but not a deodorant, 248
Alfred the Great a naval architect, 12
Allardyce's patent wind shute, 65
Alphabetical book (medical officers'), 282
Ambulance lifts, 286
— cot of Dr. Gorgas, U.S.N., 286
— hammock of the author, 287
Ammonia in the air, 48
Ancient Britons, ships of, 9
— — anchors and cables of, 10
Angle irons, 33
Angles in tubes, estimation of loss thereby, 71
Antiseptics, 248
Appendix of medical instructions and enactments, 291
Aphorisms for bathers (R. H. S. R.), 217

BIS

Apron, 22
Aqueous vapour in the air, 48
Archimedian screw, 85
Armstrong, Sir A., K.C.B., on lime-juice and scurvy, 205
Arnott's scheme of ventilation for the ragged schools, 62
— ventilating pump, 87
Articles of diet, source and mode of preparation, 179
— inspection of, 184
Artificial ventilation, 77
Atmospheric air, 45
— — composition of, 46
Axial tube in the funnel for ventilation, 90

BACTERIA in the air, 49, 50
Baneful effects of so frequently washing decks, 164
Beams, 27
— in iron ships, 40
Bearding line, 22
Beef, ship's, 180
Bellows and pump ventilators, 86
Bends or wales, 28
Berthing rail, 30
Bertin's ventilating system ('L'Annamite'), 113
Bilge, position of, 28
— water, 28
— and bilge effluvia, 243
Binding strakes, 27
Biscuit, ship's, 180
— — characters of, 184

DEO

Deodorants, 248
Desagulier's wheel, or rotatory fan, 77
Diatomaceæ with mineral particles in the air, 49
Diet, historical retrospect, 169
— present scale, 178
— and climate, 181
Disinfectants, 248
Disinfection of bedding, clothing, &c., 261
Distillation of fresh water from the sea, 140
— views and suggestions of philosophers, 140, 141
Distilling apparatus (emigrant ships), 234
Ditty-box and bag of the seaman, 200
Division of tubes, estimation of loss thereby, 73
Double bottoms, cleaning and coating, precautions to be taken, 132
Double ventilating shaft of the author, 80, 82-83
Dove-tailed score (waterway and beam), 27
Downtake cowls and shafts, 62
Drainage-holes in ships, 232
Duties and responsibilities of medical officers, 280
— of medical officers (army) in charge of troops on board ship, 333

EDGAR, reference to, 12
Edmond's, Dr., R.N., ventilating system, 95
Edward III., reference to, 12
'Egeria,' H.M.S., ventilation of (Levinge), 105-108
Eklund, Dr. F., on ship ventilation, 116
Emigrant ships (distilling apparatus), 234
Endboards (hammock netting), 36
Engineers' berth and gunroom, ventilation of, 64
Epithelial scales in the air, 49, 50
Knesdies, for seeresation, &c., 193

GRE

Expansion by heat for ventilation, 87
External planking, 28
Extraction compared with the plenum principle, 56, 57

FALSE keel, 19
Fashion pieces, 23
Filling frame, 21
Fillings of Sir Rob. Seppings, 23
Filtration, filtering media, 148
Flame for ventilation, 88
Fleet-Surgeon Eustace on nitrate of lead, 252
— — Magill on Thier's patent system of ventilation, 112
Fletcher, Dr., R.N., on the naval dietary of 1786, 171
— — proposed improvements in the scale, 173
Flour, 180
Forecastle, 41, 42
Forehoods, 19
Foreign-going steamers. measurement of, 228
Fore storeroom, ventilation of, 64
Frame in wooden ships, 21
Framing in iron ships, 35
Fresh meat, inspection of, 190
Frictional area and the forms of tubes, 75
Fumigation of ships, 262
— — with chlorine gas, 268
— — with nitrous acid, 267
— — with sulphurous acid, 262
Funnel casing, &c. (Mr. Baker), 90
Futtocks, 1st, 2nd, 3rd, 4th, &c., 21

GAMMONING piece (knee of the head), 30
Garboard strakes in wooden ships, 28
— — in iron ships, 33
Gasometer principle of pump, 87
General, and fire quarters, 284
General orders, sanitary regulations, &c., 211
Goolden's, Dr., formula for nitrate of lead, 252
'Great Harry,' H.M.S., 13

Greeks, vessels of the, 10, 11
Gripe (knee of the head), 30
Guide table of ventilation, 59
Gun deck or lower deck, 42
Gun room and engineers' berth, ventilation of, 64

HAIR bracket, 30
— Hales', Dr. S., bellows, or 'ships' lungs,' 86, 87
Half beams, 27
Half breadth plan, 15, 16
Half floors, 21
Hammock berthing, 30
— netting, 30
Harris', Captain, advice to seamen, 274
'Harry Grace de Dieu,' H.M.S., 13
Hatches and scuttles, 31
Hatchways, fore, main, and after, 31
Hawse pieces, 25
Heads and bow galleries, 246
Health of the crew affected by the type of ship, 234
— — preserved by cleanliness and dryness of the ship, 238
— bill of, form A (American), 355, 356
Hebrews, King Solomon's expeditions to Ophir and Tarshish, 11
Henry IV., perfection of the magnetic needle, introduction of cannon, 12
— V., 'Chamber,' 'Saloon,' and 'Queen's Hall,' 13
— VII., 'Great Harry,' 13
— VIII., 'Harry Grace de Dieu,' first 'Navy List, 13
Homer's account of the ship of Ulysses, 10
Home trade ships, measurement of, 229
— — — sanitary provisions in reference to, 233
Hospital and sick quarters (medical instructions), 304
Hospital ships for an army corps, 356
— — ('Victor Emanuel'), 218

INDEX. 361

LEA

Lead-poisoning in the French navy, 236
— — in cleaning and re-coating double bottoms, 236
Leading principles of ventilation, 50, 53
Leaky ships assumed to be sweet ones, 244
Leave and interchange of duties (medical officers'), 280
Ledoyen's fluid (nitrate of lead), 252
Lengthening pieces, 21
Limber boards, 28
— strakes, 28
Lime-juice, 179
— as an anti-scorbutic, 201
— early writers on its efficiency in scurvy, 203
— citric acid, and nitrate of potash, relative merits of, 204
— chemical examination of, 208
— lozenges, general remarks, 207
— and scurvy, Sir Alexander Armstrong on, 205
Long and short-armed floor, 21
Longitudinal system (Scott Russell), 35, 36
Longitudinals, 38

MAGAZINES, ventilation of, 127
Main deck, 42
— post, 22, 25
— rail, 30
Manning and arming boats, 283
Marsh water, 138
Mast-head cover in iron ships, 41
McKinnell's ventilating scheme, 56
Measurement of cubic space, 129
Medical documents required on board ship, 282
Medical instructions, 304
Middle rail, 30
'Minden,' H.M.S., ventilation of, 93
Mixed system of framing, 35, 38
Monitor ships, ventilation of, 118
Movement of troops by sea, 335
Mulguf (Egyptian), 60
Mushroom ventilators, 231

PER

NATURAL character and habits of the sailor, 272
Natural waters, 136
Natural ventilation, 59
Naval dietary for 1797, 174
— — — 1825, 174, 175, 176
— — — 1850-67, 177
— — present scale, 178
'Navy List,' the first published (Henry VIII.), 13
Necho and the Phœnicians, 11
Niger expedition, ventilation supervised by Dr. Reid, F.R.S., 80, 85, 93
Nitrate of lead *versus* permanganate of potash, 252
Nitrogen and oxygen in the air, 46
Normandy's condensing apparatus, preliminary statements, 142
— — — description of, 143

OPENINGS between the timbers turned to account for ventilation, 90
Ophir and Tarshish, allusion to, 11
Ordinate lines, 17
Orlop deck, 42
Organic matter in the air, 48
Oxygen and nitrogen in the air, 46

PAINTING or cementing compartments, &c., precautions, 132
Parkes, Professor, on the relative merits of lime juice and citric acid, 204
Partners, 27
Passenger steamers classified, 227
— — accommodation, 228
Payne, Dr. E., U.S.N., on white cap covers, 197
— — — — on shoes and underclothing, 198
Perkins' automatic ventilator (Finlayson), 108
Permanganate of potash, a deodorant, 248
— — — effect upon *bacteria*, 251
Personal cleanliness, 160

INDEX.

Peruvian bark first used on the African coast, 208
— — supplied to the West Indies in 1796, 208
Peyres' pump for ventilation, 87
Phineas Pett, naval constructor, 13
Phœnicians, shipbuilders and mariners, 9, 11
Physics of the atmosphere, 50
Physique of the sailor, 270
Pintles and braces, 25
Plain bar keel, 33
Poop-deck, 42
Pork not cured by the Government, 180
Potential energy of food, 183
— — of the naval dietary, 184
Practical application of ventilating principles, 59
Present scale of diet, 178
'Prince,' H.M.S. (James I.), 13
Prison cells, ventilation of, 64
Prophylactic power of quinine, 241
Proposed scheme for the ventilation of frigates, 101–5
Ptinus, a genus of small coleoptera often present in biscuit, 185
Pus corpuscles in the air, 49

QUARANTINE regulations, 329
Quarter-deck, 41
Queen Elizabeth ('Triumph,' H.M.S.), 13
'Queen's Hall,' H.M.S., 13
Quinine to be issued in malarious districts, 208, 209

RABBET of the keel, 19
— of the stem, 19
Rabbeted bar keels, 33
'Racoon,' ventilation of, 91, 92
Rain-water, 136
Reduction of the spirit ration, 177
Reid, Dr., F.R.S., on rotatory fans, 80
Revaccination circular, March 7, 1871, 209
— remarks thereon, 210

River water, 137
Rivets, hot, bolt, s

Routine of one d (Thursday), 277
Rudder head, 25
— port, 25
— post, 25
Rum, navy strengt
Running into a c case of yellow fe

SANITARY rul
H.M.S. 'In African coast, 21
Sanitas, 254
'Saloon,' H.M.S. (
Salt lakes, 138
Salt meat, inspectio
Salts of the ocean i
Saxons and Danes,
Scale of diet, 17 jewel'), 170
— — — 1786 (Dr. 171
Screw-alley, ventila
— port, 25
Scuppers, 31
Scurvy, definition of
— early writers on t
— conditions giving
— in the late Po 205, 206
Scuttles and hatches,
Sectional area of tu of currents, 74
Secretary Preston's s tions, 215
Segregation of the si
Selections from the regulations, 3??
Seppings', Sir R., syst 21
Shark's mouth winds
Sheer drawing, 15
— plan, 15, 16
Shelf-piece, 25

SHI

Ship of Adramyttium, St. Paul's disaster, 10
Ships, Phœnician and ancient British, 9
— structure and economy, 9
Side-bar keel, 34
Simons' pump and bellows, 87
Siphon ventilation, Mr. Tredgold and Dr. Chowne, 76
Sister keelsons, 22
Skid beams, 41
— gratings, 41
Sleeping on shore, 240, 241
Sluggish streams, 138
Small rails, 30
Sochet's ventilator, 85
Soluble chocolate, preparation of, 179
Souchou's ventilator, 85
Southerly bursters and 'brickfielders,' 49
'Sovereign of the Seas,' H.M.S., 13
Special list book (medical officers'), 283
— systems of ventilation, 90
Sperketting, 28
Spirit ration, general remarks, 176
— room, 43
Spring water, 137
Square body of the ship, 21
Stanchions, 25, 40
Standing orders, Rear-Admiral Wyman, U.N.S., 213
Starches, classification of, 189
Steam ventilation, by Dr. Edmonds, R.N., 87
Stem, 19
— piece, 25
Stems in iron ships, 35
Stemson, 22
Stepping pieces, 22, 23
Stern, 25
Sternson, 22
Stern post, 19, 25
— posts in iron ships, 35
Stringer plates, 40
Stokers, Dr. Hunter, U.S.N., on the duties of, 194
— MM. Bourel Roniere and Leroy de Mericourt on a beverage for, 195

VEL

Storage of water and watering ship, 146
Stoves for ventilation, 88
Stowage of provisions, &c., 43
Superficial area of a given deck space, measurement of, 230
Surgeon M'Carthy, R.N., on the ventilation of the 'Devastation,' 119
— Major T. M. Bleckley, M.D., C.B., on ventilation of the 'Victor Emanuel,' 114
— — — general report on the 'Victor Emanuel,' 220
— — Notter's experiments with filtering media, 148
Sutton's method of extraction by heat, 56

TAFFRAIL, 25
Terebene preparations, 253
— powder, var A, 253
— — — B, 254
— liquid, 254
Tiling the decks in cement (Anderson), 165
T-iron, 33
Top-gallant forecastle, 42
Transverse system of framing, 35, 36
'Triumph,' H.M.S. (Queen Elizabeth), 13
Trotter, Dr., on the character of the British seaman, 272
Trusses, 28
Tube and cowl ventilators, 62, 65
Twin-fan ventilator of the author, 80

ULYSSES, vessel of, Homer's account, 10
'Undaunted,' H.M.S., ventilation of, 97
Universal disinfectant, 251
Upper deck, 41
Uptake cowls and shafts, 65

VASCO DE GAMMA, 11
Velocity of currents of air and cubic delivery, 74

WALES or bends, 28
Water supply, general remarks, 134
— chemical examination, 152
— microscopical examination, 156
— physical examination of, 151
Watering ship at British stations abroad, 148
Water-ledges, 31
Water-lines, 17
Waterways, 27
Watson's ventilating system, 55, 56
Weevils (*Calandra granaria*), 185

William of Normandy, 12
Wilson, Dr., U.S.N., on racter of the seaman, 27
Windmill ventilator, 86
Wind sails, 59, 60
Wing passage, 43
— transom, 23
Wooden ships, construction

'ZEALOUS,' H.M.S., v of, 88
Zoological illustrations lating principles, 57, 58,

LANE MEDICAL LIBRARY
300 PASTEUR DRIVE
PALO ALTO, CALIFORNIA 94304

Ignorance of Library's rules does not exempt violators from penalties.

L985
.M13   MacDonald, J. D.
1881   Outlines of naval hygiene

NAME	DATE DUE

L985
M13

Lightning Source UK Ltd.
Milton Keynes UK
UKHW011356051118
331792UK00007B/1397/P